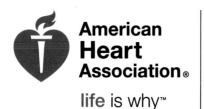

American Heart Association®

life is why™

American Academy of Pediatrics

DEDICATED TO THE HEALTH OF ALL CHILDREN™

D1597585

PEDIATRIC ADVANCED LIFE SUPPORT

INSTRUCTOR MANUAL

© 2016 American Heart Association
ISBN 978-1-61669-547-7
Printed in the United States of America
First American Heart Association Printing October 2016
5 4 3 2

Acknowledgments

The American Heart Association thanks the following people for their contributions to the development of this manual: Ricardo A. Samson, MD; Stephen M. Schexnayder, MD; Mary Fran Hazinski, RN, MSN; Reylon Meeks, RN, BSN, MS, MSN, EMT, PhD; Lynda J. Knight, MSN, RN, CPN; Allan de Caen, MD; Jonathan Duff, MD, MEd; Mary Ann McNeil, MA, NRP; Mary E. McBride, MD, MEd; Cindy Brownlee, BSN, RN; Jeffrey M. Berman, MD; Farhan Bhanji, MD, MSc(Ed); Kelly D. Kadlec, MD; Mark A. Terry, MPA, NREMT-P; Adam Cheng, MD; Aaron Donoghue, MD, MSCE; Claire R. Wells, AC-PNP; Sallie Johnson, PharmD, BCPS; Holly Capasso-Harris, PhD; and the AHA PALS Project Team.

 To find out about any updates or corrections to this text, visit **www.ahainstructornetwork.org**, navigate to the page for this course, and click on "Updates." You must be registered and confirmed as an instructor on the AHA Instructor Network to access these updates.

To access the Student Website for this course, go to **www.heart.org/eccstudent** and enter this code: pals15

Contents

Contents

Part 2
Teaching the Course   35

Part 3
Testing and Remediation

Contents

**Part 6
PALS Lesson Plans**

PALS Update Lesson Plans

HeartCode PALS Lesson Plans

PALS Instructor CD Contents

Precourse Materials

Equipment List

PALS Course Sample Agenda

PALS Update Course Sample Agenda

HeartCode PALS Course Sample Agenda

Sample Precourse Letter—Student

Sample Precourse Letter—HeartCode Student

Sample Precourse Letter—Instructor

Course Materials

PALS Lesson Plans

PALS Update Lesson Plans

HeartCode PALS Lesson Plans

PALS Course Progress Checklist

PALS Update Course Progress Checklist

Child CPR and AED Skills Testing Checklist

Infant CPR Skills Testing Checklist

Learning Station Competency Checklists

Airway Management Skills Station Competency Checklist

Rhythm Disturbances/Electrical Therapy Skills Station Competency Checklist

Vascular Access Skills Station Competency Checklist

PALS Practice Case Scenarios (16)

PALS Testing Case Scenarios (14)

Team Dynamics Debriefing Tool

PALS Case Scenario Testing Checklists (12)

Team Role Labels

PALS Systematic Approach Algorithm

PALS Systematic Approach Summary

Pediatric Recognition of Respiratory Problems Flowchart

Pediatric Management of Respiratory Emergencies Flowchart

Pediatric Recognition of Shock Flowchart

Pediatric Management of Shock Flowchart

Life Is Why™ Activity Page

PALS Instructor CD Instructions and System Requirements

Instructions

The PALS Instructor CD-ROM will auto-launch when the CD is inserted in the drive. For a Windows PC, if AutoRun has been disabled on your computer, you can double-click to launch the CD or right mouse click on the CD drive and choose "Open AutoPlay." If that option is not available, right mouse click on the CD drive and choose "Explore" or Open." Double click on "PC_start.exe" to launch the CD. For a Mac, find and click on "Mac_start.html" to start.

System Requirements

PC

- Core 2 Duo processor or equivalent AMD processor
- Windows 7 or later
- Minimum of 512 MB of RAM
- 500 MB of available hard-disk space
- Internet Explorer 8, Mozilla Firefox 3, or Chrome Web browser or later
- Screen resolution of 1024 × 768 or higher
- CD-ROM drive (8 × or faster)
- Adobe Acrobat Reader 8.0 or later

Mac

- Processor: PowerPC iMac, iBook, MacBook, Mac Pro, or faster
- Mac OS X or later
- Minimum of 512 MB of RAM
- 500 MB of available hard-disk space
- Safari 4 or Mozilla Firefox 3 Web browser or later
- Screen resolution of 1024 × 768 or higher
- CD-ROM drive (8 × or faster)
- Adobe Acrobat Reader 8.0 or later

This CD contains Adobe Acrobat (PDF) and Microsoft Word (DOC) files.

If you do not own Adobe Acrobat, you can download, for free, Adobe Acrobat Reader from Adobe's website: **http://get.adobe.com/reader/**

If you have a problem loading or using the CD, make sure your computer system meets the minimum system requirements. If your system meets the requirements and you are still having trouble, visit **www.heart.org/cprproductsupport** for additional assistance.

life is why.™

At the American Heart Association, we want people to experience more of life's precious moments. That's why we've made better heart and brain health our mission. It's also why we remain committed to exceptional training—the act of bringing resuscitation science to life—through genuine partnership with you. Only through our continued collaboration and dedication can we truly make a difference and save lives.

Until there's a world free of heart disease and stroke, the American Heart Association will be there, working with you to make a healthier, longer life possible for everyone.

Why do we do what we do?
life is why.

Life Is Why is a celebration of life. A simple yet powerful answer to the question of why we should all be healthy in heart and mind. It also explains why we do what we do: Lifesaving work. Every day.

Throughout your student manual, you will find information that correlates what you are learning in this class to **Life Is Why** and the importance of cardiovascular care. Look for the **Life Is Why** icon (shown at right), and remember that what you are learning today has an impact on the mission of the American Heart Association.

We encourage you to discover your **Why** and share it with others. Ask yourself, what are the moments, people, and experiences I live for? What brings me joy, wonder, and happiness? Why am I partnering with the AHA to help save lives? Why is cardiovascular care important to me? The answer to these questions is your **Why.**

Instructions

Please find on the back of this page a chance for you to participate in the AHA's mission and **Life Is Why** campaign. Complete this activity by filling in the blank with the word that describes your **Why**.

Share your **"_____ Is Why"** with the people you love, and ask them to discover their **Why.**

Talk about it. Share it. Post it. Live it.   **#lifeiswhy**   **#CPRSavesLives**

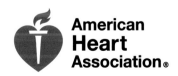

       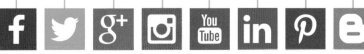

is why.

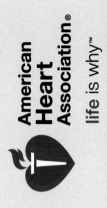

American Heart Association®

life is why™

Part 1

Preparing for the Course

Course Overview

Course Overview and Design

The Pediatric Advanced Life Support (PALS) Provider Course is designed to give students the opportunity to acquire, practice, and demonstrate proficiency in the assessment and management of critically ill pediatric patients. The primary educational methodology used in the course is that of *simulation*, whether for skill acquisition, complex medical decision making, or teamwork. Other modalities used are video demonstration and group discussion.

Students will have the opportunity to learn the following:

Skills:

- Performing child and infant cardiopulmonary resuscitation (CPR)
- Using oxygen delivery and airway management equipment
- Establishing intraosseous (IO) access and a method for giving rapid fluid boluses
- Using electrocardiogram (ECG) monitoring
- Providing defibrillation/cardioversion

Pediatric assessment: A systematic approach

Medical management:

- 4 types of acute respiratory problems
- 4 types of acute circulatory problems
- 4 types of acute cardiac problems, including cardiac arrest

Leadership: Communication and other important elements of team dynamics as they relate to resuscitation

Students will then be tested for competency in the following areas:

1. Child and infant basic life support (BLS)
2. Approach and management of 2 cases using teamwork:
   - 1 cardiac case *and*
   - 1 respiratory or 1 shock case

Course Description

The PALS Provider Course is designed for healthcare providers who either direct or participate in the management of respiratory and/or cardiovascular emergencies and cardiopulmonary arrest in pediatric patients. Precourse preparation, didactic instruction, and active participation in skills stations and simulated cases will be used to enhance the recognition and intervention of respiratory emergencies, shock, and cardiopulmonary arrest.

Course Goal

The goal of the PALS Provider Course is to improve outcomes for pediatric patients by preparing healthcare providers to effectively recognize and intervene in patients with respiratory emergencies, shock, and cardiopulmonary arrest by using high-performance team dynamics and high-quality individual skills.

Learning Objectives

Upon successful completion of this course, students will be able to:

- Perform high-quality CPR per American Heart Association (AHA) BLS recommendations
  - Child CPR and automated external defibrillator (AED) use
  - Infant CPR
- Differentiate between patients who do and do not require immediate intervention
  - Describe the systematic approach
  - Describe the evaluate-identify-intervene sequence
  - Use the Pediatric Assessment Triangle to form an initial impression of patient status
  - Apply the primary assessment, which includes airway, breathing, circulation, disability, and exposure
  - Apply the secondary assessment, which includes a SAMPLE history and a physical exam
  - Demonstrate reassessment of patients after each intervention by using the evaluate-identify-intervene sequence
- Recognize cardiopulmonary arrest early and begin CPR within 10 seconds
- Apply team dynamics
  - Describe roles and responsibilities of team
  - Describe elements of effective team dynamics
  - Demonstrate effective team dynamics in case scenarios
- Differentiate between respiratory distress and failure
  - Recognize early signs and symptoms of respiratory distress and failure
  - Describe disorders of oxygenation
  - Describe disorders of ventilation
  - Identify causes of respiratory distress and failure, including upper airway obstruction, lower airway obstruction, parenchymal disease, and disordered control of breathing

- Perform early interventions for respiratory distress and failure
  - Describe different methods of supplementary oxygen delivery
  - Demonstrate appropriate noninvasive interventions for a child in respiratory distress or failure (such as positioning and suctioning)
  - Recognize requirement for positive-pressure ventilation
  - Perform effective bag-mask ventilation
  - Use adjuncts to bag-mask ventilation (such as 2-person bag-mask ventilation and oropharyngeal airways)
  - Recognize requirement for advanced airway
  - Recommend specific diagnostic tests and treatments for various etiologies of respiratory distress and failure
- Differentiate between compensated and decompensated (hypotensive) shock
  - Recognize early signs and symptoms of shock
  - Describe the pathophysiology of shock
  - Identify causes of different types of shock, including hypovolemic, obstructive, cardiogenic, and distributive
- Perform early interventions for the treatment of shock
  - Describe indications for IO access
  - Demonstrate appropriate fluid resuscitation for different etiologies of shock
  - Recommend specific diagnostic tests and treatments for various etiologies of shock
- Differentiate between unstable and stable patients with arrhythmias
  - Identify common arrhythmias in pediatric patients
- Describe clinical characteristics of instability in patients with arrhythmias
  - Demonstrate treatment of common arrhythmias (eg, sinus tachycardia, sinus bradycardia, supraventricular tachycardia, ventricular fibrillation [VF]/pulseless ventricular tachycardia [pVT], asystole)
  - Demonstrate safe use of a manual defibrillator
  - Recommend specific diagnostic tests and treatments for various arrhythmias
- Implement post–cardiac arrest management
  - Describe the systematic approach to a patient after cardiac arrest
  - Describe initial steps of post–cardiac arrest management

Critical Role of the Instructor

The instructor is critical to successful student outcomes in this course and can facilitate this by

- Demonstrating effective case management consistent with the *2015 AHA Guidelines Update for CPR and Emergency Cardiovascular Care* (ECC)
- Modeling high-quality principles of care in PALS
- Facilitating small-group discussions with a focus on desired outcome
- Listening to students' responses and providing feedback to ensure that they understand the learning concepts
- Observing students' actions and coaching them as necessary
- Providing positive or corrective feedback
- Keeping discussions and simulations on track for optimal learning and use of time in the classroom
- Conducting structured debriefing sessions after each simulation

Educational Design

The PALS Course uses a variety of teaching methods and adult learning principles in an environment that, in some cases, will mimic (simulate) or actually be a real healthcare setting (eg, back of an ambulance, emergency department bed). From an educational perspective, the closer the simulated emergency is to a real-life case (eg, setting, equipment), the better the transfer of skills. Cognitive, psychomotor, and some affective domains will be accomplished through small-group teaching and case scenario practice on a manikin as a Team Leader and team members (ie, hands-on learning) and use of large- or small-group short video presentations with instructor-student interaction (ie, engage student in discussion).

Simulation, previously referred to as *mock codes*, has been the fundamental educational model for PALS for more than 20 years. Although the technology is more sophisticated and the science of simulation education continues to expand, the fundamentals remain the same. Simulation offers students the opportunity to learn and practice their cognitive and psychomotor skills before applying them to real patients. There is ample evidence from many disciplines to support the effectiveness of such simulation-based education in improving participant knowledge, skills, team performance, leadership, and communication. For this reason, the PALS Course continues to incorporate this model into its design.

The AHA is building a full range of experiences that will engage different types of students with various learning styles.

This course has been designed to maximize student learning and retention. Meeting audience-specific needs includes changing scenarios to fit specific locations in certain sessions with certain groups.

Two different course formats are available to accommodate the learning needs of individual students and offer flexibility for instructors:

- Instructor-led training
- Blended learning

All formats have the same learning objectives and offer the same course completion card.

Instructor-Led Training

The instructor-led training is a traditional classroom course conducted on-site at a Training Center or other facility. The course is structured as follows:

- Core concepts are presented through course videos, instructor-led discussions, and case-based scenarios around a manikin.
- Students take an exam to confirm understanding of core concepts.
- The instructor coaches students as they practice skills.
- The instructor monitors as each student demonstrates skills proficiency as outlined in the skills testing checklist.

Blended Learning

Blended learning combines the flexibility of online learning with on-site skills practice and testing.

Course Structure

A blended-learning course is structured as follows:

- Core concepts are presented in an online interactive format using the HeartCode® program (see HeartCode below). Interactivity is enhanced by video, interactive learning activities, and eSimulation. The online course is self-directed—the student controls the time, place, and pacing of the instruction.
- Students will work with an AHA Instructor at a Training Center or other location for the hands-on session.
- The hands-on session includes a skills practice, which is the practical, hands-on portion of this blended-learning course. In addition, the hands-on session has a skills testing portion that includes the same skills tests conducted in the full PALS Course and PALS Update Course. For the optional case scenario testing, at least 3 students should be present for each case scenario.

Skills Practice and Testing

Students must demonstrate that they can successfully perform each skill as outlined in the BLS Skills Testing Checklists and the PALS Skills Testing Checklist. In the blended-learning courses, skills practice and testing can be conducted by an AHA PALS Instructor.

Benefits of Blended Learning

The online component of the blended-learning experience benefits both students and instructors. Online learning accommodates many different learning styles. For example, some students prefer learning in a self-directed environment as opposed to a group setting. Also, online learning is time efficient for the following reasons:

- Students have the flexibility to take the online instruction whenever their schedules permit. Time spent at a Training Center or other facility for supervised practice and testing is reduced
- Instructors have more time to focus on students' learning needs, such as answering questions, coaching, and skills development
- Testing of core concepts is completed online, so students don't have to wait for other students to finish taking the exam

Preparing to Teach Blended-Learning Courses

To be prepared to teach a blended-learning course, we recommend that instructors take the online course for each discipline you teach. This will help you understand what students learn and are prepared to do. As with instructor-led courses, all online courses are developed by using educational principles and best practices. Course materials are presented in a way that helps students learn and retain the information. Students are required to complete all online course activities, which are designed to teach and test core concepts. The online instruction is also designed to help students transfer and apply their knowledge to skills performance.

Instructors should review all course materials, including the *PALS Instructor Manual*, skills testing checklists, critical skills descriptors, and skills sections of the course videos.

For the HeartCode PALS hands-on session, please use the following materials provided in this manual:

- Lesson Plans PALS HC Introduction through PALS HC 8
- PALS Skills Testing Checklist in Appendix A

Understanding HeartCode

The online component of the blended-learning course includes HeartCode. HeartCode is a Web-based, self-paced instructional program that uses eSimulation technology to allow students to assess and treat patients in virtual healthcare settings. In this environment, students apply their knowledge to real-time decision making and skills development. Debriefings and coaching are provided immediately after each simulation to facilitate learning.

In HeartCode PALS, the eSimulations include

- High-Quality Child and Infant BLS
- Upper Airway Obstruction
- Lower Airway Obstruction
- Lung Tissue Disease
- Disordered Control of Breathing
- Hypovolemic Shock
- Distributive Shock
- Obstructive Shock
- Cardiogenic Shock
- Bradycardia
- Supraventricular Tachycardia
- Pulseless Electrical Activity (PEA)/Asystole
- VF/Pulseless VT

Validation of Online Course Certificates

When a student has completed the online portion of any AHA course, a skills practice and testing session must be completed with an AHA Instructor.

As a PALS Instructor, you may be asked to do a skills practice and testing session for the hands-on session of HeartCode PALS. You can confirm that the certificate a student brings you is valid.

 To validate a student's online certificate or completion, go to **www.onlineaha.org/verify_certificate**.

PALS Skills

Saving a patient in cardiac arrest requires both cognitive and psychomotor skills, as listed below:

- *Cognitive skills* include rhythm recognition, prioritizing medication administration, and algorithm application.
- *Psychomotor skills* include compressions, ventilations, and basic and advanced airway management.

PALS and BLS Skills Integration

PALS interventions are add-ons to the core skills of BLS and must be integrated carefully into ongoing BLS efforts. If a student is not performing BLS effectively, there is a strong probability that his or her PALS efforts may fail.

Effective Teamwork

Students need to understand that effective teamwork and communication increase the success of resuscitation. A Team Leader is responsible for ensuring that the team accomplishes everything in the right way at the right time; team members must be proficient in skills (within their scope of practice).

Remember, you will be testing students on their performance as Team Leaders (ie, each student must demonstrate effective management of both the patient and the resuscitation team as a whole).

Each student will

- Learn and practice specific skills in learning stations
- Integrate these skills in simulated cases
- Practice and become proficient in managing a case scenario as a Team Leader

Course Videos

Although the PALS Provider Course is instructor led, multiple videos are incorporated into the course. The videos provide information, case illustrations, and demonstrations. They are designed to facilitate the instructor's ability to provide consistent delivery of course content and information.

Course Audience

Audience-Specific Course

Some evidence suggests that adding content to the course may actually decrease learning and retention. Although it is not considered a best practice to insert additional material into this course, instructors may add related topics, as long as none of the required lessons or course content is eliminated or shortened.

If you choose to add any additional topics or information, you should do this at the beginning or end of the course so that it does not disrupt the flow of the required lessons. Additional content added by the instructor will increase course time. You must inform the students of any additional information that is from non-AHA sources. Testing requirements for course completion and card issuance cannot be changed.

Course Prerequisites

Students **must prepare adequately** to enable successful completion of the PALS Provider Course. This course does not teach BLS skills, interpretation of rhythm strips, or basic PALS pharmacology. Thus, before taking the course, students must already be proficient in the following:

- Performing child and infant BLS skills by using the *2015 AHA Guidelines Update for CPR and ECC*
- Reading and interpreting ECG rhythm strips
- Knowing basic resuscitation pharmacology

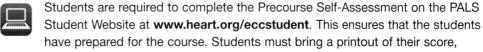 Students are required to complete the Precourse Self-Assessment on the PALS Student Website at **www.heart.org/eccstudent**. This ensures that the students have prepared for the course. Students must bring a printout of their score, which must be 70% or higher, to the PALS Course.

The following table lists additional resources for each of these requirements. **It is unlikely that students who do not complete the prerequisites and self-assessments listed below will be able to pass the PALS Provider Course.**

Prerequisite	Measurements	Resources
BLS	Demonstrate high-quality • Child CPR and AED use • Infant CPR	BLS Course *2015 AHA Guidelines Update for CPR and ECC*
ECG rhythm interpretation	Identify—on a monitor and/or paper tracing—the following rhythms and rhythm disturbances: • Normal sinus rhythm • Sinus bradycardia • Sinus tachycardia • Supraventricular tachycardia • Ventricular tachycardia • Asystole • Ventricular fibrillation	We strongly recommend that students review the ECG rhythm recognition Precourse Self-Assessment on the PALS Student Website. After this review, if students need more help to prepare for the course, we suggest they complete the AHA eLearning course on pediatric rhythms or any other appropriate ECG training program or course.
Pharmacology	Demonstrate a basic understanding of the essential drugs used in the management of • Cardiac arrest • Bradycardia • Tachycardia	We strongly recommend that students review the pharmacology Precourse Self-Assessment on the PALS Student Website. After this review, if students need more help to prepare for the course, we suggest they complete a course on pediatric pharmacology.
Combination	Be able to combine ECG rhythm recognition and pharmacology	We strongly recommend that students review the practical application in the Precourse Self-Assessment on the PALS Student Website. This section combines practical application of both rhythm recognition and pharmacology.

BLS Provider Course Completion Card

The AHA has designed its PALS courses with BLS skills as the foundation. The PALS Course does not test on all the skills for BLS and does not have the BLS exam. If a BLS Provider card is to be issued, a BLS Instructor must be present to complete the skills testing checklists and exam. The addition of testing for BLS skills and exam will add time to the PALS Course.

Precourse Self-Assessment and Checklist

 The PALS Student Website (**www.heart.org/eccstudent**) contains the following resources:

Resource	Description	How to Use
Mandatory Precourse Self-Assessment	The Precourse Self-Assessment evaluates a student's knowledge in 3 sections: rhythm recognition, pharmacology, and practical application	Complete *before the course* to help evaluate your proficiency and determine the need for additional review and practice before the course
Systematic Assessment Video	• Initial impression • Primary assessment • Secondary assessment	Review
Management of Respiratory Emergencies Video	• Basic airway management • Advanced airway management	
Management of Shock Emergencies Video	• Compensated and hypertensive shock management	
Management of Arrhythmia Video	• PALS core rhythms • Defibrillation	

 To ensure that students have prepared for the course, students must complete and pass the Precourse Self-Assessment with a score of 70% or higher. Have students print their certificate with their scores from the Precourse Self-Assessment on the PALS Student Website and bring it to class.

In addition, students should complete the Precourse Preparation Checklist that is part of the *PALS Provider Manual* and bring it to the class.

HeartCode PALS students must also complete the Precourse Self-Assessment online. After completing the Precourse Self-Assessment, HeartCode PALS students then complete the online portion of the course. Before participating in the hands-on session, students must print their online certificate of completion and bring it to the hands-on session.

Students With Special Needs

The AHA does not provide advice to Training Centers on Americans With Disabilities Act requirements or any other laws, rules, or regulations. Training Centers must determine accommodations necessary to comply with applicable laws. The AHA recommends consultation with legal counsel.

A student must be able to successfully complete all course completion requirements to receive a course completion card. Reasonable accommodations may be made, such as manikin positioning, use of a text reader, or the exam being read to the student.

If a student is unable to successfully complete skills testing because of a disability, he or she should be given written documentation of class attendance with a listing of what testing was not successfully completed.

Course Flexibility

The AHA allows instructors to tailor the PALS Course to meet audience-specific needs. Consider the following examples:

- You may choose to adapt situations to the specific location.
- You may eliminate "phone 9-1-1" for students who are emergency medical services professionals and other emergency responders.

One example of course flexibility is local protocol discussions built into some of the lessons. Also, some local protocols related to CPR can be implemented into the learning stations. The use of different protocols, such as 3 cycles of 200 continuous compressions with passive oxygen insufflation and airway adjuncts, compression-only CPR in the first few minutes after arrest, and continuous chest compressions with asynchronous ventilation once every 6 seconds with the use of a bag-mask device, are a few examples of optimizing chest compression fraction and high-quality CPR. A default compression-to-ventilation ratio of 30:2 should be used by less-trained healthcare providers or if 30:2 is the established protocol. All protocols of CPR used in the learning stations should remain within the framework of 2-minute cycles. In addition, an increased number of case scenarios for a more diverse audience and the ability to build your own scenarios further expand the flexibility to tailor the PALS Course.

Any changes to the course are in addition to the basic course contents as outlined in this manual and will add to the length of the course. Instructors may not delete course lessons or course components. Any additions or alterations to the course must be specifically identified as non-AHA material. Please refer to the section titled Non-AHA Content in this Instructor Manual for further detail.

Instructor Needs and Resources

Who Can Teach the Course

 AHA courses must be taught by AHA Instructors who have current instructor status in their specific discipline. (For detailed information about becoming an instructor, please go to **www.heart.org/cpr**, Instructor Network.)

Each AHA course must have a Course Director who is physically present throughout the course. The Course Director is responsible for course logistics and quality assurance and for ensuring that specialty faculty follow AHA guidelines in every course they teach.

An AHA Instructor in the appropriate discipline must also perform the formal assessment or testing of students.

Lead Instructor

If more than 1 instructor is teaching in a PALS Course, a Lead Instructor needs to be designated. The Lead Instructor will oversee the communication among all instructors before and during the course. The Lead Instructor will also be responsible for issuing and ensuring that students receive course completion cards from the instructor's Training Center and that all course paperwork (eg, roster, skills testing checklists, course evaluations) is supplied for the training.

The following guidelines apply to Lead Instructors for provider courses:

- Each PALS Provider Course must have a Lead Instructor physically on-site throughout the course.
- The Lead Instructor can also fill the role of instructor in the course.
- The Lead Instructor is responsible for course logistics and quality assurance.
- The Lead Instructor is assigned by the Training Center Coordinator.

Faculty Requirements

The following table lists the faculty requirements for the PALS Course. Note that one person may perform multiple roles. One instructor is needed for each of the learning stations as well as for the case scenario testing stations.

Role	Responsibilities
Course Director	• Oversees the quality of the PALS program • Must be available to answer questions during the PALS Course
PALS Instructor(s)	• One instructor is needed for the large-group interactions • One instructor is needed for each video case discussion and case scenario practice with simulations station • One instructor is needed for each of the skills stations: Airway Management, Rhythm Disturbances/Electrical Therapy, and Vascular Access • One instructor is needed for the BLS Competency Testing Station • One instructor is needed for each of the case scenario practice with simulations stations and for each of the PALS case scenario testing stations

Specialty Faculty

Specialty faculty are content experts in a particular area of the program being presented, eg, intensivists, emergency medicine physicians, and anesthesiologists. Specialty faculty are supplementary to the core staff required to teach the course (ie, they are not a substitute for the PALS Instructors). Additionally, although specialty faculty may teach in skills stations, **they may not evaluate students or be involved in the testing process.**

For further information about specialty faculty for AHA courses, please see the latest edition of the *Program Administration Manual*.

Responsibilities of specialty faculty:

• Serve as PALS content experts
• Provide necessary content while adhering to AHA guidelines
• *Do not test students or participate in the testing process*

Instructor-to-Student Ratio

The number of students allowed to participate in this course varies and usually depends on the facility, number of instructors, and available equipment.

The PALS Course has been set up for 12 students: 2 stations of 6 students each and 1 instructor for each station. The preferred ratio is 6 students to 1 learning station with 1 instructor. The station rotation schedules are designed for this ratio.

There is no absolute minimum number of students required in each station except that there must be enough students in each of the stations to actively participate in team roles. A student-to-instructor ratio of 4:1 for each station would accomplish this goal.

In some cases, a maximum learning station ratio of 8 students to 1 instructor may be permitted. The total class time, however, will increase by at least 80 minutes for *each* student over the ideal number of 6 per instructor. This is because each additional student must have practice time in each of the learning stations, additional cases need to be presented to accommodate the additional students, and additional time must be allotted for testing.

The ratio of students to instructor depends on the activity, as depicted in the table below.

Activity	Recommended Size or Ratio
Large-group interactions	The size of the group is limited by the size of the room and the number of video monitors or projection screens.
BLS station	The student-to-instructor ratio should be 6:1, with a student-to-manikin ratio of 3:1.
Skills stations and learning stations	The student-to-instructor ratio should be 6:1, up to a maximum of 8:1 (with additional time required as indicated above).
PALS case scenario testing	The student-to-instructor ratio should be a maximum of 8:1. Each student is tested as a Team Leader while the other students perform various team roles.

Student-to-Manikin Ratio

For the Airway Management and High-Quality BLS stations, there should be 1 manikin for every 3 students. For the upper airway obstruction, lower airway obstruction, lung tissue disease, disordered control of breathing, hypovolemic shock, distributive shock, obstructive shock, cardiogenic shock, bradycardia, tachycardia, PEA/asystole, and VF/pulseless VT stations, the student-to-manikin ratio is 6:1 (with a maximum ratio of 8:1, as mentioned above).

Instructor Preparation

Preparing to Teach

An essential component of teaching the PALS Provider Course is instructor preparation. Before teaching the PALS Course or the HeartCode PALS hands-on session, please take the time to read and review in detail all of the following program components:

- The *PALS Instructor Manual*
- All Lesson Plans (more information about the Lesson Plans is presented later in this manual)
- All video material
- The *PALS Provider Manual* and the Student Website

As you view the videos and the Lesson Plans (Part 6), note how the course is organized and the expectations for you and the students. Make notes on your Lesson Plans as needed.

This important preparation will enable you to teach the course more effectively and anticipate what you will need to do as the course unfolds. This is especially true for those parts of the course that require you to organize the students for practice or testing, present the video to give information, facilitate discussions, distribute equipment, conduct debriefings, and give exam or hands-on tests.

Without adequate preparation, you will not be successful teaching the PALS Course.

Course Planning and Support Materials

Determining Course Specifics

Before you teach a course, determine the course specifics:

- Student audience
- Number of students
- Special needs or equipment

You will teach both large-group and small-group sessions in this course. The small-group sessions are called *learning stations* and *testing stations*.

The following skills are tested in the testing stations:

- High-quality BLS
- Bag-mask ventilation with oropharyngeal airway
- Case scenarios

Use the sample course outlines and agendas shown in Part 2 of this manual and the Lesson Plans in Part 6 to guide you.

Please review the *PALS Instructor Manual* and the *PALS Provider Manual* as part of this process.

Templates

The *PALS Instructor Manual* and Instructor CD contain templates for letters, forms, and other materials to help you prepare to teach the course. You will need to customize some of these materials, including the precourse letter.

Sample Precourse Letter to Students (Classroom Course)

We recommend that you send a letter to students before the course. A sample letter is shown below and can also be found on the Instructor CD or on the Instructor Network; please modify the letter to suit your needs or those of your Training Center.

(Date)

Dear PALS Course Student:

Welcome to the Pediatric Advanced Life Support (PALS) Provider Course.

When and Where the Class Will Be Given:

Dates: _____

Times: _____

Location: _____

Please plan to arrive on time, because it will be difficult for late students to catch up once we start. Students are expected to attend and participate in the entire course.

What We Sent You

We have enclosed the agenda and your copy of the *PALS Provider Manual,* which includes access to a Student Website.

How to Get Ready

The PALS Course is designed to teach you the lifesaving skills required to be both a team member and a team leader in either an in-hospital or an out-of-hospital setting. Because the PALS Course covers extensive material in a short time, you will need to prepare for the course beforehand.

Precourse Requirements

You should prepare for the course by doing the following:

1. Complete the precourse checklist that came with your *PALS Provider Manual.* Bring the checklist with you to the course.
2. Review the course agenda and note course activities where you might need to supplement your knowledge before attending the course.
3. Be prepared to pass the Child CPR and AED Skills Testing Checklist and Infant CPR Skills Testing Checklist. You will not be taught how to do CPR or how to use an AED during the course. The resuscitation scenarios require that your BLS skills and knowledge are current. Review and understand all 2015 BLS guidelines, especially as they relate to pediatric patients. You may find this information in the *BLS Provider Manual* or in other publications based on the *2015 AHA Guidelines Update for Cardiopulmonary Resuscitation and Emergency Cardiovascular Care* (see **www.heart.org/cpr**).
4. Review and understand the information in your *PALS Provider Manual* and on the Student Website. Pay particular attention to the systematic approach to pediatric assessment, the evaluate-identify-intervene sequence, and the management of respiratory and circulatory abnormalities.

(continued)

(continued)

5. Review, understand, and complete the Precourse Self-Assessment (mandatory) on the Student Website (**www.heart.org/eccstudent**). You will find the code to access the Student Website in the beginning of the *PALS Provider Manual*. This test consists of 3 sections: ECG rhythm identification, pharmacology, and practical application. Use this assessment to identify areas where you need to increase your knowledge.

6. *Print your Precourse Self-Assessment score:* A passing score of 70% or above is required for the Precourse Self-Assessment. You can take the Precourse Self-Assessment as many times as needed to achieve a passing score. Bring the printout of your score with you to the PALS Course.

7. Be familiar with the PALS algorithms and flowcharts so that you can apply them to clinical scenarios. Note that the PALS Course does not present the details of each algorithm.

What This Course Does Not Cover

The PALS Course does not teach CPR, ECG rhythm identification, PALS pharmacology, or algorithms. *If you do not review CPR and if you do not learn and understand the ECG and pharmacology information in the Precourse Self-Assessment, it is unlikely that you can successfully complete the PALS Course.* You will not be taught how to read or interpret ECG rhythm strips in the course, nor will you be taught details about PALS pharmacology.

It is essential that you bring your *PALS Provider Manual* to class; you will need it during each lesson in the course.

You may refer to the *2015 Handbook of Emergency Cardiovascular Care for Healthcare Providers* (optional), and you may bring it to the course to use as a reference during some of the stations in the course.

What to Wear

Please wear loose, comfortable clothing to class. You will be practicing skills that require you to work on your hands and knees, and the course requires bending, standing, and lifting. If you have any physical conditions that might prevent you from engaging in these activities, please tell an instructor. The instructor may be able to adjust the equipment if you have back, knee, or hip problems.

We look forward to welcoming you on (day and date of class). If you have any questions about the course, please call (name) at (telephone number).

Sincerely,

(Name), Lead Instructor

Sample Precourse Letter to Students (HeartCode PALS)

The letter below is a sample you may modify and send to students completing HeartCode PALS.

(Date)

Dear HeartCode PALS Course Student:

Welcome to the HeartCode PALS Course. This course has 2 components: an online portion and an instructor-led classroom portion referred to as the *hands-on session*. You must complete the online portion first.

Your course key to access the online portion is (key number).

The online portion includes an exam. You will have access to your *PALS Provider Manual* online during the exam.

Important: You must print the certificate of completion at the end of the online portion. You will need to give this to your instructor when you attend the classroom portion. It is necessary to show that you completed the online portion and passed the exam. If you do not have your certificate of completion, you will not be able to complete the skills practice and testing of the course.

The classroom portion is scheduled for

Date: _____

Time: _____

Location: _____

What to Expect
Please wear loose, comfortable clothing. You will be practicing skills that require working on your hands and knees, bending, standing, and lifting. If you have physical conditions that might prevent you from participating in the course, please tell one of the instructors when you arrive for the course. The instructor will work to accommodate your needs within the stated course completion requirements. In the event that you are ill, please notify your instructor to reschedule your training.

We look forward to welcoming you on (day and date of class). If you have any questions about the course, please call (name) at (telephone number).

Sincerely,

(Name), Lead Instructor

Sample Precourse Letter to Instructors (Classroom Course)

(Date)

Dear PALS Course Instructor:

Thank you for being available to teach the PALS Course. Attendance on your date of instruction is critical. You are scheduled as an instructor for the following class:

Dates: _____

Times: _____

Location: _____

Preparing to Teach the Course

Adequate preparation is essential. Review the course agenda with list of groups, numbers, and rotation assignments. Study the Lesson Plans carefully. All lessons should be taught *exactly* as detailed on the Lesson Plans. Review the *PALS Instructor Manual, PALS Provider Manual*, and PALS Student Website.

Faculty Assignments

See the Lesson Plans for an explanation of how to conduct your assigned lessons. Faculty assignments are as follows:

Lesson Number	Course Event	Who Has This Assignment?
Introduction	Course Introduction	
1	Life Is Why™ Activity (Optional)	
2	Course Overview	
3	Science of Pediatric Resuscitation	
4A	Learning/Testing Station: Child High-Quality BLS Practice	
4B	Learning/Testing Station: Child High-Quality BLS Testing—Testing Details	
5A	Learning/Testing Station: Infant High-Quality BLS Practice	
5B	Learning/Testing Station: Infant High-Quality BLS Testing—Testing Details	
6	Learning/Testing Station: Child and Infant Choking (Optional)	
7A	Overview of Systematic Approach Model	
7B	Secondary Assessment	
8	Team Dynamics	
9A	Management of Respiratory Emergencies	
9B	Respiratory Video Case Discussion	

(continued)

(continued)

Lesson Number	Course Event	Who Has This Assignment?
9C	Learning Station: Airway Management	
10A	Management of Shock Emergencies	
10B	Shock Video Case Discussions	
10C	Learning Station: Vascular Access	
11A	Management of Arrhythmia Emergencies	
11B	Arrhythmia Video Case Discussions	
11C	Learning Station: Rhythm Disturbances/ Electrical Therapy	
12	Management of Post–Cardiac Arrest Care	
13	Learning Station: Coping With Death (Optional)	
14	Case Scenario Practice With Simulations	
15	Case Scenario Testing	
16	Exam	

If you have any questions about your assignment, please call (name) at (telephone number). Thanks again for your commitment to serve as faculty for this PALS Provider Course.

Sincerely,

(Name), Lead Instructor

Notice of Courses

For US-based instructors aligned with the AHA Instructor Network, the AHA offers the My Courses tool, where instructors can enter and maintain the classes they offer to the general public. These are displayed to customers searching for scheduled classes at the AHA's CPR & First Aid website, **www.heart.org/cpr**. Before entering classes, check with your Training Center to determine what policies your Training Center may have regarding instructors entering their classes. As an instructor, you can still add your classes for display through My Courses even if your Training Center is not participating in listing through My Courses.

For instructors based outside the United States, inform your International Training Center of courses open to the public so that they can send inquiries for classes to you.

Instructor Network

The AHA provides the Instructor Network as a resource to instructors. Here, instructors can access up-to-date resources and reference information about AHA ECC Programs and science.

AHA Instructor Network
www.ahainstructornetwork.org

All AHA Instructors are required to register on the Instructor Network and be aligned with a Training Center. Alignment must be approved by that Training Center before access to content is available. Acceptance of the user agreement is required during registration.

Once registered and approved, you will receive an instructor identification number. This number will be placed on your instructor card and is the same for all disciplines. This number stays the same if you change Training Centers. It is used on all course completions cards for classes that you teach.

The AHA reserves the right to delete or deny alignments on the Instructor Network.

Full Code Pro App

A program that can be useful in the team resuscitation activity and in your clinical practice is the AHA's Full Code Pro. This is a free, easy-to-use, mobile application that allows healthcare providers to quickly document critical interventions during cardiac arrest resuscitation events or training sessions in real time. This allows providers to focus on the patient without sacrificing proper documentation.

You can find information and a link to this app on the AHA CPR & First Aid website, **www.heart.org/cpr**, CPR under Healthcare Providers.

Ordering Materials

To help with the distribution of ECC materials, the AHA has partnered with companies in the United States and all international territories that provide high-quality customer service and support. Current lists of distributors for your country are available on the AHA's CPR & First Aid website, **www.heart.org/cpr**.

As an instructor, you can order books and other support materials directly from any AHA distributor, but only a Training Center Coordinator can order course completion cards from an authorized AHA distributor. Work with your Training Center Coordinator to ensure cards are issued to the students of the classes you teach.

Copyright of AHA Materials

The AHA owns the copyright to AHA books and other training materials. These materials may not be copied, in whole or in part, without the prior written consent of the AHA.

For more information and to request permission to reprint, copy, or use portions of ECC textbooks or other materials, go to **copyright.heart.org**.

Exam Security

To prevent possible compromise, exams are distributed to Training Center Coordinators only. You will need to contact your Training Center Coordinator for the specific exams you will need for a course.

Exam security is of the utmost importance:

- Ensure that all exams are kept secure and not copied or distributed outside the classroom.
- Exams cannot be edited, and only AHA-translated exams can be used.*
- Course exams may not be posted to any learning management system, Internet, or intranet site.
- Always use the current exams to determine successful course completion.
- Each exam should be accounted for and returned to the instructor at the end of the testing period.
- If receiving the exams electronically from your Training Center Coordinator, they must be sent to an email address that only you can access.

*Exams are translated into multiple languages. If a translated exam is needed for a course you are teaching, have your Training Center Coordinator contact the ECC Customer Support Center to see if the needed translation is available.

Room Requirements

You can teach a typical course—for example, with 12 students and 2 to 3 instructors—in 1 large room and 1 or 2 small rooms. The large room should comfortably hold at least 20 people. The smaller rooms must hold up to 8 students plus the instructor(s) and required manikins and equipment.

Please see below for additional details.

An average PALS Course consists of 12 students divided into 2 smaller groups of 6 during the case simulations. To accommodate 12 students, there should be 1 large room that seats 12 to 15 people comfortably. Because case scenarios can be conducted with 7 people, smaller rooms should accommodate up to 8 people (7 students and 1 instructor) along with equipment.

Both the large and small rooms should have

- Good acoustics
- Bright lighting that can be adjusted for video presentations
- An instructor-controlled video player and a monitor or screen large enough to be viewed by all the students (although a TV may be acceptable for small classes with only a few groups, larger classes with several manikins may require a large-screen TV or a computer and LCD projector)
- A chair for each student
- A table for completing the exam

Smoking Policy

The Training Center must prohibit smoking in classrooms and training facilities during all AHA ECC training programs.

Sample Floor Plan

The following graphic shows a sample small-group room layout for the case scenario practice with simulation discussions and case scenario testing portions of the PALS Provider Course.

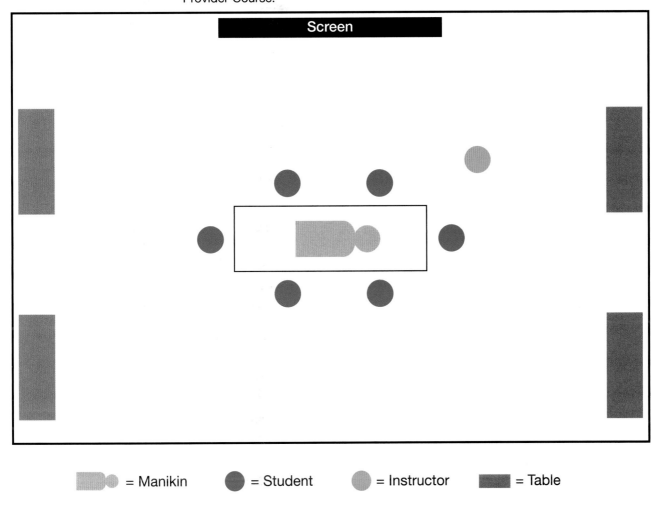

= Manikin   = Student   = Instructor   = Table

Core Curriculum

Each AHA course must follow the guidelines and core curriculum in the most current editions of the *PALS Provider Manual* and *PALS Instructor Manual*. Current editions of AHA course materials must serve as the primary training resources during the course.

PALS instructor materials include the following course support materials:

- Instructor Manual
- Student Website
- Instructor CD
- Course video
- Lesson Plans
- Cases scenarios
- Posters
- Checklists
- Algorithms and flowcharts
- *2015 Handbook of ECC for Healthcare Providers* (ECC Handbook)
- Equipment list

PALS Instructor Manual and CD

The Instructor CD contains copies of many of the important materials included in the *PALS Instructor Manual*, eg, Lesson Plans, case scenarios, and testing checklists. By having the material available in 2 formats, instructors and Course Coordinators have flexibility in retrieving the information.

Lesson Plans

Located in Part 6, Lesson Plans are full-color, 2-sided, 3-hole–punched information pages used to guide the instructor through each lesson. The Lesson Plans will guide you in teaching each lesson in the course.

Case Scenarios

A repository of instructor case scenarios has been created for each of the case scenarios to allow instructors to challenge students related to their scope of practice and level of experience. The case scenarios contain the information that you will need to facilitate the case discussions and case simulations. Each page includes a debriefing tool on the back that is specific to that particular scenario. Scenarios are grouped from least complex to most complex.

Posters (Optional)
- PALS Systematic Approach Algorithm
- PALS Systematic Approach Summary
- Pediatric Cardiac Arrest Algorithm—2015 Update
- Pediatric Bradycardia With a Pulse and Poor Perfusion Algorithm
- Pediatric Tachycardia With a Pulse and Adequate Perfusion Algorithm
- Pediatric Tachycardia With a Pulse and Poor Perfusion Algorithm
- Pediatric Septic Shock Algorithm
- PALS Management of Shock After ROSC Algorithm
- Pediatric Management of Respiratory Emergencies Flowchart
- Pediatric Management of Shock Flowchart

Place the posters in a prominent location, or have students use other AHA materials that contain the AHA algorithms in each of the learning stations in the course to guide and reinforce skills practice. Also place such materials in common areas of the workplace or organization (eg, kitchen, work room, break room) to remind employees and staff of steps to take in an emergency.

Case Scenario Testing Checklists
- Upper Airway Obstruction
- Lower Airway Obstruction
- Lung Tissue Disease
- Disordered Control of Breathing
- Hypovolemic Shock
- Obstructive Shock
- Distributive Shock
- Cardiogenic Shock
- Supraventricular Tachycardia
- Bradycardia
- Asystole/PEA
- VF/Pulseless VT

Learning Station Competency Checklists
- Airway Management
- Rhythm Disturbances/Electrical Therapy
- Vascular Access

Algorithms and Flowcharts
Use these algorithms and flowcharts during the learning stations:
- PALS Systematic Approach Algorithm
- PALS Systematic Approach Summary
- Pediatric Cardiac Arrest Algorithm—2015 Update
- Pediatric Bradycardia With a Pulse and Poor Perfusion Algorithm
- Pediatric Tachycardia With a Pulse and Adequate Perfusion Algorithm
- Pediatric Tachycardia With a Pulse and Poor Perfusion Algorithm
- Pediatric Septic Shock Algorithm
- Pediatric Recognition of Respiratory Problems Flowchart
- Pediatric Management of Respiratory Emergencies Flowchart
- Pediatric Recognition of Shock Flowchart
- Pediatric Management of Shock Flowchart

ECC Handbook (Optional)

The ECC Handbook may be purchased (optional) through the website at **www.heart.org**. Students may use the ECC Handbook during all learning stations and the exam, with the following stipulations:

- A student may use the ECC Handbook to check a drug dose during the learning and testing stations.
- A student may not spend a significant amount of time looking up details of case management in the ECC Handbook.

PALS Provider Manual
The *PALS Provider Manual* is designed to be both a stand-alone publication and a complement to the PALS Course. We strongly recommend that both instructors and students review the appropriate sections before each course session. Students should keep their manuals with them during all course activities.

Refer to the manual often during each class session.

The *PALS Provider Manual* also includes access to the PALS Student Website, where the Precourse Self-Assessment is located. The Precourse Self-Assessment tests students' knowledge of ECG rhythm identification, pharmacology, and practical application.

PALS Course Videos

The PALS Course videos cover the following topics:
- Course Overview
- Life Is Why (Optional)
- Science of Pediatric Resuscitation
- Child High-Quality BLS
- Infant High-Quality BLS
- Systematic Approach
- Secondary Assessment
- Team Dynamics
- Management of Respiratory Emergencies
- PALS Respiratory Video Case Discussions
- Management of Shock Emergencies
- PALS Shock Video Case Discussions
- IO Access
- Management of Arrhythmia Emergencies
- PALS Arrhythmia Video Case Discussions
- Management of Post–Cardiac Arrest Care
- Coping With Death (Optional)

Encourage students to follow along in their *PALS Provider Manual* while watching the PALS Course videos.

Precourse Self-Assessment

Student preparation is essential for participating in and completing the PALS Course. The mandatory Precourse Self-Assessment certificate is required for entrance into the course. This assessment allows the student to understand any gaps in knowledge needed to participate in and successfully complete the course. A student who enters the PALS Course without basic arrhythmia, pharmacology, high-quality BLS, and bag-mask ventilation knowledge and skills will not be able to function in the learning and testing stations and is unlikely to successfully complete the PALS Course.

Students should prepare for the PALS Course by doing the following:
1. Complete the Precourse Preparation Checklist that came with their *PALS Provider Manual*, and bring the checklist with them to the course.
2. Review the course agenda.
3. Review and understand the information in their *PALS Provider Manual*.

4. Review, understand, and complete the Precourse Self-Assessment on the Student Website (**www.heart.org/eccstudent**).
5. Students must print their scores (certificate) for the Precourse Self-Assessment and bring them to class. A score of 70% or above is needed to pass the assessment. A student can take the Precourse Self-Assessment as many times as needed to achieve a passing score.
   - Should a student fail to provide a printed copy of his or her certificate, advise the student to log back into the Student Website and print the certificate.
   - If the student is unable to validate a score of 70% with the instructor, have the student reschedule to complete the PALS Course.

Ordering Course Completion Cards

Only a Training Center Coordinator, or another authorized Training Center representative designated by the Training Center Coordinator, can use the confidential security code to order course completion cards for approved disciplines. The Training Center Coordinator should keep this code confidential. Training Center Coordinators cannot order course completion cards without this code.

The Training Center Coordinator has final responsibility to the AHA for the security code. The Training Center Coordinator must notify the AHA Account Manager or the ECC Training Network Support Center *immediately* if the security code is suspected as lost, stolen, disclosed, or used without authorization.

The AHA may change the code if deemed necessary to maintain the confidentiality of the code.

Misuse of the confidential security code could result in termination of the Training Center Agreement.

For more information on course completion cards, refer to the Course Card Reference Guide on the Instructor Network.

Non-AHA Content

As an instructor, you can best serve your students when you can adapt to meet the needs of a specific audience. As discussed earlier, some course flexibility has been added to the AHA courses in the form of a wider range of scenarios, set agenda time for discussion of local protocols, and tools to help lead those discussions. If you find that your students will be better served by adding location-specific information, equipment, or specialty-specific content and you plan to discuss that non-AHA content in class or distribute handouts, follow these rules:

- None of the required AHA lessons or course content can be eliminated or shortened.
- Any changes to the course are in addition to the basic content as outlined in your Instructor Manual.
- Adding additional content will add time to the course.
- Any location-specific protocols or procedures that do not comply with AHA processes (eg, substituting new medications, specialized techniques) should be identified to the audience as location specific.
- Any non-AHA content must be identified as not approved or reviewed by the AHA, and the source of the information must be provided to the students.
- Supplementary materials that you use need to be approved by the PALS Lead Instructor or the Course Director for advanced courses, as well as your Training Center Coordinator.
- A copy of a revised agenda, and any print material shared in class must be part of the permanent course file.
- Your students cannot be tested on non-AHA content. If they complete the AHA-defined course completion requirements, they must be issued an AHA course completion card or eCard.

 For questions about adding location-specific information or specialty-specific content, contact **resuscitationlearning@heart.org**.

Course Equipment

All AHA ECC courses require that manikins and equipment allow demonstration of the core skills of the course being taught (eg, airway management, correct hand placement, compression depth, chest recoil).

The AHA neither endorses nor recommends a particular brand of manikin or other equipment. The decision of which brand or model of equipment to use is the responsibility of the Training Center. The AHA does strongly encourage the use of manikins that provide audiovisual feedback to help aid both students and instructors on psychomotor skills performance.

Equipment List

Equipment required for each class held is listed in the table below. All equipment used must be clean and in proper working order and good repair.

The table lists the equipment and supplies needed to optimally conduct this course. This includes a code cart for in-hospital providers and a jump kit and defibrillator unit for prehospital providers. The code cart/jump kit should contain the equipment and supplies listed in the table.

Equipment and Supplies	Quantity Needed	Learning/Testing Station Equipment Needed
Paperwork		
Precourse letter	1/student	Precourse
Course roster	1/course	Beginning of course
Name tags	1/student and instructor	All
Course agenda	1/student and instructor	End of course
Course completion card	1/student	All
PALS Provider Manual	1/student and instructor	All
PALS Instructor Manual with Lesson Plans	1/instructor	All
Instructor case scenarios	1/instructor	All
Team role labels	1 set/station to identify team role for each student	All small group stations
Skills station competency checklists	1/student and instructor	BLS and skills stations
PALS Course Progress Checklist	1/instructor	All
Cardiac, shock, and respiratory practice scenario checklists	1/student	Airway Management Learning Station, Vascular Access Learning Station, and Rhythm Disturbances/Electrical Therapy Learning Station
Child and infant BLS skills testing checklists	1 of each/student	Child and Infant High-Quality BLS
ECC Handbook (optional)	1/student and instructor	Optional; all
PALS algorithms/flowcharts	1 set/station	All
PALS Exam	1/student	Exam
Blank exam answer sheet	1/student	Exam
Exam answer key/annotated answer key	1/course	Exam
Algorithm posters	1/course	Cardiac case scenario discussions, Rhythm Disturbances/Electrical Therapy Learning Station

(continued)

(continued)

Equipment and Supplies	Quantity Needed	Learning/Testing Station Equipment Needed
Institution-based documentation form	1/course	Cardiac case scenario discussions
Learning station competency checklists	1/student	Child and Infant High-Quality BLS, Airway Management Learning Station, Rhythm Disturbances/Electrical Therapy Learning Station, Vascular Access Learning Station
Audiovisual Equipment		
TV with DVD player or computer with video player and projection screen	1/station	Course Overview, Overview of PALS Science, Child and Infant High-Quality BLS Practice and Testing, Airway Management Learning Station, Rhythm Disturbances/Electrical Therapy Learning Station, Vascular Access Learning Station, Systematic Approach, Team Dynamics
Course video	1	Course Overview, Overview of PALS Science, Child and Infant High-Quality BLS Practice and Testing, Airway Management Learning Station, Rhythm Disturbances/Electrical Therapy Learning Station, Vascular Access Learning Station, Systematic Approach, Team Dynamics
CPR and AED Equipment		
BLS feedback device recommended*	1/station	Child and Infant High-Quality BLS Practice and Testing, Rhythm Disturbances/Electrical Therapy Learning Station, cardiac case scenario discussions
Child CPR manikin with shirt*	1/every 3 students	Child and Infant High-Quality BLS Practice and Testing, Rhythm Disturbances/Electrical Therapy Learning Station, cardiac case scenario discussions, shock case scenario discussions
Infant CPR manikin*	1/every 3 students	Child and Infant High-Quality BLS Practice and Testing, Management of Cardiac Emergencies Learning Station, cardiac case scenario discussions, shock case scenario discussions
Child airway manikin or intubation head	1/every 3 students	Airway Management Learning Station, respiratory case scenario discussions
Infant airway manikin or intubation head	1/every 3 students	Airway Management Learning Station, respiratory case scenario discussions
Stopwatch/timing device	1/instructor	High-Quality BLS Practice and Testing
Countdown timer	1/instructor	High-Quality BLS Practice and Testing

(continued)

(continued)

Equipment and Supplies	Quantity Needed	Learning/Testing Station Equipment Needed
AED trainer with adult and child AED training pads	1/every 3 students	High-Quality BLS Practice and Testing, Rhythm Disturbances/Electrical Therapy Learning Station, cardiac case scenario discussions
CPR backboard	1/every 3 students	High-Quality BLS Practice and Testing, cardiac case scenario discussions
Stools to stand on for CPR	1/every 3 students	High-Quality BLS Practice and Testing, cardiac case scenario discussions
Airway and Ventilation		
Infant airway manikin or intubation head	1/every 3 students	Airway Management Learning Station, respiratory case scenario discussions
Child pocket mask and infant pocket mask	1/every 3 students or 1/student	High-Quality BLS Practice and Testing, respiratory case scenario discussions
1-way valve	1/student	High-Quality BLS Practice and Testing, respiratory case scenario discussions
Bag-mask devices • 450 to 500 mL for infants and young children • 1000 mL or larger for older children and adolescents	1/every 3 students	High-Quality BLS Practice and Testing, Rhythm Disturbances/Electrical Therapy Learning Station, respiratory case scenario discussions, shock case scenario discussions
Nonrebreathing mask with reservoir	1/station	Airway Management Learning Station, respiratory case scenario discussions, shock case scenario discussions
Nasal cannula	1/station	Airway Management Learning Station, respiratory case scenario discussions
High-flow nasal cannula (optional)	1/station	Airway Management Learning Station, respiratory case scenario discussions
Simple oxygen mask	1/station	Airway Management Learning Station, respiratory case scenario discussions
Suction catheters	1 set of multiple sizes/station	Airway Management Learning Station, respiratory case scenario discussions
Nebulizer setup	1 set/station	Airway Management Learning Station, respiratory case scenario discussions
Waveform capnography equipment*	Pictures can be used to represent this technology	Airway Management Learning Station, Rhythm Disturbances/Electrical Therapy Learning Station, respiratory case scenario discussions, cardiac case scenario discussions, shock case scenario discussions
Stethoscope	1/every manikin	Airway Management Learning Station, respiratory case scenario discussions, shock case scenario discussions

(continued)

(continued)

Equipment and Supplies	Quantity Needed	Learning/Testing Station Equipment Needed
Color-coded length-based resuscitation tape	1/station	Airway Management Learning Station, Rhythm Disturbances/Electrical Therapy Learning Station, respiratory case scenario discussions, cardiac case scenario discussions, shock case scenario discussions, Vascular Access Learning Station
Towel	1/every 3 students	Airway Management Learning Station, respiratory case scenario discussions
Exhaled CO_2 detector: adult, child, and infant	1/station	Airway Management Learning Station, respiratory case scenario discussions, shock case scenario discussions
Tube holder or tape, pediatric	1/every manikin	Airway Management Learning Station, respiratory case scenario discussions
Rhythm Recognition and Electrical Therapy		
Cardiac monitor with ECG leads, electrodes, and pads (infant, child/adult)	1 set/station	Rhythm Disturbances/Electrical Therapy Learning Station, cardiac case scenario discussions
Rhythm generator	1/course	Rhythm Disturbances/Electrical Therapy Learning Station, cardiac case scenario discussions
AED trainer	1/station	Rhythm Disturbances/Electrical Therapy Learning Station, cardiac case scenario discussions
Color-coded length-based resuscitation tape		Rhythm Disturbances/Electrical Therapy Learning Station
BLS feedback devices recommended*		Rhythm Disturbances/Electrical Therapy Learning Station
Waveform capnography recommended		Rhythm Disturbances/Electrical Therapy Learning Station
Equipment and Medications		
IO manikin	1 (with replacement bones)	Vascular Access Learning Station, shock case scenario discussions
IO drill and needles recommended	1 drill, various needle sizes	Vascular Access Learning Station, shock case scenario discussions
IO manual needles	3/station	Vascular Access Learning Station, shock case scenario discussions

(continued)

(continued)

Equipment and Supplies	Quantity Needed	Learning/Testing Station Equipment Needed
Respiratory medications: resuscitation drugs or drug cards • Albuterol • Ipratropium • Epinephrine 1 mg/mL racemic (2.25%) • IM epinephrine 1 mg/mL	1/student	Respiratory case scenario discussions
Cardiac medications: resuscitation drugs or drug cards • Adenosine • Amiodarone • Atropine sulfate • Epinephrine 0.1 mg/mL • Glucose • Lidocaine • Magnesium sulfate		Cardiac case scenario discussions
Shock medications: resuscitation drugs or drug cards • Atropine sulfate • Epinephrine 0.1 mg/mL • Fluids • Glucose • Inotropes • Vasopressors		Shock case scenario discussions
Fluid bag	1	Vascular Access Learning Station, shock case scenario discussions
3-way stopcock	1	Vascular Access Learning Station, shock case scenario discussions
60-cc locking syringe	1	Vascular Access Learning Station, shock case scenario discussions
Syringes	2-3/station	Vascular Access Learning Station, shock case scenario discussions
Advanced Airways (must choose endotracheal tube and at least 1 supraglottic device)		
Oropharyngeal airways	Various infant/child sizes/1 each	High-Quality BLS Practice and Testing, respiratory case scenario discussions, Airway Management Emergencies Learning Station
Supraglottic airways	Various samples sizes	Airway Management Learning Station, respiratory case scenario discussions
MDI, spacers, and mouth piece/mask	1 set/station	Airway Management Learning Station, respiratory case scenario discussions
Water-soluble lubricant	1/station	Airway Management Learning Station, respiratory case scenario discussions
Laryngoscope handle	1 adult and 1 child size/ every 3 students	Airway Management Learning Station, respiratory case scenario discussions

(continued)

(continued)

Equipment and Supplies	Quantity Needed	Learning/Testing Station Equipment Needed
Laryngoscope blades	Multiple straight and curved blades	Airway Management Learning Station, respiratory case scenario discussions
Endotracheal tubes, cuffed and uncuffed with stylet	Various sizes that fit airway manikin	Airway Management Learning Station, respiratory case scenario discussions
Safety		
Sharps container (if using real needles)	1/station	Vascular Access Learning Station, shock case scenario discussions
Cleaning Supplies for Use Between Student Practice and After Course		
Manikin cleaning supplies	As needed between students	High-Quality BLS Practice and Testing, Airway Management Learning Station, Rhythm Disturbances/Electrical Therapy Learning Station, Vascular Access Learning Station, respiratory case scenario discussions, cardiac case scenario discussions, shock case scenario discussions

*Directive feedback devices.

Equipment and Manikin Cleaning

Infection Control

It is your responsibility as an instructor to ensure that a safe, clean environment is maintained in your class. You need to inform your students in advance that training sessions involve close physical contact with manikins and that they will be close to other students.

In your welcome letter that is sent with course materials, students should be told about not attending class if they know they have an infectious disease, feel sick, or have open sores or cuts on their hands, mouth, or areas around their mouth.

You also need to advise other instructors teaching with you to refrain from coming to class if they are ill.

Equipment and Manikin Cleaning

To reduce the risk of potential disease transmission, all manikins and training equipment need to be thoroughly cleaned after each class. Manikins used for CPR practice and testing require special actions to be taken between each student. The AHA strongly recommends that you follow manufacturers' recommendations for manikin use and maintenance. In the absence of manufacturers' recommendations, the guidelines below may be used during and after courses.

During Class

- Students and instructors should practice good hygiene with proper hand-washing techniques.
- When individual protective face shields are used, all decontamination recommendations listed for cleaning manikins during and after a course should still be followed. In addition, to reduce the risks to each user for exposure to contaminants, ensure that all students consistently place the same side of the face shield on the manikin during use.
- If you are not using face shields during the course, manikins should be cleaned after use by each student with a manikin wipe that has an antiseptic with 70% ethyl alcohol:
  - Open the packet, and take out and unfold the manikin wipe.
  - Rub the manikin's mouth and nose vigorously with the wipe.
  - Wrap the wipe snugly over the mouth and nose.
  - Keep the wipe in place for 30 seconds.
  - Dry the manikin's face with a clean paper towel or something similar.
  - Continue with the ventilation practice.

After Class

- Manikins should be taken apart as directed by the manufacturer. Anyone taking apart and decontaminating manikins should wear protective gloves and wash his or her hands when finished.
- Any part of the manikin that came in contact with potentially infectious body fluids during training should be cleaned as soon as possible at the end of each class to prevent contaminants from drying on manikin surfaces.
- If manikins are stored for more than 24 hours before cleaning, follow these steps:
  - All surfaces, reusable protective face shields, and pocket masks should be washed thoroughly with warm, soapy water and brushes.
  - All surfaces should be moistened with a sodium hypochlorite solution having at least 500 ppm free available chlorine (one quarter cup of liquid household bleach per gallon of tap water) for 10 minutes. This solution must be made fresh for each class and discarded after each use. Using a concentration higher than one quarter cup has not been proven to be more effective and may discolor the manikins.
  - All surfaces should be rinsed with fresh water and allowed to air dry before storing.
  - Some manufacturers have recommendations for cleaning manikin parts in a dishwasher. Check with the manufacturer of the manikins being used to determine if this is an acceptable method. Some manikin materials could be damaged in a dishwasher.
- Disposable airway equipment must be replaced at the end of each day of class.
- Manikin clothing and the manikin carrying case should be cleaned periodically or when soiled.
- Other equipment used in class needs to be maintained according to hospital policy. Surfaces touched by students should be wiped with antiseptic solution.

Exposure

Participants and instructors should postpone CPR training if they are known to be in the active stages of an infectious disease, have reason to believe they have been exposed to an infectious disease, or have open sores or cuts on their hands, mouth, or area around the mouth.

Part 2

Teaching the Course

Interacting With Students

Greeting Students

Be sure to greet each student as he or she arrives so that everyone feels welcome and comfortable with you as the instructor.

During the Course

Throughout the course, try to get to know each student, observe each person's strengths and weaknesses, and work with each individual to ensure that learning is taking place. As the course progresses, share information about each student with other instructors so that each student has an opportunity for coaching, feedback, and encouragement from all instructors.

Importance of High-Quality CPR

High-quality CPR, comprised of manual chest compressions and ventilations, is the foundation of lifesaving resuscitation for cardiac arrest victims. Advanced interventions in resuscitation (such as administering medication) will not be effective without chest compressions and effective breaths. This is because chest compressions are needed to deliver the medication to vital organs and the body's tissues.

Too often, CPR is not performed or is performed with too many interruptions during out-of-hospital and in-hospital arrests. Studies of CPR skills retention have shown patterns of significant erosion of CPR skills in the days, weeks, and months after CPR training.

All PALS students will have the opportunity to learn and practice high-quality CPR and then be able to demonstrate these lifesaving skills during the course assessment.

Components of high-quality CPR for infants or children in cardiac arrest include the following:

- Push hard, at least 2 inches (5 cm) in adolescents, at least one third the antero-posterior diameter of the chest (about 2 inches [5 cm]) in children, and at least one third the anteroposterior diameter of the chest (about 1½ inches [4 cm]) in infants; when a feedback device is available, adjust to a maximum depth of 2.4 inches (6 cm) in adolescents, because excessive compression depth has been shown to cause injuries during CPR.
- Push fast: compress at a rate of 100 to 120 per minute.
- Minimize interruptions in compressions to less than 10 seconds.
- Allow for complete chest recoil between compressions (do not lean on the chest between compressions).
- Avoid excessive ventilation, delivering breaths over 1 second that produce visible chest rise.
- Switch compressors about every 2 minutes or earlier if fatigued.

35

High-Performance Teamwork

With resuscitation teams, high-performance teamwork is a critical element of providing high-quality CPR. Resuscitation skills competency is most often verified on an individual basis despite the fact that successful patient outcome for cardiac arrest depends on a team.

Students learn about high-performance teamwork in the PALS Course. They will practice it in the PALS Course and in the classroom portion of HeartCode PALS.

Teams function differently in different facilities and in all out-of-hospital settings. Knowing the policies and procedures and the local protocols of your classroom audience is essential to instructor preparation.

Learning Stations and Skills Practice

Introduction

During the learning stations, you will review specific skills and case scenarios with the students. There are several case scenarios for each of the learning and testing stations; both out-of-hospital and in-hospital scenarios are provided in Appendix A.

It is critical that every student has a role in each case and that every student has an opportunity to be the Team Leader 2 times in the course. Assigned student roles may vary depending on the number of students in the station. Extra students may be given roles as additional recorders or as a second person managing the airway. Instructors are not required to present cases in any specific sequence, but assigned student roles should not be changed. Case order in subsequent learning stations rotates students so that no one student always goes first in the station.

During the full PALS Course, a student must take the role of Team Leader 2 times in the following stations:

- Upper Airway Obstruction
- Lower Airway Obstruction
- Lung Tissue Disease
- Disordered Control of Breathing
- Hypovolemic Shock
- Obstructive Shock
- Distributive Shock
- Cardiogenic Shock
- Bradycardia
- SVT
- Asystole/PEA
- VF/Pulseless VT

During the PALS Update Course, a student must take the role of Team Leader at least 1 time:

- Case Scenario Practice With Simulations
- Case Scenario Testing

Preparing for Learning Stations

Teach the learning stations:

- Airway Management
- Vascular Access
- Rhythm Disturbances/Electrical Therapy
- Case Scenario Practice With Simulations

The sample agendas provided can be modified based on the needs of the Training Center. The first 3 lessons should be done in order, and the BLS and Airway Management testing should be accomplished early on day 1, as they are the foundation for the PALS Course.

To prepare for the learning stations, carefully review all the material for each station in the Lesson Plans (Part 6) in this manual and in the *PALS Provider Manual*. Preparation includes practicing components of a learning station. For the first few times, it may be helpful for you and other instructors to rehearse with each other. The practice sessions will make you familiar with the materials and which instructor can best cover particular sections of the content.

Additional preparation includes the following:

- Set up your learning station—make sure you have all the necessary equipment and supplies and that everything works properly.
- Confirm that you have enough supplies.
- Confirm that batteries are fully charged and backups are available.
- Confirm that you can properly operate the simulators and manikins.
- Review the Lesson Plans.
- Review the ECC Handbook (optional) and the *2015 AHA Guidelines Update for CPR and ECC*.

Three categories of case scenarios are presented in the learning stations. The student is to use the systematic approach outlined in the Systematic Approach Algorithm for each case. This approach includes the **evaluate-identify-intervene** sequence.

You need to understand the Systematic Approach Algorithm to effectively facilitate the case discussions and case scenario simulations. Please read "Part 3: Systematic Approach to the Seriously Ill or Injured Child" in the *PALS Provider Manual* for a detailed explanation of this core concept.

Each 10-minute *case discussion* begins with a short video clip of a seriously ill or injured infant or child. Students form their initial impression of the child's condition by assessing appearance, breathing, and color. This guides the next steps. If the child is unresponsive and not breathing (or only gasping), CPR should be immediately initiated. If the child has a pulse of greater than 60/min with normal breathing, students may proceed with the evaluate-identify-intervene sequence. The second portion of the video provides information to help students evaluate the child's condition. Evaluation includes the primary assessment, secondary assessment, and diagnostic assessment. From that information, students can begin to identify the type (respiratory, circulatory, or both) and severity of the clinical condition more specifically. Each case discussion ends with a video summary of key findings. **Do not discuss treatment during the case discussions.**

During the *case scenario simulations,* students perform important interventions on a manikin. Each case has a designated Team Leader who directs the team members in actions to manage the case. As the instructor, use the case scenarios to conduct the simulation and create a realistic environment that engages the students in hands-on management of the simulated patient. While the team is managing the patient, make observations and note the actions in preparation for the debriefing section of the simulation scenario. Be careful to limit the case simulation to no longer than 10 minutes and follow immediately with the debriefing. The debriefing is a critical component of the case simulations and should last 10 minutes (use a stopwatch or timer). Conduct a thorough debriefing with both of the debriefing tools printed on the case scenarios. Remember to give feedback phrased in a positive, constructive manner rather than in a negative way and to avoid criticizing the performance of the Team Leader or members. Because the learning stations are designed to help students learn from the case simulations, the instructor should strive to make them positive experiences, avoiding any resemblance to a testing experience.

Review the Lesson Plans for detailed instructions on how to conduct each learning station.

To prepare for the skills and learning stations, carefully review all the material for each learning station in the *PALS Provider Manual*, this manual, the Lesson Plans, and the case scenarios.

- In the case simulation stations, identify students' team roles by using team role labels.
- Use the stopwatch (not a wristwatch) to time the simulation section (10 minutes) and the debriefing section (10 minutes).
- If the station includes a case scenario, read the scenario lead-in for the case. Be prepared to provide key information about the case as it unfolds in case discussion and case simulations. Use the patient information on the case scenarios for the case. Do not deviate from the information provided.
- *During case scenario simulations, give answers to requests for case information only after a team member performs the appropriate assessment-related action on the manikin.* For example, when asked for the child's blood pressure, provide it only after the blood pressure cuff is in place and a team member simulates taking the blood pressure.
- If the group strays from the learning station objectives, encourage the Team Leader to guide them back to the objectives. You can give hints or advice, but let the Team Leader and the students work through the evaluate-identify-intervene sequence.
- Encourage students to work together as a team. Positively reinforce team skills and appropriate behaviors for Team Leaders and team members.
- Do not spend the entire case simulation in practice and make sure to provide adequate time for the debriefing discussion at the end of each case. Remember, although it is important to complete this clinical scenario, it is equally important to allow adequate time for debriefing/discussion.
- Debriefing starts with you asking the Team Leader how the case went, followed by asking the Timer/Recorder, and then asking the team members (see Lesson Plans).

Be positive and encouraging. If you observe actions that are inappropriate or incorrect, suggest better ways to perform appropriate interventions. Do not critique the Team Leader or team members in a negative way. Instead, state in a positive way the specific action that should be refined or changed.

Case Scenarios for the Learning Stations

Case scenarios can be customized for your learners. A wide variety of case scenarios have been developed for each case to allow you to challenge students related to their scope of practice and level of experience. To help further engage student learning in the PALS Course, the case scenarios include the following topics: respiratory, shock, and cardiac.

The case scenarios contain the information that you will need to facilitate the case discussions and case simulations. Each page includes a debriefing tool on the back that is specific to that particular scenario. Select 1 of the case scenarios in Appendix A for each student.

Respiratory:

- Upper Airway Obstruction
- Lower Airway Obstruction
- Lung Tissue Disease
- Disordered Control of Breathing

Shock:

- Hypovolemic Shock
- Obstructive Shock
- Distributive Shock
- Cardiogenic Shock

Cardiac:

- Bradycardia
- SVT
- Asystole/PEA
- VF
- pVT

Review of Technology and Equipment

Before conducting the learning stations, be sure each student is familiar with all equipment and is able to operate the monitor/defibrillator and any other necessary equipment:

- Review the available resuscitation equipment.
- Review how to use the monitor/defibrillator at the station, including pacing and cardioversion.
- Give each student an opportunity to push the buttons on the defibrillator and become comfortably familiar with its use.
- Emphasize the importance of safety.
- Familiarize students with pacing and cardioversion.

Be sure each student is familiar with the proper use of an AED and the transition to a manual defibrillator. Emphasize the following:

- Remedies for pads-connector incompatibility (use an adapter or switch pads as quickly as possible)
- The importance of continuous, uninterrupted chest compressions, including providing compressions during the charging of a manual defibrillator if the charge time is greater than 10 seconds

Conducting Learning Stations/Case Scenarios

When conducting the learning stations, introduce yourself (if necessary) as students enter the room. Describe the objectives of the learning stations. Remember that time for hands-on practice by students is essential in the learning stations.

Your responsibility is to coach the students, not lecture them about specific skills.

Facilitate skills practice in the stations and demonstrate only when indicated on the Lesson Plans for the station.

If the station includes a case-based scenario, give the Team Leader and other team members information about the case. (See the figure below for suggested locations for the Team Leader and team members during the case scenario.)

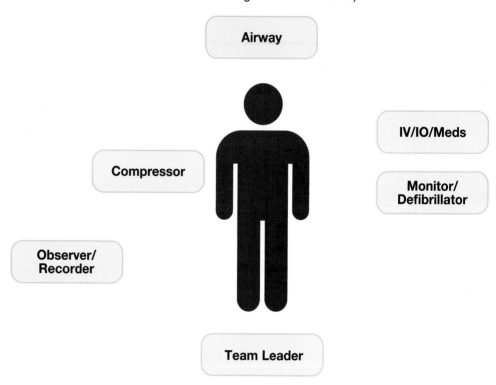

Suggested locations for the Team Leader and team members during case simulations.

Be prepared to provide key information about the case as it unfolds. If the group strays from the learning station objectives, guide them back to the objectives. You can give hints or advice, but let the students work through the algorithms and surveys under the direction of the student acting as Team Leader.

If you are a new instructor or are teaching for the first time, you may want to watch and work with an experienced PALS Instructor before conducting a learning station on your own. Do not spend all the time in case practice; be sure to provide adequate time for a debriefing after each case. It is not necessary to resolve each case clinically during the case practice; rather, end the case in a timely way to provide sufficient opportunity for discussion.

Gloves can be worn during learning station simulations just as they would be used in a real emergency. Donning gloves should not delay the initiation of chest compressions.

Systematic Approach to Assessment and Management

Experienced providers use a systematic approach to the assessment and management of seriously ill or injured children. This course gives students an opportunity to learn and practice these important skills:

- **Evaluate:** Evaluate the child by using a systematic approach to pediatric assessment.
- **Identify:** Determine the type and severity of the clinical condition and make medical decisions about appropriate management.
- **Intervene:** Provide treatments and interventions.

Ensure that all students have ample opportunity to demonstrate proficiency in their systematic approach to the assessment and management of a critically ill child.

Practice High-Performance Teamwork and Local Protocols

Successful resuscitations are the result of not only medical expertise and mastery of resuscitation skills, but also effective communication and teamwork. This course teaches students effective team behaviors and gives them an opportunity to apply what they have learned through practice in simulated cases.

Instructors should discuss team dynamics as part of the debriefing portion of each learning scenario (simulation) and emphasize the importance of effective team dynamics in influencing positive patient outcomes. See figure "Roles and Responsibilities of Team Dynamics" in Lesson 8: Team Dynamics in Part 6 for more information.

Educational Model and Principles

Case scenario simulation, previously referred to as *mock codes*, has been the fundamental educational model for PALS for more than 20 years. Although the technology is more sophisticated and the science of simulation education continues to expand, the fundamentals remain the same. Simulation offers students the opportunity to learn and practice their cognitive and psychomotor skills before applying them to real patients. There is ample evidence from many disciplines to support the effectiveness of such simulation-based education in improving participant knowledge, skills, team performance, leadership, and communication. For this reason, the PALS Course continues to incorporate this model in its design.

In addition to using simulation-based educational methods, the PALS Course uses other adult learning principles in its structure:

- Principle: Adults learn best when they actively participate in the learning process. A top priority in this course is to actively and consistently engage the student.
- Principle: Instructors are most effective when they act as facilitators as opposed to lecturers. The majority of the course is composed of 3 categories of case discussions and simulations with debriefing. The role of the instructor is to facilitate student discussion and coach students to perform appropriate management actions.
- Principle: Adults learn best when they feel safe from intimidation and ridicule. Instructors should do their best to ensure a safe, harm-free learning environment for all PALS students.

All PALS Instructors should strive to adhere to these principles, whether it is during the students' learning of skills using specific equipment (eg, intraosseous [IO] infusion model) or during the learning of medical assessment and decision making in specific scenarios.

The role of the PALS Instructor is to create an environment for the learner that simulates an emergency situation as realistically as possible, observe what the learner does, and then facilitate a review of the learner's actions and thought process, providing constructive feedback. Although sophisticated technology can help to create a realistic environment, the learning process is probably more dependent on the skill of facilitation of the discussion afterward. This facilitation process is called *debriefing*.

Instructor Teaching Materials

Understanding Icons   The icons used in the Lesson Plans, in this manual, and in the course video are there to remind you of what specific action needs to be taken at that point in the course. The icons used throughout the course are as follows:

Icon	Action
	Play video.
	Pause video.
	Students **practice while watching** video.
	Discussion
	Students practice
	Rotate the students between 2 stations.
	Exam or skills test
	Life Is Why™

Understanding Lesson Plans   All AHA ECC Instructor Manuals include Lesson Plans. The purposes of Lesson Plans are to

- Help you as an instructor to facilitate your courses
- Ensure consistency from course to course
- Keep you focused on the main objectives for each lesson
- Explain your responsibilities during the course

Lesson Plans are meant to be used only by you as the instructor. They are your tools to guide you, so make notations on them and make them your own.

The following illustration is a sample Lesson Plan:

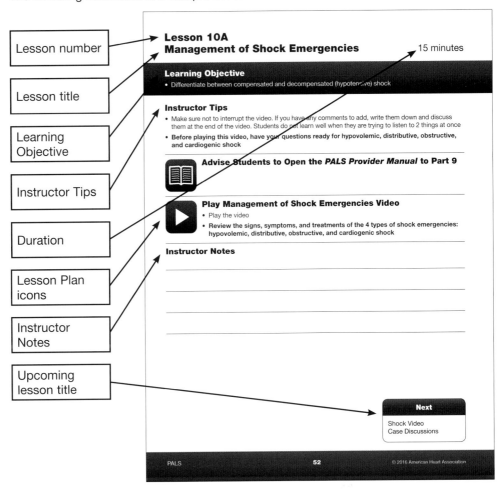

Lesson number

Lesson title

Learning Objective

Instructor Tips

Duration

Lesson Plan icons

Instructor Notes

Upcoming lesson title

Lesson 10A
Management of Shock Emergencies   15 minutes

Learning Objective
• Differentiate between compensated and decompensated (hypotensive) shock

Instructor Tips
• Make sure not to interrupt the video. If you have any comments to add, write them down and discuss them at the end of the video. Students do not learn well when they are trying to listen to 2 things at once
• Before playing this video, have your questions ready for hypovolemic, distributive, obstructive, and cardiogenic shock

Advise Students to Open the *PALS Provider Manual* to Part 9

Play Management of Shock Emergencies Video
• Play the video
• Review the signs, symptoms, and treatments of the 4 types of shock emergencies: hypovolemic, distributive, obstructive, and cardiogenic shock

Instructor Notes

Next
Shock Video
Case Discussions

PALS   52   © 2016 American Heart Association

Using Lesson Plans

Your Lesson Plans were created to be used before and during courses and during skills practice and testing sessions.

When	How to Use
Before the course	Review your Lesson Plans to understand • Objectives for each lesson • Your role for each lesson • Resources that you need for each lesson Make notes of things you want to remember or add.
During the course	• Follow each Lesson Plan as you conduct the course. • Remind students what they will see in each video segment. • Make sure you have all the resources, equipment, and supplies ready for each lesson. • Help the students achieve the objectives identified for each lesson.
During practice before a skills test	A student may have a question about a certain part of skills they will be tested on. The Lesson Plans serve as a resource for you when answering those questions.

Course Videos

Although the PALS Course is instructor led, multiple videos are incorporated into the course. These videos provide information, case illustrations, and demonstrations. They also ensure consistent delivery of course content and information.

Understanding Skills Stations

The skills stations are designed to give students an opportunity to practice and demonstrate competency in specific resuscitation skills, such as bag-mask ventilation or IO access. Skills stations in the PALS Course are

- Airway Management
- Vascular Access
- Rhythm Disturbances/Electrical Therapy

Evaluate each skill listed on the skills station competency checklist for each student. Indicate evaluation results on the PALS Course Progress Checklist.

Review the Lesson Plans for detailed instructions on how to conduct each skills station.

Using the Skills Station Competency Checklists

	How to Use
Student	• Review before the station to determine areas that need improvement • Use during practice as a reference to required skills • Use to make notes of how to improve skills
Instructor	• Use to evaluate competency of each skill listed on the checklist for each student

Using the PALS Course Progress Checklist

The instructor will use the PALS Course Progress Checklist to indicate whether or not each student has actively participated in and completed all required activities in each station as described in the table below:

Station Abbreviation	Indicate on the checklist whether each student has...
Skills Stations	
BLS test	Successfully passed the required BLS skills tests
Respiratory	Demonstrated competency in all the skills listed on the Airway Management Skills Station Competency Checklist
Vascular	Demonstrated competency in all of the skills listed on the Vascular Access Skills Station Competency Checklist
ECG	Demonstrated competency in all of the skills listed on the Rhythm Disturbances/Electrical Therapy Skills Station Competency Checklist
Case Scenarios	

(continued)

(continued)

Station Abbreviation	Indicate on the checklist whether each student has...
Group 1 • Hypovolemic shock • Lower airway obstruction • Upper airway obstruction • Asystole/PEA **Group 2** • Parenchymal lung disease • Septic/distributive shock • SVT • VF/pVT **Group 3** • Obstructive shock • Cardiogenic shock • Disordered control of breathing • Bradycardia	Actively participated as a Team Leader or a team member in the case scenario practice with simulation stations
Tests	
Cardiac Case Scenario	Passed the PALS case scenario 1 test
Respiratory/Shock Case Scenario	Passed the PALS case scenario 2 test
Exam	Passed the exam with a score of 84% or better

This checklist is for internal use only. It allows the instructor, Course Director, and course coordinator to see each individual student's progress throughout the course. Use this checklist to identify and remediate student deficiencies early in the course.

Using the Learning Station Competency Checklists

	How to Use
Student	• Review before the course to familiarize yourself with criteria used for evaluation during case scenario simulations and case scenarios • Use during case simulations when assigned the role of Timer/Recorder to check off actions performed by the team and to guide your report during debriefing
Instructor	• Use as a reference during case simulations in addition to the case scenarios

Understanding Case Scenarios

The PALS Course case scenarios have been carefully designed by experts in pediatric resuscitation. Meeting audience-specific needs may include changing scenarios to fit specific locations in certain sessions with certain groups. Although the scenario lead-ins are easily modified, the instructor should use caution when modifying details contained in the scenarios.

A set of case scenarios is provided. The scenarios are divided into 3 categories from least complex to most complex. The 3 categories are:

Group 1
1. Hypovolemic Shock
2. Lower Airway Obstruction
3. Upper Airway Obstruction
4. Asystole/Pulseless Electrical Activity

Group 2
1. Parenchymal Lung Disease
2. Septic/Distributive Shock
3. Supraventricular Tachycardia
4. Ventricular Fibrillation/Pulseless Ventricular Tachycardia

Group 3
1. Obstructive Shock
2. Cardiogenic Shock
3. Disordered Control of Breathing
4. Bradycardia

Case Scenario Layout

- The first page provides a lead-in and vital signs to each scenario.
- The front provides the scenario overview and scenario-specific objectives.
- The students are taken through the steps of the evaluate-identify-intervene sequence of emergency response.
- The back of each scenario contains a debriefing tool.
- The top of the debriefing tool shows the general and scenario-specific learning objectives for each case.
- General debriefing principles are provided.
- The bottom of the debriefing tool contains the materials to help guide the gather-analyze-summarize discussions.

Sample Case Scenario

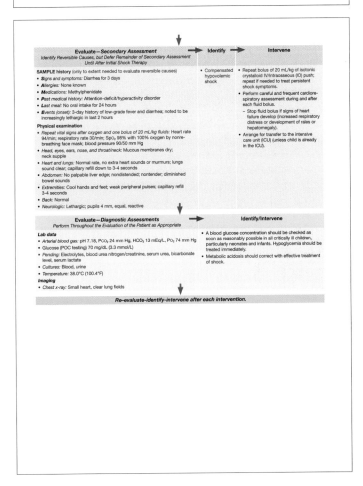

Testing Case Scenario 1

Hypovolemic Shock
(Child)

American Heart Association® · life is why™

American Academy of Pediatrics · DEDICATED TO THE HEALTH OF ALL CHILDREN®

Scenario Lead-in

Prehospital: You have been dispatched to transport a 5 year old with a 3-day history of fever and diarrhea. She has been increasingly lethargic in the last 2 hours.

ED: You are asked to assess and manage a 5 year old with a 3-day history of fever and diarrhea. She has been increasingly lethargic in the last 2 hours. Efforts for a peripheral intravenous access have been unsuccessful.

General Inpatient Unit: You are called to assess a 5 year old who has been admitted to the ward with a 3-day history of fever and diarrhea. She has been increasingly lethargic in the last hour and has had severe ongoing diarrhea. Her intravenous access is no longer functioning.

ICU: You are called to the bedside of a 5 year old who has been admitted to the intensive care unit with a 3-day history of fever and diarrhea. She has been increasingly lethargic in the last 2 hours and has had severe ongoing diarrhea. Her intravenous access is no longer functioning.

Vital Signs	
Heart rate	140/min
Blood pressure	100/80 mm Hg
Respiratory rate	36/min
SpO$_2$	92% on room air
Temperature	38.0°C (100.4°F)
Weight	21 kg
Age	5 years

Scenario Overview and Learning Objectives

Scenario Overview	Scenario-Specific Objectives
Emphasis in this scenario should be on identification of compensated hypovolemic shock. Priorities include oxygen, immediate establishment of intravenous (IV) access, and administration of fluid bolus of isotonic crystalloid, repeated as needed to treat shock signs. Reassessment of cardiorespiratory status is needed during and after each fluid bolus. Glucose concentration should be checked early in this lethargic child.	• **Recognizes signs of compensated and hypotensive shock;** this case illustrates compensated hypovolemic shock (key indicators include anxiety, tachypnea without abnormal labor, tachycardia, cool and mottled skin, delayed capillary refill, and normotension) • **Summarizes signs and symptoms of hypovolemic shock;** in this scenario, the child has a 3-day history of diarrhea and fever, signs of shock, and poor skin turgor • **Demonstrates correct interventions for hypovolemic shock;** the most important interventions in this scenario include oxygen administration, administration of one or more boluses of isotonic crystalloid, and careful reassessment during and after each fluid bolus • **Summarizes how to evaluate systemic (end-organ) perfusion;** indirect indicators of end-organ perfusion include skin temperature/color, level of consciousness, and urine output

Evaluate—Initial Impression (Pediatric Assessment Triangle)	→	Identify	→	Intervene
Appearance • Anxious, restless **Breathing** • Fast rate, increased respiratory effort **Circulation** • Pale, dry, and significant mottling, especially in hands and feet		• Immediate intervention needed		• Activate the emergency response system. Emergency medical services requests additional assistance if needed. • Administer 100% oxygen by nonrebreathing face mask. • Apply cardiac monitor. • Apply pulse oximeter.

Evaluate—Primary Assessment Focused on Assessment Needed to Support Airway, Oxygenation, Ventilation, and Perfusion	→	Identify	→	Intervene
• **Airway:** Patent; no audible abnormal airway sounds (no stridor, no audible wheezing) • **Breathing/Ventilation:** Respiratory rate about 36/min; minimal intercostal retractions; SpO$_2$ 92% on room air, increases to 100% with 100% oxygen; lungs clear on auscultation • **Circulation/Perfusion:** Central pulses fair, peripheral pulses weak; heart rate 140/min; blood pressure 100/80 mm Hg; capillary refill about 4 seconds; cool, mottled hands and feet *Remainder of Primary Assessment performed if airway, ventilation, and perfusion are adequately supported* • **Disability:** Poor skin turgor • **Exposure:** Temperature 38.0°C (100.4°F); weight 21 kg		• Compensated shock • Sinus tachycardia		• Obtain vascular access (child has compensated shock, so initial attempt should focus on IV access). • Administer a fluid bolus of 20 mL/kg of isotonic crystalloid rapidly via IV. – Assess perfusion and monitor cardiorespiratory status closely during and immediately after each fluid bolus. – Stop fluid bolus if signs of heart failure develop (eg, increased respiratory distress or development of rales or hepatomegaly). • Check point-of-care (POC) glucose concentration and treat hypoglycemia, if needed. • Assess response to oxygen administration.

© 2016 American Heart Association

Evaluate—Secondary Assessment Identify Reversible Causes, but Defer Remainder of Secondary Assessment Until After Initial Shock Therapy	→	Identify	→	Intervene
SAMPLE history (only to extent needed to evaluate reversible causes) • **Signs and symptoms:** Diarrhea for 3 days • **Allergies:** None known • **Medications:** Methylphenidate • **Past medical history:** Attention-deficit/hyperactivity disorder • **Last meal:** No oral intake for 24 hours • **Events (onset):** 3-day history of low-grade fever and diarrhea; noted to be increasingly lethargic in last 2 hours **Physical examination** • *Repeat vital signs after oxygen and one bolus of 20 mL/kg fluids:* Heart rate 94/min; respiratory rate 30/min; SpO$_2$ 98% with 100% oxygen by nonrebreathing face mask; blood pressure 90/50 mm Hg • *Head, eyes, ears, nose, and throat/neck:* Mucous membranes dry; neck supple • *Heart and lungs:* Normal rate, no extra heart sounds or murmurs; lungs sound clear; capillary refill down to 3-4 seconds • *Abdomen:* No palpable liver edge; nondistended; nontender; diminished bowel sounds • *Extremities:* Cool hands and feet; weak peripheral pulses; capillary refill 3-4 seconds • *Back:* Normal • *Neurologic:* Lethargic; pupils 4 mm, equal, reactive		• Compensated hypovolemic shock		• Repeat bolus of 20 mL/kg of isotonic crystalloid IV/intraosseous (IO) push; repeat if needed to treat persistent shock symptoms. • Perform careful and frequent cardiorespiratory assessment during and after each fluid bolus. – Stop fluid bolus if signs of heart failure develop (increased respiratory distress or development of rales or hepatomegaly). • Arrange for transfer to the intensive care unit (ICU) (unless child is already in the ICU).

Evaluate—Diagnostic Assessments Perform Throughout the Evaluation of the Patient as Appropriate	→	Identify/Intervene	
Lab data • *Arterial blood gas:* pH 7.18, PCO$_2$ 24 mm Hg, HCO$_3$ 13 mEq/L, PO$_2$ 74 mm Hg • *Glucose* (POC testing) 70 mg/dL (3.3 mmol/L) • *Pending:* Electrolytes, blood urea nitrogen/creatinine, serum urea, bicarbonate level, serum lactate • *Cultures:* Blood, urine • *Temperature:* 38.0°C (100.4°F) **Imaging** • *Chest x-ray:* Small heart, clear lung fields		• A blood glucose concentration should be checked as soon as reasonably possible in all critically ill children, particularly neonates and infants. Hypoglycemia should be treated immediately. • Metabolic acidosis should correct with effective treatment of shock.	

Re-evaluate-identify-intervene after each intervention.

Using the Provider Manual

Each student must have the current *PALS Provider Manual* readily available for use before, during, and after the course.

Students will need to do the following with the Provider Manual:

- Read it before coming to class
- Bring it to class to use as a resource during the exam
- Refer to it after the course to maintain knowledge

The Lesson Plans tell you when to refer students to specific sections of the Provider Manual.

The Provider Manual is designed for individual use and is an integral part of the student's education. Students may reuse their manuals during renewals or updates until new science guidelines are published.

Students taking the HeartCode PALS course have access to the *PALS Provider Manual* and other reference materials within the eLearning course. They may access the reference materials for up to 2 years from the date of key activation. Students should be allowed to bring electronic devices into the classroom to access these electronic materials.

Effective Use of Simulation

Preparing Students for Simulation-Based Learning

Because some students may be new to simulation-based learning, the instructor should give a short introduction to this type of learning before starting any simulated scenarios. The following should be included:

- *Description of simulation-based learning:* Emphasize that simulation-based learning allows trainees to learn and practice in a realistic environment without causing any potential harm or danger to the patient. Mistakes are used as learning opportunities.
- *Performance expectations during the simulation:* Encourage the trainees to "suspend disbelief," pretend that things are real, and actively immerse themselves in the simulation. Tell them that this will enhance the learning experience.
- *Orientation to the simulated environment:* Briefly introduce the students to the physical properties of the simulator manikin (whether high fidelity or low fidelity) or task trainer before beginning the simulations. This allows them to understand what procedures can be done and what cues the manikin might provide. For example, students should be shown where to insert an IO needle and where to place the paddles when defibrillating the simulator manikin.
- *Description of debriefing:* Let the students know that after each simulation, there will be a debriefing session facilitated by an instructor. The purpose of the debriefing session is to reflect openly on their performance in the simulation to identify ways to improve care in the future.

High-Fidelity vs Low-Fidelity Simulation

Simulators have been used to teach BLS for decades. They give students the opportunity to practice and improve the clinical skills needed for resuscitation of real patients.

Improvements in technology have provided healthcare professionals with a broader array of monitor displays, procedural options, and remote control, thus facilitating the observation of pathophysiologic signs. The variety of simulators has expanded considerably. Some are as simple and old-fashioned as the use of an orange to practice intramuscular injections. Others are highly sophisticated, employing a computer-guided mechanical device to create a very realistic look and feel of specific procedures. Improved plastics have made task trainers (eg, airway practice models) more versatile and realistic, and many manikins are "high fidelity," with lifelike features and enhancements.

While the term *high fidelity* has been used as a synonym for *high technology*, *fidelity* actually refers to the level of realism as this relates to specific learning objectives. Thus, high fidelity implies a very realistic simulation, while low fidelity implies that the student must use his or her imagination to fill in the gaps. This definition is based on the experience of the student rather than the device itself.

For example, a case scenario might require needle decompression. A high-tech patient simulator with numerous realistic features—eg, breathing, blinking, talking, heart sounds, and physiologic monitors arranged to mimic an emergency department—could be used to create a high-fidelity simulation for the goal of diagnosing and deciding to treat a pneumothorax. However, if the goal is to learn and practice needle decompression, the same manikin would have very low fidelity for the specific skills required for needle decompression. In fact, a simple task trainer with a realistic chest could be a much higher-fidelity mechanism for that particular learning experience.

Although advanced technology and high-fidelity simulation are appealing and may result in higher learner satisfaction, they increase costs substantially without necessarily enhancing learning compared with more basic simulators. In fact, none of the available products is truly realistic compared with real human beings.

You may find high-fidelity manikins useful for teamwork and skills integration, but it is not certain which specific aspects of the scenario are improved by a higher degree of realism. Having a more pertinent case and setting for particular students—or matching the equipment to that used by the learners—may be more important than a high-fidelity manikin for transferring the learning process into clinical practice.

There is some evidence that the "realism that matters" is the part that conveys the story—that is, once students understand the situation from the cues provided, better technology or high fidelity may not add much to the actual experience of learning.

Thus, while use of highly realistic manikins is acceptable, it is not required for teaching PALS or BLS.

As an instructor, you can tailor your approach by using the resources available to create a high-fidelity environment that both satisfies students and achieves the desired learning objectives.

Debriefing After Practice

Definition of Debriefing

During the learning stations in the PALS Course, you will debrief students on what happened, how issues were addressed, and outcomes.

Structured and supported debriefing is an organized, evidence-based, student-focused process that takes place in a nonthreatening environment. It is a method of assisting students in thinking about what they did, when they did it, why and how they did it, and how they can improve.

In an effective debriefing session, instructors ask questions and encourage students to analyze their own performance rather than offer only the instructor's perspective. Because this approach is focused on what the student thinks and does rather than on the instructor's viewpoint, students are more likely to remember and apply the lessons in their practice.

 For more about debriefing, refer to the Structured and Supported Debriefing Course at **OnlineAHA.org**.

Feedback vs Debriefing

Instructors should include structured and supported debriefing after each case in the learning stations as a technique to facilitate learning, particularly when covering high-performance team concepts.

Simple feedback is typically geared toward correcting student actions the instructor has observed—an approach that can sometimes have the unintended consequence of fixing one mistake only to create others. Effective debriefing, on the other hand, focuses more on understanding why students acted a certain way, which allows correction of their thinking. Students typically do things for a reason that makes sense to them. Good debriefing helps students review their own performance and achieve a deeper understanding.

Although debriefing takes longer than simply giving feedback, reframing students' understanding will make the lesson more applicable to real life and will have a more lasting impact on future performance.

Effective Debriefing Characteristics

The characteristics of an effective debriefing session include

- Active participation
- Learner discussion
- Self-analysis
- Application
- Thorough processing of information

With effective debriefing, students should

- Analyze and evaluate what happened
- Recognize how tools can help them manage situations
- Develop the habit of self-critique

The AHA recommends using structured and supported debriefing—a learner-centered debriefing model that focuses on what the student knows and thinks. This approach draws on evidence-based findings from behavioral science to focus on critical thinking and encourage students to analyze their motivations and performance. It is an efficient and organized process to help students think about what they did; why, how, and when they did it; and how they can improve.

Structured and supported debriefing follows a simple, 3-step format to achieve a comprehensive and effective debriefing:

- *Gather* information about the events
- *Analyze* the information by using an accurate record
- *Summarize* the attainment of objectives for future improvement

Structured elements include the 3 specific phases mentioned above, while supported elements include both interpersonal support and the use of protocols, algorithms, and best evidence.

Be sure to allow enough time (at least 8 minutes per simulation) to conduct a debriefing session after each case scenario.

For your convenience, Appendix A includes a debriefing tool for each case scenario in which debriefing should be performed.

Structured and Supported Debriefing Process

Phase	Goal	Actions
Gather	Listen to students to understand what they think and how they feel about the simulation.	• Request a narrative from the Team Leader. • Request clarifying or supplementary information from the team.
Analyze	Facilitate students' reflection on and analysis of their actions.	• Review an accurate record of events. • Report observations (both correct and incorrect steps). • Assist students in thoroughly reflecting on and examining their performance during the simulation as well as on their perceptions during the debriefing. • Direct and/or redirect students during the debriefing to ensure continuous focus on session objectives.
Summarize	Facilitate identification and review of the lesson learned.	• Summarize comments or statements from students. • Have students identify positive aspects of team or individual behaviors. • Have students identify areas of team or individual behaviors that require change or correction.

You should view yourself as a facilitator whose goals are to enhance learning during the training session and encourage students to critique themselves and reflect on future clinical encounters. This promotes continued self-improvement and will have a long-lasting effect well beyond any individual course.

A good facilitator effectively uses the key skills of listening, genuine inquiry, and open-ended questions to determine how the student understood the situation and what he or she was thinking. Correcting a particular action will have an impact on only a single behavior; correcting an approach will affect the student's actions in a variety of situations.

Appropriate pauses and silence can give students the time they need to formulate their thoughts. Demonstrating the usefulness of protocols and algorithms is also part of an effective facilitation.

Structured and Supported Debriefing can help facilitate learning the skills and techniques needed for clinical practice. It is also important that you model and encourage good debriefing techniques because debriefing of actual resuscitation events can be a useful strategy to help healthcare providers improve future performance in clinical practice.

For PALS debriefing, follow these steps:

- Step 1: Start the debriefing by asking the Team Leader to critique his or her own performance along with the team's performance in the scenario that just concluded.
- Step 2: Move to the Timer/Recorder for accurate information about what happened in the scenario, and accommodate any other team members who want to comment on the team's performance.
- Step 3: After other team members have had a chance to comment on the case, summarize the correct actions, and make sure the team understands the areas for improvement so that the next Team Leader can correct those actions.

The entire team will learn from the debriefing and apply it to the next case.

 The AHA recommends that all PALS Instructors take the AHA Structured and Supported Debriefing Course online at **OnlineAHA.org**.

Key Debriefing Principles

Key principles to keep in mind:

- Debriefing sessions are 9 minutes long
- Address all learning objectives
- Summarize key messages at the end of the debriefing

Encourage

- Students to self-reflect
- Engagement of all participants

Avoid

- Mini-lectures and closed-ended questions
- Dominating the discussion

Tools for Debriefing

Debriefing Tool
Testing Case Scenario 1
Hypovolemic Shock (Child)

General Debriefing Principles

- Use the table below to guide your debriefing; also refer to the **Team Dynamics Debriefing Tool.**

[callout] Begin by reviewing the General Debriefing Principles before getting started. Be attentive to the time allotted.

...he end of the debriefing.

...ipants
...d questions
Dominating the discussion

General Management Objectives

- Uses the PALS Systematic Approach Algorithm to assess and
- ...y CPR (including the use of a feedback ...
- Demonstrates basic airway maneuvers and use of relevant airway device as appropriate
- Demonstrates application of cardiac and respiratory monitors

- Identifies the cardiac rhythm
- Applies appropriate PBLS or PALS algorithms
- Summarizes general indications, contraindications, and doses of relevant drugs
- Discusses principles of family-centered care in pediatric cardiac arrest
- Applies the 8 elements of effective team dynamics
- Performs frequent reassessment

[callout] Review the General Management Objectives.

Action	Gather	Analyze	Summarize
	Student Observations	**Done Well**	**Student-Led Summary**
- Assesses ABCDE, including vital signs - Administers 100% oxygen - Applies cardiac monitor and pulse oximeter - Recognizes signs and symptoms of hypovolemic shock	- Can you describe the events from your perspective? - How well do you think your treatments worked? - Can you review the events of the scenario (*directed to the Timer/Recorder*)? What could you have improved? What did the team do well?	- How were you able to [*insert action here*]? - Why do you think you were able to [*insert action here*]? - Tell me a little more about how you [*insert action here*].	- What are the main things you learned? - Can someone summarize the key points made? - What are the main take-home messages?
...loid; monitors for signs of heart failure during and after fluid bolus - Reassesses patient during and in response to interven... particularly during and each fluid bolus - Repeats fluid bolus as ... to treat shock - Checks glucose with ... care testing	**Instructor Observations** - I noticed that [*insert action here*]. - I observed that [*insert action here*]		messages are... - What are the therapeutic end points during shock management? (Answer: Normalized heart rate; improved peripheral perfusion, mental status, and urine output; normalized blood pressure; correction of metabolic/lactic acidosis) - Which are the indirect signs of improved end-organ function? (Answer: Improved skin blood flow, increased responsiveness/improved level of consciousness, increased urine output, correction of lactic acidosis)

[callout] Use the Action column to help guide your observation of required critical actions.

[callout] Use the Gather column to help start off discussion; this can be a student-based observation or something that you noticed as an instructor.

[callout] Use the Analyze column to determine if an action was done or needs improvement, and use the suggested wording to help guide discussion to close performance gaps.

[callout] Use the Summarize column to summarize at the end of each debriefing session; this may be student or instructor led.

See some examples in the table below:

Action	Gather	Analyze	Summarize
Student Observations			
• Administers 100% oxygen	• How do you think your treatments worked?	• What prevented you from administering 100% oxygen in a timely fashion?	• Let's summarize what we learned about administering 100% oxygen.
Instructor Observations			
• Directs IV or IO access	• I noticed that you were unable to gain IO access.	• Why do you think that occurred?	• Let's summarize what we learned about administering IO access.

A Team Dynamics Debriefing Tool has been developed to help facilitate discussion of leadership, communication, and other team dynamics–related issues. This tool is meant to be used for each of the case scenarios. Use the tool in the same manner as the Medical Management Debriefing Tool. Take a team dynamics–related action (blue box) and ask questions of the student by using the gather-analyze-summarize principles (moving from left to right).

Team Dynamics Debriefing Tool

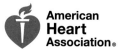 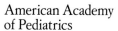

American **Heart** Association®

life is why™

American Academy of Pediatrics

DEDICATED TO THE HEALTH OF ALL CHILDREN™

Instructions

- Use the table below to guide your debriefing.
- Observe and record elements of team dynamics.
- Identify 2 or 3 elements of team dynamics to discuss per debriefing session.

Action	Gather	Analyze	Summarize
Closed-Loop Communication	***Student Observations***	***Done Well***	***Student-Led Summary***
• Orders acknowledged and confirmed when given • Orders announced when executed	• Can you describe the events from your perspective? • How well do you think your treatments worked? • Can you review the events of the scenario? (*directed to the Timer/Recorder*) • What could you have improved? • What did the team do well?	• How were you able to [*insert action here*]? • Why do you think you were able to [*insert action here*]? • Tell me a little more about how you [*insert action here*].	• What are the main things you learned? • Can someone summarize the key points made? • What are the main take-home messages?
Clear Messages			
• Team members speak clearly • Orders are questioned when doubt exists			
Clear Roles			
• All team members have appropriate roles • Roles are reallocated when appropriate	***Instructor Observations***	***Needs Improvement***	***Instructor-Led Summary***
Knowing One's Limitations	• I noticed that [*insert action here*]. • I observed that [*insert action here*]. • I saw that [*insert action here*].	• Why do you think [*insert action here*] occurred? • How do you think [*insert action here*] could have been improved? • What was your thinking while [*insert action here*]? • What prevented you from [*insert action here*]?	• Let's summarize what we learned… • Here is what I think we learned… • The main take-home messages are…
• Calls for assistance • Seeks advice when appropriate			
Knowledge Sharing			
• Sharing information between team members • Asks for ideas and suggestions			
Constructive Intervention			
• Identifies priorities • Questions colleagues who make mistakes			
Reevaluation and Summarizing			
• Reevaluates patient • Summarizes patient condition and treatment plan			
Mutual Respect			
• Speaks in a professional, friendly tone of voice • Provides positive feedback			

Course Outlines and Agendas

PALS Course Outline and Agenda

The PALS Course is made up of 24 lessons plus the exam. The course was designed with a ratio of 6 students to 1 instructor to 1 manikin or station. The High-Quality BLS Practice and Testing Station and Airway Management Station require 1 instructor and 2 manikins for 6 students per station.

The ratio of students to instructors in an AHA PALS Course may not exceed 8 students to 1 instructor. Adding a seventh or eighth student will cause the total course time to increase by approximately 80 minutes *per student*.

The following pages provide outlines and sample agendas for the PALS Course and PALS Update Course. Please note that times given in the chart below are approximate and may vary from class to class. Moreover, the Course Director will need to factor in transition times between activities and rooms.

Outline for PALS Course

Approximate course duration: 13 hours 40 minutes (without breaks)
(Student-instructor ratio for learning stations is 6:1)

Lesson	Course Event	Estimated Time (in Minutes)	Lesson Plan Actions
Introduction	Course Introduction	10	
1 (optional)	Life Is Why Activity	5	
2	Course Overview	5	
3	Science of Pediatric Resuscitation	10	
4A	Learning/Testing Station: Child High-Quality BLS Practice	25	
4B	Learning/Testing Station: Child High-Quality BLS Testing—Testing Details	15	
5A	Learning/Testing Station: Infant High-Quality BLS Practice	20	
5B	Learning/Testing Station: Infant High-Quality BLS Testing—Testing Details	15	

Lesson	Course Event	Estimated Time (in Minutes)	Lesson Plan Actions
6 (optional)	Learning/Testing Station: Child and Infant Choking	20	
7A	Overview of Systematic Approach Model	45	
7B	Secondary Assessment	15	
8	Team Dynamics	15	
9A	Management of Respiratory Emergencies	15	
9B	Respiratory Video Case Discussions	25	
9C	Learning Station: Airway Management	20	
10A	Management of Shock Emergencies	15	
10B	Shock Video Case Discussions	25	
10C	Learning Station: Vascular Access	20	
11A	Management of Arrhythmia Emergencies	15	
11B	Arrhythmia Video Case Discussions	20	
11C	Learning Station: Rhythm Disturbances/ Electrical Therapy	25	
12	Management of Post–Cardiac Arrest Care	15	

Lesson	Course Event	Estimated Time (in Minutes)	Lesson Plan Actions
13 (optional)	Learning Station: Coping With Death	20	
14	Case Scenario Practice With Simulations Refer to case scenarios Group 1 • Hypovolemic shock • Lower airway obstruction • Upper airway obstruction • Asystole/PEA	80	
14	Case Scenario Practice With Simulations Refer to case scenarios Group 2 • Parenchymal lung disease • Septic/distributive shock • SVT • VF/pVT	80	
14	Case Scenario Practice With Simulations Refer to case scenarios Group 3 • Obstructive shock • Cardiogenic shock • Disordered control of breathing • Bradycardia	80	
15	Case Scenario Testing	120	
16	Exam	60	
REM	Remediation	Variable	

Total instructional time with 6:1 student-to-instructor ratio:
approximately 820 minutes or 13 hours 40 minutes (not counting breaks and transition times)

Outline for PALS Update Course

Approximate course duration: 7 hours 40 minutes (without breaks)
(Student-instructor ratio for learning stations is 6:1)

Lesson	Course Event	Estimated Time (in Minutes)	Lesson Plan Actions
Introduction	Course Introduction	10	
1 (optional)	Life Is Why Activity	5	
2	Science of Pediatric Resuscitation	15	
3A	Learning/Testing Station: Child High-Quality BLS Practice	25	
3B	Learning/Testing Station: Child High-Quality BLS Testing—Testing Details	15	
4A	Learning/Testing Station: Infant High-Quality BLS Practice	20	
4B	Learning/Testing Station: Infant High-Quality BLS Testing—Testing Details	15	
5 (optional)	Learning/Testing Station: Child and Infant Choking	20	
6	Overview of Systematic Approach Model	15	
7	Team Dynamics	15	
8	Management of Post–Cardiac Arrest Care	15	
9 (optional)	Learning Station: Coping With Death	20	

Lesson	Course Event	Estimated Time (in Minutes)	Lesson Plan Actions
10	Case Scenario Practice With Simulations Refer to case scenarios Learning Stations One case scenario per student	120	
11	Case Scenario Testing	120	
12	Exam	60	
REM	Remediation	Variable	

Total instructional time with 6:1 student-to-instructor ratio: approximately 460 minutes or 7 hours 40 minutes (not counting breaks and transition times)

Outline for HeartCode PALS

Approximate course duration: 2 hours 30 minutes (without optional lessons)
and 5 hours (with optional lessons)
(Student-instructor ratio for learning stations is 6:1)

Lesson	Course Event	Estimated Time (in Minutes)	Lesson Plan Actions
Introduction	Course Introduction	10	
1 (optional)	Life Is Why Activity	5	
2A	Learning/Testing Station: Child High-Quality BLS Practice	25	
2B	Learning/Testing Station: Child High-Quality BLS Testing—Testing Details	15	
3A	Learning/Testing Station: Infant High-Quality BLS Practice	20	
3B	Learning/Testing Station: Infant High-Quality BLS Testing—Testing Details	15	
4 (optional)	Learning/Testing Station: Child and Infant Choking	20	
5	Learning Station: Airway Management	20	
6	Learning Station: Vascular Access	20	
7	Learning Station: Rhythm Disturbances/ Electrical Therapy	25	
8 (optional)	Case Scenario Testing	120	

Total instructional time with 6:1 student-to-instructor ratio:
approximately 150 minutes or 2 hours 30 minutes (not counting breaks and transition times or optional lessons); 295 minutes or 5 hours (not counting breaks and transition times and including optional lessons)

Sample Agenda for PALS Course

18 Students, 3 PALS Instructors
Approximately 17 hours 15 minutes with breaks

Day 1			
8:00-8:10	**Course Introduction**		
8:10-8:15	**Lesson 1:** Life Is Why Activity (Optional)		
8:15-8:20	**Lesson 2:** Course Overview		
8:20-8:30	**Lesson 3:** Science of Pediatric Resuscitation		
Divide class into 2 groups	**Lessons 4-6** Learning/Testing Stations: Child and Infant High-Quality BLS*	**Lessons 7-8** Overview of Systematic Approach Model; Secondary Assessment; Team Dynamics	
8:30-9:45	Group A	Group B	
9:45-10:00	**Break**		
10:00-11:15	Group B	Group A	
Divide class into 3 groups	**Lesson 9** Management of Respiratory Emergencies; Respiratory Video Case Discussions; Learning Station: Airway Management	**Lesson 10** Management of Shock Emergencies; Shock Video Case Discussions; Learning Station: Vascular Access	**Lesson 11** Management of Arrhythmia Emergencies; Arrhythmia Video Case Discussions; Learning Station: Rhythm Disturbances/ Electrical Therapy
11:15-12:15	Group A	Group B	Group C
12:15-1:00	**Lunch**		
1:00-2:00	Group B	Group C	Group A
2:00-2:15	**Break**		
2:15-3:15	Group C	Group A	Group B
3:15-3:30	**Lesson 12:** Management of Post–Cardiac Arrest Care		
3:30-3:50	**Lesson 13:** Learning Station: Coping With Death (Optional)		
3:50-4:15	**End-of-Day Debriefing**		

Day 2			
Divide class into 3 groups	**Lesson 14** Case Scenario Practice With Simulations Category 1	**Lesson 14** Case Scenario Practice With Simulations Category 1	**Lesson 14** Case Scenario Practice With Simulations Category 1
8:00-9:20	Group A	Group B	Group C
Divide class into 3 groups	**Lesson 14** Case Scenario Practice With Simulations Category 2	**Lesson 14** Case Scenario Practice With Simulations Category 2	**Lesson 14** Case Scenario Practice With Simulations Category 2
9:20-10:40	Group A	Group B	Group C
10:40-11:00	**Break**		
Divide class into 3 groups	**Lesson 14** Case Scenario Practice With Simulations Category 3	**Lesson 14** Case Scenario Practice With Simulations Category 3	**Lesson 14** Case Scenario Practice With Simulations Category 3
11:00-12:20	Group A	Group B	Group C
12:20-12:45	**Lunch**		
12:45-2:45	**Lesson 15:** Case Scenario Testing		
2:45-3:00	**Break**		
3:00-4:00	**Lesson 16:** Exam		
4:00-5:00	**Class Ends/Remediation**		

*Lesson 6: Learning/Testing Station: Child and Infant Choking (Optional) (20 minutes) may be facilitated in this time slot.

Sample Agenda for PALS Update Course

18 Students, 3 PALS Instructors
Approximately 9 hours with breaks

8:00-8:10	**Course Introduction**
8:10-8:15	**Lesson 1:** Life Is Why Activity (Optional)
8:15-8:30	**Lesson 2:** Science of Pediatric Resuscitation
8:30-9:30	**Lessons 3-5:** Learning/Testing Stations: Child and Infant High-Quality BLS*
9:30-9:45	**Lesson 6:** Overview of Systematic Approach Model
9:45-10:00	**Lesson 7:** Team Dynamics
10:00-10:15	**Lesson 8:** Management of Post–Cardiac Arrest Care
10:15-10:35	**Lesson 9:** Learning Station: Coping With Death (Optional)
10:35-10:45	**Break**
10:45-11:45	**Lesson 10:** Case Scenario Practice With Simulations[†]
11:45-12:15	**Lunch**
12:15-1:15	**Lesson 10:** Case Scenario Practice With Simulations[†]
1:15-3:15	**Lesson 11:** Case Scenario Testing
3:15-4:15	**Lesson 12:** Exam
4:15-5:00	**Class Ends/Remediation**

*Lesson 5: BLS Learning/Testing Station: Child and Infant Choking (Optional) (20 minutes) may be facilitated in this time slot.

[†]See Update Lesson 10 for an explanation of which category each student should practice.

Sample Agenda for HeartCode PALS Without Optional Lessons

Student-instructor ratio 6:1
Approximately 2 hours 30 minutes

8:00-8:10	**Course Introduction**
8:10-9:25	**Lessons 2-3:** Learning/Testing Stations: Child and Infant High-Quality BLS
9:25-9:45	**Lesson 5:** Learning Station: Airway Management
9:45-10:05	**Lesson 6:** Learning Station: Vascular Access
10:05-10:30	**Lesson 7:** Learning Station: Rhythm Disturbances/Electrical Therapy
10:30-11:30	**Class Ends/Remediation**

Sample Agenda for HeartCode PALS With Optional Lessons

Student-instructor ratio 6:1
Approximately 5 hours

8:00-8:10	**Course Introduction**
8:10-8:15	**Lesson 1:** Life Is Why Activity (Optional)
8:15-9:30	**Lessons 2-3:** Learning/Testing Stations: Child and Infant High-Quality BLS
9:30-9:50	**Lesson 4:** Learning/Testing Station: Child and Infant Choking (Optional)
9:50-10:10	**Lesson 5:** Learning Station: Airway Management
10:10-10:30	**Lesson 6:** Learning Station: Vascular Access
10:30-10:55	**Lesson 7:** Learning Station: Rhythm Disturbances/Electrical Therapy
10:55-12:55	**Lesson 8:** Case Scenario Testing (Optional)
12:55-1:55	**Class Ends/Remediation**

Part 3

Testing and Remediation

Testing for Course Completion

The AHA requires successful completion of skills tests and an exam for a student to receive a PALS Provider course completion card. Additional information about testing and criteria for completion is presented throughout this chapter.

The prompt and accurate delivery of PALS skills and knowledge is critically important for patient survival. Accurate, objective, and uniform testing reinforces these lifesaving skills and knowledge and is critical for the consistent delivery of the PALS Provider Course content by all instructors.

All PALS Instructors are expected to maintain high standards of performance for all PALS skills tests, as discussed below.

Important: Students must demonstrate competency during PALS testing without any assistance, hints, or prompting from the instructor.

Course Completion Requirements

To receive a course completion card, students taking the full course must attend and participate in all lessons of the course, pass all skills tests, and pass the exam.

The recommended update or renewal interval for all AHA courses is 2 years. Students who intend to take an update course must show a valid provider card to enroll in an update or renewal course. At the discretion of the Training Center Coordinator, Course Director, or Lead Instructor, exceptions may be allowed. The Training Center Coordinator has the final authority and responsibility for allowing a student to take an update course if he or she does not have a current AHA Provider card. Students who present an expired provider card or do not possess a provider card may be allowed to take an update course but will not be given the option of remediation. These students will need to complete the entire provider course if they cannot successfully meet the course completion requirements when tested. If the student fails any skills test, he or she should be referred back to the full PALS Course. At the instructor's discretion, students who wish to take the PALS Update Course (who have a current PALS card) have the option of taking the required tests instead of attending classes.

In addition, HeartCode PALS students must participate in the hands-on session, which includes skills practice and skills testing. Students must pass all skills tests with an AHA Instructor after completing the online portion.

Explain clearly to the students which actions, if not performed correctly, will result in a "no pass" and require remediation (eg, failure to confirm airway placement, shocking a perfusing rhythm).

It will be the student's responsibility to be familiar with the *2015 AHA Guidelines Update for CPR and ECC*.

Students who meet all course prerequisites and are eligible to receive a course completion card must do the following:

Skills Testing Requirements	Exam Requirements
Students must successfully pass these skills tests: • Child CPR and AED Skills Test • Infant CPR Skills Test • PALS Case Scenario Test 1—cardiac • PALS Case Scenario Test 2—respiratory or shock	Students must score at least 84% on the exam

Completion Requirements for the PALS Update Course

To successfully complete the PALS Update Course and receive a course completion card, a student must do the following:

• Pass the Child CPR and AED and Infant CPR Skills Tests (see High-Quality BLS Testing)
• Actively participate in, practice, and complete all learning stations
• Complete the open-book exam with a minimum score of 84%
• Pass 2 PALS case scenarios (1 cardiac and 1 respiratory or shock) as a Team Leader by providing appropriate medical treatment and demonstrating effective team dynamics

Completing HeartCode PALS

The HeartCode PALS online portion is a self-directed learning program that uses eSimulation technology videos and interactive learning activities.

Course completion consists of 2 parts: the computer-based cognitive online portion and the hands-on session, which includes a skills practice portion and a skills testing portion. The hands-on session must be completed with an AHA PALS Instructor.

Course completion requirements to receive an AHA course completion card by using HeartCode PALS are as follows:

1. Successful completion of all cases in the HeartCode PALS online portion
2. Achieving a score of 84% or better on the online exam
3. Successful completion of the required BLS skills test administered by an AHA PALS Instructor
4. Active participation in, practice, and completion of all learning stations
5. Optional: Successful completion of 1 PALS case scenario test per student is highly encouraged but not required

Each student must individually demonstrate the psychomotor skills of managing a respiratory emergency. Instructors will use the Airway Management Skills Station Competency Checklist found on the PALS Instructor CD to evaluate this skill. This skill evaluation can be incorporated into the PALS case scenario tests if desired.

Each student must individually discuss the indications and contraindications for IO access and demonstrate the psychomotor skills of IO access. Instructors will use the Vascular Access Skills Station Competency Checklist found on the PALS Instructor CD to evaluate this skill. This skill evaluation can be incorporated into the PALS case scenario tests if case scenario tests are used.

Each student must individually demonstrate the psychomotor skills of rhythm disturbances/electrical therapy. Instructors will use the Rhythm Disturbances/Electrical Therapy Skills Station Competency Checklist found on the PALS Instructor CD to evaluate this skill. This skill evaluation can be incorporated into the PALS case scenario tests if desired.

Students who do not successfully complete any of the skills testing requirements should receive remediation and be retested by using the same guidelines for remediation provided in the *PALS Instructor Manual* for classroom courses.

Bag-Mask Ventilation Skills Testing

All PALS students must participate in the lesson on Airway Management and must pass the Bag-Mask Ventilation Skills Test. Students will be asked to perform effective bag-mask ventilation for 1 minute during a respiratory arrest scenario, including inserting an oropharyngeal airway (see the checklist in Appendix B).

High-Quality BLS Skills Testing

All students in the PALS Course must participate in the lessons on High-Quality BLS practice and testing and must pass the Child CPR and AED and Infant CPR Skills Tests regardless of the method of preparation or prior CPR training.

Skills Testing

As part of the emphasis on better teaching and learning, the AHA developed CPR skills tests to ensure that there is a uniform and objective approach for testing CPR skills. The skills testing checklists help instructors evaluate each student's CPR skills. The AHA-approved voice-assisted manikin is designed to align with the skills testing checklists. As a result of the course design and skills tests, the AHA expects that students in CPR classes will learn more effectively and instructors will work with students to achieve higher levels of CPR skills competency.

CPR competency is critical to victim survival. It is important that you use the skills testing checklists to evaluate each student's performance and to ensure consistent testing and learning across all AHA PALS courses. Your adherence to these testing procedures will enhance the CPR competency of your students.

You must keep a copy of completed skills testing checklists for students who are unsuccessful.

Skills Testing of eLearning Students

Instructors may need to conduct the hands-on session of the eLearning course. Specific content from the PALS Course has been incorporated into the hands-on session for a blended-learning solution. The hands-on session includes skills practice and skills testing (see HeartCode Lesson Plans). The skills testing portion of the hands-on session should be conducted the same as in an instructor-led course. A minimum of 3 students should be present to conduct the case scenario tests.

Overview of Skills Testing

This section details how to conduct the BLS skills tests.

These descriptions provide the detailed information you need to evaluate student performance during the skills tests.

Here is a summary of the forms you will need and how to use them.

Form	Use
BLS Skills Testing Checklist	• To record the student's results • Before testing to facilitate student practice • During testing to indicate additional practice needed
Skills Testing Critical Skills Descriptors	• To determine if the student performs each step of the skill correctly

Using a Stopwatch/ Timing Device

To achieve accuracy during the skills practice and testing, a stopwatch is used to measure the rate of compressions. Follow these rules when using a stopwatch:

- Start your stopwatch when the student first compresses the sternum.
- Stop your stopwatch at the end of the 30th compression.
- Mark the step correct if the number of seconds is between 15 and 18.

Using the Skills Testing Checklists and Critical Skills Descriptors

Use the skills testing checklists to document the student's performance during the skills testing portion of the course. The skills testing checklist should be filled out while the student is performing the skills. Use the skills testing critical skills descriptors to determine if a student has demonstrated each step of the skill correctly.

- If the student successfully completes a step, place a check (✓) in the box to the right of the step on the skills testing checklist.
- If the student is unsuccessful, leave the box next to the step blank on the skills testing checklist. Circle the step under the critical skills descriptor that the student did not complete successfully.

If a student demonstrates each step of the skills test successfully, mark the student as passing that skills test on the skills testing checklist. If a student does not receive checks in all boxes, refer the student to the remediation lesson at the end of the course for further testing in that skill. Also, discuss with the student the areas that you circled on the critical skills descriptors and how to correctly perform each skill that was circled.

You should be very familiar with all of the critical skills descriptors to be able to test BLS skills correctly.

Skills Testing Checklist Rules

When using the skills testing checklists, remember the rules listed in the chart that follows:

Rule	Reminder
Check only the steps that the student performs correctly.	• On the BLS skills testing checklist, put a check in the box next to a specific step if the student performs that step correctly based on the critical skills descriptor. • If the student does not perform that step correctly, do not mark the checklist for that step. • Once the student has correctly performed all steps, the student has passed the skills test.

(continued)

(continued)

Rule	Reminder

Do not give hints during the test.	• Do not tell the student any specific information about the assessment steps. For example, do not say "no breathing" as the student checks for breathing.
	• Do not comment on the skills performance of the student during the test. This ensures that
	  – The student relies on his or her own assessments of the "victim," makes decisions about what to do, and performs CPR *independent of the instructor*
	  – The test more accurately reflects a real-life CPR situation; *this is an important criterion to determine skills competency in CPR*

Refer to the critical skills descriptors for detailed information about what to observe.	• Do not interpret or read into the critical skills descriptors or evaluate anything not specifically identified in the skills descriptions for each skill.
	• Determine whether the student has performed a step exactly as the description indicates.
	  – If yes, place a "correct" check on the checklist for that step.
	  – If no, leave the checklist blank for that step.

Stop the test when the BLS skills testing checklist indicates.	• Mark the student's skills test as "Pass" or "NR" (needs remediation).
	• For those with a mark of NR
	  – Check the steps that need more practice on the student's practice sheet
	  – Tell the student to practice those steps before retesting later in the course
	  – Conduct additional practice and retesting as part of the remediation lesson later in the course

If a student does not pass, you may retest the student during the BLS testing station, if time permits, or during the remediation lesson.	• If the student stops the test before the stop point indicated on the checklist
	  – Mark the student as "NR"
	  – Refer the student for more practice

Retest the entire skill.	• When retesting a student during the remediation lesson, you must test the *entire* skill.

Understanding the Child CPR and AED Skills Testing Checklist

Section	How to Use
Assessment and Activation	The steps in this box do not have to be completed in a specific order; the student only needs to complete all of the steps before beginning compressions. In addition, the student must take no less than 5 seconds and no more than 10 seconds to check breathing and check a pulse (ideally these checks should be done at the same time). **Script** Once the student shouts for help, the instructor should say, "Here's the barrier device. I am going to get the AED."
Child Compressions	During this section, evaluate the student's ability to perform high-quality chest compressions. High-fidelity manikins are optimal feedback devices and are highly recommended to objectively evaluate chest compressions. Compressions should be initiated within 10 seconds of recognition of cardiac arrest. **Hand Placement** Evaluate the student to ensure that hand placement is on the lower half of the breastbone (sternum) and that the heel of the hand is used. When the student uses 2 hands, the second hand is placed on top of or grasping the wrist of the first hand. **Rate** Compression rate should be evaluated by using a stopwatch. To achieve a rate of 100 to 120 compressions per minute, students should deliver 30 compressions in 15 to 18 seconds. **Depth and Recoil** Evaluating depth and recoil in the absence of a feedback device or a manikin is unreliable. To increase the validity and reliability of the test, you can use commercial feedback devices or manikins that have the capability to objectively evaluate depth and recoil. High-fidelity manikins, with lights or an electronic display that indicates correct depth and recoil, are highly recommended. Manikins with a depth indicator that makes a clicking sound when compressions are deep enough are acceptable. *Tip:* To help students achieve adequate compression depth and to minimize fatigue, instruct them to perform chest compressions with their elbows locked and their shoulders over the victim.

(continued)

(continued)

Section	How to Use
Child Breaths	**Breaths** Breaths should be given with a barrier device, such as a pocket mask or face shield. The device used should be similar to what the students will be using in their workplace. If the type of device is unknown, instructors should provide students with the device they used in training. In some circumstances, a workplace may only have a bag-mask device available. In these instances, students may complete their skills test with a bag-mask device. Instructors should emphasize that in the clinical setting, a rescuer will not be able to deliver 2 breaths within 10 seconds when using a bag-mask device during 1-rescuer CPR. **Each Breath Given Over 1 Second** Students should open the victim's airway by using the head tilt–chin lift. Each student should deliver 2 breaths. Each breath should be given over 1 second while the student observes for chest rise. **Visible Chest Rise** Students should deliver just enough air for visible chest rise. *Tip:* If students are having difficulty providing breaths, ensure they have a proper seal and that the airway is open. You might need to help students with their hand placement on the pocket mask or bag-mask device so that they can get a proper seal. **Minimizing Interruptions** The pause from the end of the last compression in a cycle to the beginning of the first compression of the next cycle should be no more than 10 seconds. This can be challenging to achieve with a bag-mask device.
Child Cycle 2	Students should deliver another set of 30 compressions and 2 breaths. Evaluate students with the same criteria as in Cycle 1.

(continued)

(continued)

Section	How to Use
Child AED	The second rescuer (either another student or the instructor) may participate in the delivery of CPR or bring the AED. The instructor or a second student can arrive with an AED and hand it to the first student. The second student or instructor can take over compressions. If a second student is not available, the instructor can hand the student the AED and instruct the student to use the AED. The instructor can tell the student that another rescuer is providing chest compressions. It is important that students understand that the attachment of AED pads should not interrupt chest compressions. The student should turn the AED on as required for his or her specific device; this may require the student to push the power button on the AED, or the AED may turn on automatically when the case is opened. Students should attach the AED pads to the manikin by following the pictures on the pads. Students should follow the prompts of the AED they are using. Instructors should be aware that some of the AED steps outlined on the skills testing checklist might not be completely applicable to all devices. Some AEDs require the patient to be cleared during the analysis and charging cycle, and some AEDs allow compressions to be continued while the device is charging. Once the AED is ready to deliver a shock, the student should clear the patient both verbally and visually. Once everyone is clear, the student should press the shock button. The student should resume compressions immediately. *Note:* An AED is not used in infant testing.
Resumes Compressions	The student being evaluated can begin compressions immediately after the shock is delivered or tell the instructor to begin compressions immediately after the shock is delivered. Evaluate the student's ability to begin compressions immediately after the shock delivery. Evaluate students with the same criteria for compressions as in Cycle 1; if the student resumes compressions or directs the instructor to begin compressions immediately, stop the test.
Test Results	If the student successfully performs all of the skills, circle "Pass" on the student's skills testing checklist. If the student does not successfully perform all of the skills, circle "NR" for *needs remediation*. The instructor should retest (reevaluate) the student on the skills that were not performed correctly by using a new skills testing checklist. If remediation is needed, both the skills testing checklist that indicated the need for remediation and the new skills testing checklist indicating that the student passed should be stored with the course records. Provide your initials, your instructor ID, and the date in the box at the end of the checklist.

Pediatric Advanced Life Support
Child CPR and AED
Skills Testing Checklist

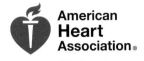

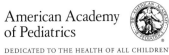

American Heart Association®

life is why™

American Academy of Pediatrics

DEDICATED TO THE HEALTH OF ALL CHILDREN™

Student Name _____   Date of Test _____

Hospital Scenario: "You are working in a hospital or clinic, and you see a child who has suddenly collapsed in the hallway. You check that the scene is safe and then approach the patient. Demonstrate what you would do next."

Prehospital Scenario: "You arrive on the scene for a child who is not breathing. No bystander CPR has been provided. You approach the scene and ensure that it is safe. Demonstrate what you would do next."

Assessment and Activation

☐ Checks responsiveness   ☐ Shouts for help/Activates emergency response system/Sends for AED
☐ Checks breathing   ☐ Checks pulse

Once student shouts for help, instructor says, "Here's the barrier device. I am going to get the AED."

Cycle 1 of CPR (30:2)   *CPR feedback devices preferred for accuracy*

Child Compressions

☐ Performs high-quality compressions*:

- Hand placement on lower half of sternum
- 30 compressions in no less than 15 and no more than 18 seconds
- Compresses at least one third the depth of the chest, about 2 inches (5 cm)
- Complete recoil after each compression

Child Breaths

☐ Gives 2 breaths with a barrier device:

- Each breath given over 1 second
- Visible chest rise with each breath
- Resumes compressions in less than 10 seconds

Cycle 2 of CPR (repeats steps in Cycle 1)   *Only check box if step is successfully performed*

☐ Compressions   ☐ Breaths   ☐ Resumes compressions in less than 10 seconds

Rescuer 2 says, "Here is the AED. I'll take over compressions, and you use the AED."

AED (follows prompts of AED)

☐ Powers on AED   ☐ Correctly attaches pads   ☐ Clears for analysis   ☐ Clears to safely deliver a shock
☐ Safely delivers a shock

Resumes Compressions

☐ Ensures compressions are resumed immediately after shock delivery

- Student directs instructor to resume compressions *or*
- Student resumes compressions

STOP TEST

Instructor Notes

- Place a ✓ in the box next to each step the student completes successfully.
- If the student does not complete all steps successfully (as indicated by at least 1 blank check box), the student must receive remediation. Make a note here of which skills require remediation (refer to Instructor Manual for information about remediation).

Test Results	Circle **PASS** or **NR** to indicate pass or needs remediation:	**PASS**	**NR**
Instructor Initials _____	Instructor Number _____	Date _____	

Child CPR and AED
Skills Testing Critical Skills Descriptors

1. **Assesses victim and activates emergency response system (this *must* precede starting compressions) within a maximum of 30 seconds. After determining that the scene is safe:**
   - Checks for responsiveness by tapping and shouting
   - Shouts for help/directs someone to call for help *and* get AED/defibrillator
   - Checks for no breathing or no normal breathing (only gasping)
     - Scans from the head to the chest for a minimum of 5 seconds and no more than 10 seconds
   - Checks carotid pulse
     - Can be done simultaneously with check for breathing
     - Checks for a minimum of 5 seconds and no more than 10 seconds

2. **Performs high-quality chest compressions (initiates compressions immediately after recognition of cardiac arrest)**
   - Correct hand placement
     - Lower half of sternum
     - 2-handed (second hand on top of the first or grasping the wrist of the first hand) or 1-handed
   - Compression rate of 100 to 120/min
     - Delivers 30 compressions in 15 to 18 seconds
   - Compression depth and recoil—compresses at least one third the depth of the chest, about 2 inches (5 cm)
     - Use of a commercial feedback device or high-fidelity manikin is highly recommended
     - Complete chest recoil after each compression
   - Minimizes interruptions in compressions
     - Delivers 2 breaths so less than 10 seconds elapses between last compression of one cycle and first compression of next cycle
     - Compressions resumed immediately after shock/no shock indicated

3. **Provides 2 breaths by using a barrier device**
   - Opens airway adequately
     - Uses a head tilt–chin lift maneuver or jaw thrust
   - Delivers each breath over 1 second
   - Delivers breaths that produce visible chest rise
   - Avoids excessive ventilation
   - Resumes chest compressions in less than 10 seconds

4. **Performs same steps for compressions and breaths for Cycle 2**

5. **AED use**
   - Powers on AED
     - Turns AED on by pushing button or lifting lid as soon as it arrives
   - Correctly attaches pads
     - Places proper-sized pads for victim's age in correct location
   - Clears for analysis
     - Clears rescuers from victim for AED to analyze rhythm (pushes analyze button if required by device)
     - Communicates clearly to all other rescuers to stop touching victim
   - Clears to safely deliver shock
     - Communicates clearly to all other rescuers to stop touching victim
   - Delivers a shock
     - Resumes chest compressions immediately after shock delivery
     - Does *not* turn off AED during CPR

6. **Resumes compressions**
   - Ensures that high-quality chest compressions are resumed immediately after shock delivery
   - Performs same steps for compressions

Understanding the Infant CPR Skills Testing Checklist

Section	How to Use
Assessment and Activation	The steps in this box do not have to be completed in a specific order; the student only needs to complete all of the steps before beginning compressions. In addition, the student must take no less than 5 seconds and no more than 10 seconds to check breathing and check a pulse (ideally these checks should be done at the same time). **Script** Once the student shouts for help, the instructor should say, "Here's the barrier device."
Infant Compressions	During this section, evaluate the student's ability to perform high-quality chest compressions. High-fidelity manikins are optimal feedback devices and are highly recommended to objectively evaluate chest compressions. Compressions should be initiated within 10 seconds of recognition of cardiac arrest. **Finger Placement, Cycles 1 and 2 (1-Rescuer CPR)** Evaluate the student to ensure that finger placement is in the center of the chest and 2 fingers are placed just below the nipple line. **Finger Placement, Cycle 3 (2-Rescuer CPR)** Evaluate the student's 2 thumb–encircling hands technique for infant compressions during 2-rescuer CPR. Ensure that the student's 2 thumbs are placed on the lower half of the breastbone, just below the nipple line. **Rate, Cycles 1 and 2 (1-Rescuer CPR)** Compression rate should be evaluated by using a stopwatch. To achieve a rate of 100 to 120 compressions per minute, students should deliver 30 compressions in 15 to 18 seconds. **Rate, Cycle 3 (2-Rescuer CPR)** Compression rate should be evaluated by using a stopwatch. To achieve a rate of 100 to 120 compressions per minute, students should deliver 15 compressions in 7 to 9 seconds. **Depth and Recoil** Evaluating depth and recoil in the absence of a feedback device or a manikin is unreliable. To increase the validity and reliability of your testing experience, use commercial feedback devices that have the capability to objectively evaluate depth and recoil. High-fidelity manikins, with lights or an electronic display that indicates correct depth and recoil, are highly recommended. Manikins with a depth indicator that makes a clicking sound when compressions are deep enough are acceptable.

(continued)

(continued)

Section	How to Use
Infant Breaths	**Breaths** Breaths should be given with a barrier device, such as a pocket mask or face shield. The device used should be similar to what the students would be using in their workplace. If the type of device is unknown, instructors should provide students with the device they used in training. In some circumstances, a workplace may have only a bag-mask device available. In these instances, students may complete their skills test with a bag-mask device. Instructors should emphasize that in the clinical setting, a rescuer will not be able to deliver 2 breaths within 10 seconds when using a bag-mask device during 1-rescuer CPR. **Breaths, Cycle 4 (2-Rescuer CPR)** Breaths should be given with a bag-mask device. **Each Breath Given Over 1 Second** Students should open the victim's airway by using the head tilt–chin lift. Each student should deliver 2 breaths. Each breath should be given over 1 second while the student observes for chest rise. **Visible Chest Rise** Students should deliver just enough air for visible chest rise. *Tip:* If students are having difficulty providing breaths, ensure they have a proper seal and that the airway is open. You might need to help students with their hand placement on the pocket mask or bag-mask device so that they can get a proper seal. **Minimizing Interruptions** The pause from the end of the last compression in a cycle to the beginning of the first compression of the next cycle should be no more than 10 seconds. This can be challenging to achieve with a bag-mask device.
Infant Cycle 2	Students should deliver another 30 compressions and 2 breaths. Evaluate students with the same criteria as in Cycle 1.

(continued)

(continued)

Section	How to Use
Infant Cycle 3	The student being evaluated continues compressions while the second rescuer (either another student or the instructor) gets in position to provide breaths with a bag-mask device. The student being evaluated should provide compressions with the 2 thumb–encircling hands technique, with the 2 thumbs placed on the lower half of the breastbone, just below the nipple line.

The test will end once the student has paused after 15 compressions so that the second rescuer can deliver 2 breaths.

Note: The students will switch roles at the end of this cycle, before Cycle 4. |
| **Infant Cycle 4** | The second student can continue compressions while the student being evaluated gets in position to provide breaths with a bag-mask device. After a cycle of 15 compressions, the student being evaluated should provide 2 breaths by using a bag-mask device. Each breath should be delivered over 1 second. Each breath should result in visible chest rise. There should be no more than a 10-second pause in compressions for the breaths to be delivered. |
| **Test Results** | If the student successfully performs all of the skills, circle "Pass" on the student's skills testing checklist. If the student does not successfully perform all of the skills, circle "NR" for *needs remediation*. The instructor should retest (reevaluate) the student on the skills that were not performed correctly by using a new skills testing checklist. If remediation is needed, both the skills testing checklist that indicated the need for remediation and the new skills testing checklist indicating that the student passed should be stored with the course records. Provide your initials, your instructor ID, and the date in the box at the end of the checklist. |

Pediatric Advanced Life Support
Infant CPR
Skills Testing Checklist (1 of 2)

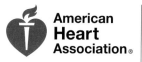 **American Heart Association®**

life is why™

 American Academy of Pediatrics

DEDICATED TO THE HEALTH OF ALL CHILDREN™

Student Name _____   Date of Test _____

Hospital Scenario: "You are working in a hospital or clinic when a woman runs through the door, carrying an infant. She shouts, 'Help me! My baby's not breathing.' You have gloves and a pocket mask. You send your coworker to activate the emergency response system and to get the emergency equipment."

Prehospital Scenario: "You arrive on the scene for an infant who is not breathing. No bystander CPR has been provided. You approach the scene and ensure that it is safe. Demonstrate what you would do next."

Assessment and Activation
☐ Checks responsiveness   ☐ Shouts for help/Activates emergency response system   ☐ Checks breathing
☐ Checks pulse

Once student shouts for help, instructor says, "Here's the barrier device."

Cycle 1 of CPR (30:2)   *CPR feedback devices preferred for accuracy*

Infant Compressions
☐ Performs high-quality compressions*:
- Placement of 2 fingers in the center of the chest, just below the nipple line
- 30 compressions in no less than 15 and no more than 18 seconds
- Compresses at least one third the depth of the chest, about 1½ inches (4 cm)
- Complete recoil after each compression

Infant Breaths
☐ Gives 2 breaths with a barrier device:
- Each breath given over 1 second
- Visible chest rise with each breath
- Resumes compressions in less than 10 seconds

Cycle 2 of CPR (repeats steps in Cycle 1)   *Only check box if step is successfully performed*
☐ Compressions   ☐ Breaths   ☐ Resumes compressions in less than 10 seconds

Rescuer 2 arrives with bag-mask device and begins ventilation while Rescuer 1 continues compressions with 2 thumb–encircling hands technique.

Cycle 3 of CPR

Rescuer 1: Infant Compressions
☐ Performs high-quality compressions*:
- 15 compressions with 2 thumb–encircling hands technique
- 15 compressions in no less than 7 and no more than 9 seconds
- Compress at least one third the depth of the chest, about 1½ inches (4 cm)
- Complete recoil after each compression

Rescuer 2: Infant Breaths
This rescuer is not evaluated.

(continued)

Pediatric Advanced Life Support
Infant CPR
Skills Testing Checklist (2 of 2)

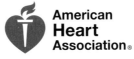

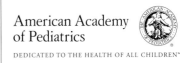

Student Name _____   Date of Test _____

Cycle 4 of CPR

Rescuer 2: Infant Compressions

This rescuer is not evaluated.

Rescuer 1: Infant Breaths

☐ Gives 2 breaths with a bag-mask device:
- Each breath given over 1 second
- Visible chest rise with each breath
- Resumes compressions in less than 10 seconds

STOP TEST

Instructor Notes
- Place a ✓ in the box next to each step the student completes successfully.
- If the student does not complete all steps successfully (as indicated by at least 1 blank check box), the student must receive remediation. Make a note here of which skills require remediation (refer to Instructor Manual for information about remediation).

Test Results	Circle **PASS** or **NR** to indicate pass or needs remediation:	**PASS** **NR**

Instructor Initials _____   Instructor Number _____   Date _____

Infant CPR
Skills Testing Critical Skills Descriptors

1. **Assesses victim and activates emergency response system (this *must* precede starting compressions) within a maximum of 30 seconds. After determining that the scene is safe:**
   - Checks for responsiveness by tapping and shouting
   - Shouts for help/directs someone to call for help *and* get emergency equipment
   - Checks for no breathing or no normal breathing (only gasping)
     - Scans from the head to the chest for a minimum of 5 seconds and no more than 10 seconds
   - Checks brachial pulse
     - Can be done simultaneously with check for breathing
     - Checks for a minimum of 5 seconds and no more than 10 seconds

2. **Performs high-quality chest compressions during 1-rescuer CPR (initiates compressions within 10 seconds of identifying cardiac arrest)**
   - Correct placement of hands/fingers in center of chest
     - 1 rescuer: 2 fingers just below the nipple line
   - Compression rate of 100 to 120/min
     - Delivers 30 compressions in 15 to 18 seconds
   - Adequate depth for age
     - Infant: at least one third the depth of the chest (about 1½ inches [4 cm])
     - Use of a commercial feedback device or high-fidelity manikin is highly recommended
   - Complete chest recoil after each compression
   - Appropriate ratio for age and number of rescuers
     - 1 rescuer: 30 compressions to 2 breaths
   - Minimizes interruptions in compressions
     - Delivers 2 breaths so less than 10 seconds elapses between last compression of one cycle and first compression of next cycle

3. **Provides effective breaths with bag-mask device during 2-rescuer CPR**
   - Opens airway adequately
   - Delivers each breath over 1 second
   - Delivers breaths that produce visible chest rise
   - Avoids excessive ventilation
   - Resumes chest compressions in less than 10 seconds

4. **Switches compression technique at appropriate interval as prompted by the instructor (for purposes of this evaluation). Switch should take no more than 5 seconds.**

5. **Performs high-quality chest compressions during 2-rescuer CPR**
   - Correct placement of hands/fingers in center of chest
     - 2 rescuers: 2 thumb–encircling hands just below the nipple line
   - Compression rate of 100 to 120/min
     - Delivers 15 compressions in 7 to 9 seconds
   - Adequate depth for age
     - Infant: at least one third the depth of the chest (about 1½ inches [4 cm])
   - Complete chest recoil after each compression
   - Appropriate ratio for age and number of rescuers
     - 2 rescuers: 15 compressions to 2 breaths
   - Minimizes interruptions in compressions
   - Delivers 2 breaths so less than 10 seconds elapses between last compression of one cycle and first compression of next cycle

Retesting Students

If time permits during skills testing, you may retest a student 1 additional time if the student did not pass. Additional retesting is done at the end of the course during the remediation lesson. (See Remediation section in this manual.)

In every retesting case, test the student in the entire skill.

In some cases, you may defer retesting to a later time after the course. For example, if remediation is not successful, you might develop a plan of improvement and schedule retesting once the student completes the plan. If a student needs substantial additional remediation, you may recommend that the student repeat a PALS Provider Course. The exam measures the mastery of cognitive skills and is an open-resource exam.

In some self-directed learning courses, the exam is included in the eLearning course. Students can print a certificate upon successful completion of the online portion of the course.

Instructors may read the exam to a student who has a learning disability or language barrier.

Each student must score at least 84% on the exam.

Case Scenario Testing

Passing the Case Scenario Tests

You will complete a case scenario testing checklist during the evaluation of each student.

To pass, a student must complete the entire case scenario test with a "correct" check for every critical performance step.

If the student does not perform a critical performance step successfully, the test result will be NR (needs remediation).

Objective and Uniform Testing of Students

Take the following steps to ensure that the evaluation of each student during the case scenario testing is objective and uniform:

Step	Description
Use the case scenario testing checklist.	• Follow the case scenario testing checklist. The basic criteria for each step of the case scenario testing checklist are the content, principles, and actions that are taught in the PALS Course. Students should avoid performing steps or skills that are not part of the PALS Course. • Observe carefully and mark only those skills that you see the student demonstrate. Skills can be demonstrated through either appropriate oral directions to the team or appropriate actions with the team. • Record student performance on the case scenario testing checklist during the test, not afterward. Do not rely on your memory to determine what the student did or did not do during the test. • To pass, a student must successfully perform *all* critical performance steps on the case scenario testing checklist.

(continued)

(continued)

Step	Description
Do not coach or give hints.	• Do not coach, guide, or lead a student through the case scenario test. • Do not answer questions or give hints about what the student should do or not do during the case scenario test. • You may, however, ask a leading question to prompt a student to verbalize a required critical performance step when indicated on the case scenario testing checklist.
Do not permit a student to excessively rely on team members.	• Team members should be directed to help the student manage the case, but not to provide suggestions for care. • Permit the student to get help from team members, but do not permit the student to depend on the team to manage most or all of the case. • If you see a student who is hesitating consistently or who is asking the team for significant guidance throughout the test, the student should receive remediation.
Make sure team members play roles realistically.	• Make sure that all students play their roles realistically during the test (eg, compressions should be done and not simulated). Confirm that students understand this before you start the test.
Allow actions that are within team members' scope of practice.	• Allow the Team Leader to direct actions that are appropriate to the scope of practice of the team members. For example, insertion of an advanced airway is not required to pass the case scenario test, but if it is ordered by the Team Leader and is within the scope of practice of the team member managing the airway, it may be done as long as interruption of chest compressions is minimized.
Make the test realistic.	• Do not allow the case scenario test to become a conversation about what is being done or should be done. Make the test a realistic scenario with hands-on skills demonstrated or simulated in real time.
Do not pause the test or allow the student to start over.	• If the student pauses during the test, remind the student that recommendations for testing do not permit a pause in the actions required to resuscitate the patient. • Do not allow a student to progress through a part of the test and then start over. If a student is not doing well, it is appropriate to stop the test, give private feedback about performance deficiencies, and refer the student for remediation. • Do not pause the test, provide feedback, and then restart the test.
Avoid misdirecting the student.	• Avoid deliberate misdirection of the student. Do not subvert the student's performance. If someone is doing very well, allow the case to continue to a reasonable end point without trying to see how much more the student knows or whether the student can handle more difficult aspects of the case.

(continued)

(continued)

Step	Description
Stop the test at the correct point.	• Stop the test when the student has demonstrated all critical actions or when it is evident that the student needs remediation. For testing purposes, it is not necessary to bring each case scenario to a realistic ending.
Do not retest during this station.	• Do not retest a student during the case scenario testing station. If a student needs retesting, do so during the remediation lesson.
Give feedback privately.	• When giving feedback to the student after the test, do so privately, out of view and range of hearing of the other students. • Testing feedback should not be given by other students. Only the instructor should give feedback about case scenario testing performance. • Do not consult other students about whether they think a student has successfully completed the case scenario testing or needs remediation. This avoids conflict between what students may say and what you may say about a test performance. This also ensures that only your feedback is used to evaluate the student's performance.
Be fair and consistent.	• Be fair, consistent, and as objective as possible when testing. • Pass students who correctly manage the case according to the case scenario testing checklist; refer students who do not to the remediation lesson. • Remember, the consistency and quality of a PALS Course are often measured by the fairness and objectivity of testing.

When to Give Exams

You will test students as outlined in the Lesson Plans.

The skills testing can be administered during the course or at the end at the discretion of the instructor. Please refer to the Lesson Plans for when to administer skills testing.

The exam is administered at the conclusion of the PALS Course. Students who complete HeartCode PALS will complete the exam within the online portion.

Exam

The exam measures the mastery of cognitive skills. Each student must score at least 84% on the exam to meet course completion requirements.

As part of the new education methodologies, the AHA has adopted an open-resource policy for exams administered online through an eLearning course and in a classroom-based course.

Open resource means that students may use resources as reference while completing the exam. Resources could include the Provider Manual either in printed form or as an eBook on personal devices, any notes the student took during the provider course, the ECC Handbook, *2015 AHA Guidelines Update for CPR and ECC*, posters, etc. Open resource does not mean open discussion with other students or the instructor.

In the welcome letter sent to students with their course materials, emphasize the importance of their bringing their books to class for use during the exam.

When you administer the exam in a classroom-based course, remember that the students may not interact with each other during the exam. When a student completes the exam, grade it and answer any questions.

Students who score less than 84% need immediate remediation. During remediation, make sure that the students understand why their answers were incorrect.

In providing remediation to a student who did not pass the exam, you must confirm knowledge acquisition and understanding. That can be done by having the student take a second exam, or by doing a verbal remediation. If you give the student a second exam, review the first exam with the student, allowing time for the student to study the questions he or she got wrong. If you provide verbal remediation, ask the student to verbally answer the questions that he or she answered incorrectly, and document on the answer sheet whether the student correctly answered each question. It needs to be documented on the answer sheet that the remediation was successful and that the student achieved a passing score.

If you have a student who has difficulty reading or understanding the written questions, you may read the exam to the student. You must read the exam as written and in a manner that does not indicate the correct answer. You may verbally translate the exam if needed.

Online courses have the exam incorporated into the online portion, so the exam does not need to be given to students when they attend the classroom portion.

Remediation

Provider Course Student Remediation

At times, you will have to provide remediation to a student who is unable to perform satisfactorily in portions of the course. This is often resource-intensive and may require considerable expertise in communication and educational creativity.

The fundamental principle is that every student who is not able to master the required skills during the course is still able to have remediation. The instructor should be committed to finding and using the proper remediation techniques that will be effective for a particular student. Adult learning principles coupled with debriefing techniques usually make for an effective combination. Here are some suggestions:

- Review the objectives for a particular scenario or skills station with the student.
- Give positive feedback when desired actions are observed; ask open-ended questions when nonpreferred actions are observed to determine the learner's thought process.
- Use the same scenario repeatedly if necessary until the student accomplishes the objectives.

Consider using another instructor to remediate, because that instructor might be a better fit for the student.

At the time of the course, some students might not have successful remediation through particular sections of the course (or exam or test). When this happens, the student may arrange for a separate remediation session. A student must meet all learning objectives to the satisfaction of the Course Director or Lead Instructor before receiving a course completion card.

Students must complete all remediation sessions, including exams, tests, and skills stations, within 30 days of the last day of the original course. The remediation date will be listed as the issue date on the course completion card.

If a student does not achieve remediation within 30 days, the course is considered incomplete and a course completion card will not be issued.

Remediation Concepts for Instructors

Remediation is a learning process in which the instructor provides additional opportunities for the student to master the required skills of the course.

Informal remediation occurs throughout the course and is part of the learning process.

Formal remediation occurs after a student has been formally tested in a skills or case scenario testing station and has been unable to demonstrate mastery.

It is important to communicate the need for formal remediation in a private, sensitive, and objective debriefing immediately after the testing has taken place by using the scenario critical action objectives as a guide.

- Every student, with rare exceptions, should be able to receive successful remediation.
- The instructor should be committed to providing remediation to students who have difficulties learning the skills and principles in the PALS Course the first time through.
- Instructor styles of facilitating and student styles of learning may not match; therefore, a change of instructor may be necessary.
- Instructors should not assume that poor performance is associated with a lack of knowledge. There may be other factors (eg, personal or work-related issues) that are influencing the student's performance.
- If an instructor has difficulty providing successful remediation to a student, the instructor may need to examine his or her own style of remediation.
- The role of the instructor is to facilitate learning.
- The instructor should always be respectful, courteous, positive, professional, and diplomatic when performing remediation with the student.

Additional materials to assist in remediation will be provided in a later section of the manual.

Informal and Formal Remediation

Informal Remediation

- Use the performance checklist to help identify weaknesses and areas for review.
- Communicate with other instructors throughout the course to identify students who are having difficulty.
- Identify knowledge deficits via subjective assessments during case scenario practice with simulations.

Assist students during breaks, lunchtime, or at the end of the day to help them succeed with skills or understand medical management better. Every effort should be taken by instructors during the course to correct knowledge and skill deficits. By doing so, the instructor will minimize the chances of having to provide formal remediation to students at the end of the course.

Formal Remediation

Have the student work one-on-one with an instructor to assess areas for improvement in performing a skill. Then, encourage the student to practice and, when ready, to indicate when he or she wishes to be tested.

Steps to Successful Remediation

If a student requires formal remediation, communicate that information in a private, sensitive, and objective debriefing as soon as possible after the testing has taken place.

Follow these steps to provide successful remediation to a student.

1	Be respectful, courteous, positive, professional, and diplomatic when performing remediation.
2	Review the objectives for a particular scenario or skills station with the student.
3	Give positive feedback when desired actions are observed; ask open-ended questions when nonpreferred actions are observed to determine the learner's thought process.
4	Use the same scenario repeatedly, if necessary, until the student accomplishes the objectives.
5	Don't assume that poor performance is associated with a lack of knowledge. There may be other factors (eg, personal or work-related issues) that are influencing the student's performance.
6	Instructor styles of facilitating and student styles of learning may not match; therefore, a change of instructor may be necessary.
7	If an instructor has difficulty providing successful remediation to a student, the instructor may need to examine his or her own style of remediation.

Skills Remediation

Have the student work one-on-one with an instructor to assess areas for improvement in performing a skill. Then, encourage the student to practice and, when ready, to indicate when he or she wishes to be tested.

Case Scenario Remediation

The following is the recommended way to provide remediation to a student for a case scenario:

1. Review the critical action steps that the student did not perform satisfactorily.
2. Using open-ended questions (debriefing tool), assess the student's thought process and correct it if necessary.
3. Identify whether other factors might have affected the student's performance (eg, performance anxiety).
4. Use the same or a similar scenario for retesting the student (eg, if the initial case scenario was a respiratory case, use a respiratory case again for the retest).
5. Use other students who need remediation or other instructors to help form a team to manage the case scenario.
6. If performance anxiety or an instructor-student personality clash is a factor, use another instructor to conduct the remediation.

In the rare case in which a student is unable to perform satisfactorily in the core testing scenarios after several remediation attempts, the following steps should be taken:

1. Ensure that the Course Director is aware,
2. Use another instructor to assess learning deficits and facilitate a case scenario test, and/or
3. Consider having the student attend part or all of another PALS course

Taking HeartCode PALS as an alternative to obtain a course completion card after failing the case scenario testing station in a PALS course is not recommended.

Exam Remediation

If the student misses 1 or 2 questions beyond what is required for a passing score (84%), a discussion and assessment of student understanding may be sufficient to achieve successful remediation and pass the student.

If a student misses more than 1 or 2 questions beyond what is required for a passing score (84%), it is likely that the student does not have sufficient knowledge. The instructor should encourage the student to review the *PALS Provider Manual* and then return to take another version of the exam at a later date.

Students who consistently demonstrate flawed reasoning in judgment and knowledge will be considered to have failed the course.

After the Course

Program Evaluation

Ongoing evaluation and improvement of AHA materials and instructors are important to the AHA. An opportunity to evaluate the class should be given to each student. As an instructor, it is your responsibility to provide that opportunity. There are several options on how a course evaluation can be provided.

- A paper-and-pencil evaluation can be used. A template is available on the Instructor Network in multiple languages. Make enough copies for all of your students. Have them complete the evaluation at the end of the course and return it to you. Review the feedback, and then send the completed forms to your Training Center Coordinator.
- If you are an instructor with a US Training Center and your Training Center is issuing eCards, your students will complete an evaluation online before they claim their course completion card.
- If you are an instructor with an International Training Center, your students will complete an evaluation online before they can claim their CPRverify™ certificate; in addition, instructors can also have students complete the paper evaluation provided by the AHA.

Issuing Provider Cards/eCards

Each student who successfully completes the AHA PALS course completion requirements is to be issued an AHA PALS course completion card or an AHA PALS eCard. Only your Training Center Coordinator can provide you with the needed cards or eCards. Check with your Training Center Coordinator about the process at your Training Center for obtaining and issuing cards to your students.

By submitting your rosters or signing your name as an assisting instructor, you are verifying that those students have successfully met all the requirements for course completion.

No AHA course completion card or eCard is issued without hands-on manikin skills practice and testing by an AHA PALS Instructor.

Continuing Education Qualifications

The PALS Course was designed to meet the following continuing education criteria:

- The course focuses on
  - Providing instructionally sound learning principles
  - Identifying and presenting the affective domain
- Learners are engaged by using
  - Dramatizations
  - Simulations
  - Additional case-based scenarios
- Activity evaluation, outcomes, and noneducation follow-up strategies and tools include
  - Pretesting
  - Skills testing
  - Course evaluation
- Additional educational tools available include
  - AHA Guidelines
  - AHA exams
  - AHA Science Highlights

Application for Continuing Education/ Continuing Medical Education Credit for Courses

Some AHA classroom courses provide continuing education (CE) credit. Training Centers are encouraged to offer CE credit whenever possible for ECC courses.

In addition, some advanced-level online AHA courses do qualify for CE, continuing education units (CEU), or continuing medical education (CME) credit for doctors, nurses, and EMS professionals.

For	Go to
Continuing education opportunities	**OnlineAHA.org**
Additional professional education opportunities	**learn.heart.org**

The AHA is contracted to offer EMS students Continuing Education Hours (CEHs) through the Commission on Accreditation for Pre-Hospital Continuing Education (CAPCE) for several classroom-based provider courses. Note: CAPCE accreditation does not represent that the content conforms to any national, state, or local standard or best practice of any nature.

Due to contractual obligations in making CAPCE credit available to all EMS professionals, Training Centers are required to collect and submit information requested on the AHA Instructor Network for every EMS professional who completes the activity. The AHA does not require students to accept the CE offering. The AHA recognizes that not all students will need the credit nor will all of the licensing agencies accept the credit.

When a provider completes one of these courses, the Training Center will make the credits available to that provider.

If you would like to offer CE credit to other professionals who attend your classroom-based courses, you will need to work with your Training Center or employer to apply for credit through the appropriate authorizing body.

CE credit is not the same as and does not replace a course completion card. Visit the Instructor Network or contact the ECC Training Network Support Center for more information.

PALS Skills

Saving a patient in cardiac arrest requires both cognitive and psychomotor skills, as listed below:

- *Cognitive skills* include rhythm recognition; what medication to provide, including dose and timing; and algorithm application.
- *Psychomotor skills* include compressions, ventilations, basic and advanced airway management, IV/IO insertion, medication administration, and other skills.

Provider Renewal

Renewal Timeline

The current recommended timeline for renewal of the PALS course completion card is every 2 years. Although there is insufficient evidence to determine the optimal method and timing of retaking the PALS Course, research on skills retention and training show the following:

- There is growing evidence that BLS knowledge and skills decay rapidly after initial training.
- Studies have demonstrated the deterioration of BLS skills in as little as months after initial training.
- Studies examining the effect of brief, more-frequent training sessions demonstrated improvement in chest compression performance and shorter time to defibrillation.
- Studies also found that students reported improved confidence and willingness to perform CPR after additional or high-frequency training.

Given how fast BLS skills decay after training, and with the observed improvement in skill and confidence among students who train more frequently, students should be encouraged to periodically review their Provider Manual and practice CPR and AED skills whenever possible.

Part 4

Additional Resources

Science Update Information

 Science and education updates occur periodically. The AHA provides the following resources so that you can access these updates as they are released:

- The AHA Instructor Network, which includes the *ECC Beat* (**www.ahainstructornetwork.org**)
- The AHA website (**www.heart.org/cpr**)

For full details of all changes that were made to the resuscitation guidelines, the AHA strongly recommends that each instructor purchase his or her own copy of the *2015 AHA Guidelines Update for CPR and ECC* or access a copy online, available at **www.heart.org/eccguidelines**.

Instructor Training and Renewal

Recruiting and Mentoring Instructors

As a current AHA Instructor, you may have students in your course who want to become an AHA PALS Instructor. The AHA encourages you to take a moment to pass along the information below to all students who are interested in becoming an instructor after they successfully complete the provider course.

An AHA Instructor course teaches the methods needed to effectively instruct others in PALS Courses. The AHA requires that instructors be at least 16 years of age to attend a PALS instructor course.

Instructor Candidate Selection

The ideal instructor candidate

- Is motivated to teach
- Is motivated to facilitate learning
- Is motivated to ensure that students acquire the skills necessary for successful course completion
- Views student assessment as a way to improve individual knowledge and skills

Instructor Course Prerequisites

Prospective participants in an AHA Instructor course must

- Have current provider status in the discipline they wish to teach
- Have completed an Instructor Candidate Application (obtained from the Training Center Coordinator)

Maintaining Instructor Status

Your instructor status must be renewed by a Training Center Faculty or Regional Faculty. You can renew your status by meeting all of the following criteria or by successfully completing all requirements for a new instructor:

- Maintain current provider status. You can do this by maintaining a current provider card or by demonstrating exceptional provider skills to a Training Center Faculty or Regional Faculty and by successfully completing the provider exam.
- If you choose the demonstration route, successful completion must be documented on the Instructor/Training Center Faculty Renewal Checklist. A new provider card may be issued at the discretion of the Training Center or if you request one, but it is not required by the AHA.
- Earn 4 credits during each 2 years of your instructor recognition by doing any combination of the following:
  - Teach an instructor-led PALS Course (1 credit per course).
  - Each day of BLS skills practice and testing sessions counts as 1 credit.
  - Conduct the classroom portion for a blended-learning course. Each day of HeartCode PALS skills practice and testing sessions counts as 1 credit. All 4 credits can be earned this way.
- Attend updates as required within the previous 2 years. Updates may address new course content or methodology and review Training Center, regional, and national ECC information.
- Be monitored while teaching before your instructor status expires. The first monitoring after the initial instructor course does not satisfy this requirement.

Special Exceptions to Teaching Requirements

The requirement for instructors to teach a minimum of 4 courses in 2 years to renew instructor status may be waived or extended under special circumstances. These circumstances include, but are not limited to, the following:

- Call to active military duty (for an instructor who is in the military reserve or National Guard). Monitoring during duty may be waived if Military Training Network Faculty members are not available
- Illness or injury that has caused the instructor to take a leave from employment or teaching duties
- A limited number of courses offered in an area because of lack of audience or delay of course materials

The Training Center Coordinator, in consultation with the assigned Regional Faculty and Training Center Faculty, may decide to waive the teaching requirements for the discipline. Consideration should be given to the amount of time an instructor is away from normal employment, the length of delay in release of materials, and the number of courses taught in relation to the number of teaching opportunities.

Documentation supporting the decision must be maintained in the instructor's file.

All other requirements for renewal must be met as stated above.

Issuing an Instructor Card

Your instructor card is issued by your primary Training Center for that discipline. That may not be the same Training Center where you took your training or monitoring.

All instructor cards are issued for 2 years.

If you are a new instructor:

- You must be monitored teaching your first course within 6 months of completing the classroom portion of your training. A current Training Center Faculty for your discipline must monitor you while you are teaching a provider course, or an update or renewal course. It is your responsibility to schedule this monitoring, working with the Training Center Faculty who conducted your course or with the Training Center Coordinator of your Training Center.

- You will receive your instructor card from your primary Training Center once you have successfully completed all monitoring requirements. The expiration date will be 2 years from the month you completed all requirements, including monitoring.

- You must register on the Instructor Network with your primary Training Center so that you receive your instructor ID number. This number is placed on the back of your card, so you need it before your card can be issued. Any questions about receiving your instructor card should be directed to your Training Center Coordinator.

If you are an existing instructor:

- Your new instructor card will be issued by your primary Training Center when you have completed and documented all renewal requirements. It is your responsibility to see that all requirements are met. If you believe that you will not be able to meet a requirement, or you will not be able to teach the required number of classes, notify your Training Center Coordinator *before* your expiration date. There are times when exceptions can be made or extensions given. However, this is at the discretion of your Training Center Coordinator.

- You must register on the Instructor Network. It is a requirement that all instructor cards have the instructor ID number on the back and that all provider cards issued must have the ID number of the instructor listed.

Part 5

Appendixes

PALS Provider Course Item Locations

Item	Location
Precourse Materials	
Sample precourse letter to instructors	*PALS Instructor Manual,* Part 1; Instructor CD
Sample precourse letter to students	*PALS Instructor Manual,* Part 1; Instructor CD
Sample precourse letter to HeartCode students	*PALS Instructor Manual,* Part 1; Instructor CD
Sample course agendas	*PALS Instructor Manual,* Part 2; Instructor CD
Equipment list	*PALS Instructor Manual,* Part 1; Instructor CD
Manikin cleaning instructions	*PALS Instructor Manual,* Part 1
All Stations	
PALS Lesson Plans	*PALS Instructor Manual,* Part 6
PALS Course Progress Checklist	Instructor CD
PALS Update Lesson Plans	*PALS Instructor Manual,* Part 6
HeartCode PALS Lesson Plans	*PALS Instructor Manual,* Part 6
PALS Update Course Progress Checklist	Instructor CD
BLS Competency Testing	
Child CPR and AED Skills Testing Checklist; Skills Testing Critical Skills Descriptors	*PALS Instructor Manual,* Appendix A
Infant CPR Skills Testing Checklist; Skills Testing Critical Skills Descriptors	*PALS Instructor Manual,* Appendix A
Skills Stations	
Airway Management Skills Station Competency Checklist	*PALS Instructor Manual,* Appendix A; Instructor CD

(continued)

(continued)

Item	Location
Rhythm Disturbances/Electrical Therapy Skills Station Competency Checklist	*PALS Instructor Manual,* Appendix A; Instructor CD
Vascular Access Skills Station Competency Checklist	*PALS Instructor Manual,* Appendix A; Instructor CD
Case Discussions/Simulations	
Instructor case scenarios/debriefing tools for case scenarios	*PALS Instructor Manual,* Appendix B
Learning station competency checklists for case scenarios	*PALS Provider Manual,* Appendix; Instructor CD
Team Dynamics Debriefing Tool	*PALS Instructor Manual,* Appendix B; Instructor CD
Algorithms and Flowcharts	
PALS Systematic Approach Algorithm	*PALS Provider Manual,* Part 3; Instructor CD
PALS Systematic Approach Summary	Instructor CD
Pediatric Cardiac Arrest Algorithm	*PALS Provider Manual,* Part 4
Pediatric Bradycardia With a Pulse and Poor Perfusion Algorithm	*PALS Provider Manual,* Part 11
Pediatric Tachycardia With a Pulse and Adequate Perfusion Algorithm	*PALS Provider Manual,* Part 11
Pediatric Tachycardia With a Pulse and Poor Perfusion Algorithm	*PALS Provider Manual,* Part 11
Pediatric Septic Shock Algorithm	*PALS Provider Manual,* Part 9
Pediatric Recognition of Respiratory Problems Flowchart	*PALS Provider Manual,* Part 6; Instructor CD
Pediatric Management of Respiratory Emergencies Flowchart	*PALS Provider Manual,* Part 7; Instructor CD
Pediatric Recognition of Shock Flowchart	*PALS Instructor Manual,* Part 8; Instructor CD
Pediatric Management of Shock Flowchart	*PALS Instructor Manual,* Part 9; Instructor CD
Evaluations	
PALS case scenario testing checklists	*PALS Instructor Manual,* Appendix A; Instructor CD
Course evaluation	Instructor Network

Appendix **A**

Skills Testing Checklists, Skills Station Competency Checklists, and PALS Case Scenario Testing Checklists

Pediatric Advanced Life Support
Child CPR and AED
Skills Testing Checklist

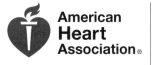 **American Heart Association®**
life is why™

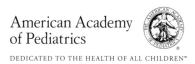 American Academy of Pediatrics
DEDICATED TO THE HEALTH OF ALL CHILDREN™

Student Name _____   Date of Test _____

Hospital Scenario: "You are working in a hospital or clinic, and you see a child who has suddenly collapsed in the hallway. You check that the scene is safe and then approach the patient. Demonstrate what you would do next."

Prehospital Scenario: "You arrive on the scene for a child who is not breathing. No bystander CPR has been provided. You approach the scene and ensure that it is safe. Demonstrate what you would do next."

Assessment and Activation
- ☐ Checks responsiveness
- ☐ Checks breathing
- ☐ Shouts for help/Activates emergency response system/Sends for AED
- ☐ Checks pulse

Once student shouts for help, instructor says, "Here's the barrier device. I am going to get the AED."

Cycle 1 of CPR (30:2)   *CPR feedback devices preferred for accuracy*

Child Compressions
- ☐ Performs high-quality compressions*:
  - Hand placement on lower half of sternum
  - 30 compressions in no less than 15 and no more than 18 seconds
  - Compresses at least one third the depth of the chest, about 2 inches (5 cm)
  - Complete recoil after each compression

Child Breaths
- ☐ Gives 2 breaths with a barrier device:
  - Each breath given over 1 second
  - Visible chest rise with each breath
  - Resumes compressions in less than 10 seconds

Cycle 2 of CPR (repeats steps in Cycle 1)   *Only check box if step is successfully performed*
- ☐ Compressions
- ☐ Breaths
- ☐ Resumes compressions in less than 10 seconds

Rescuer 2 says, "Here is the AED. I'll take over compressions, and you use the AED."

AED (follows prompts of AED)
- ☐ Powers on AED
- ☐ Correctly attaches pads
- ☐ Clears for analysis
- ☐ Clears to safely deliver a shock
- ☐ Safely delivers a shock

Resumes Compressions
- ☐ Ensures compressions are resumed immediately after shock delivery
  - Student directs instructor to resume compressions *or*
  - Student resumes compressions

STOP TEST

Instructor Notes
- Place a ✓ in the box next to each step the student completes successfully.
- If the student does not complete all steps successfully (as indicated by at least 1 blank check box), the student must receive remediation. Make a note here of which skills require remediation (refer to Instructor Manual for information about remediation).

Test Results	Circle **PASS** or **NR** to indicate pass or needs remediation:	**PASS**	**NR**

Instructor Initials _____   Instructor Number _____   Date _____

Child CPR and AED
Skills Testing Critical Skills Descriptors

1. **Assesses victim and activates emergency response system (this *must* precede starting compressions) within a maximum of 30 seconds. After determining that the scene is safe:**
   - Checks for responsiveness by tapping and shouting
   - Shouts for help/directs someone to call for help *and* get AED/defibrillator
   - Checks for no breathing or no normal breathing (only gasping)
     - Scans from the head to the chest for a minimum of 5 seconds and no more than 10 seconds
   - Checks carotid pulse
     - Can be done simultaneously with check for breathing
     - Checks for a minimum of 5 seconds and no more than 10 seconds

2. **Performs high-quality chest compressions (initiates compressions immediately after recognition of cardiac arrest)**
   - Correct hand placement
     - Lower half of sternum
     - 2-handed (second hand on top of the first or grasping the wrist of the first hand or 1-handed)
   - Compression rate of 100 to 120/min
     - Delivers 30 compressions in 15 to 18 seconds
   - Compression depth and recoil—compresses at least one third the depth of chest, about 2 inches (5 cm)
     - Use of a commercial feedback device or high-fidelity manikin is highly recommended
     - Complete chest recoil after each compression
   - Minimizes interruptions in compressions
     - Delivers 2 breaths so less than 10 seconds elapses between last compression of one cycle and first compression of next cycle
     - Compressions resumed immediately after shock/no shock indicated

3. **Provides 2 breaths by using a barrier device**
   - Opens airway adequately
     - Uses a head tilt–chin lift maneuver or jaw thrust
   - Delivers each breath over 1 second
   - Delivers breaths that produce visible chest rise
   - Avoids excessive ventilation
   - Resumes chest compressions in less than 10 seconds

4. **Performs same steps for compressions and breaths for Cycle 2**

5. **AED use**
   - Powers on AED
     - Turns AED on by pushing button or lifting lid as soon as it arrives
   - Correctly attaches pads
     - Places proper-sized pads for victim's age in correct location
   - Clears for analysis
     - Clears rescuers from victim for AED to analyze rhythm (pushes analyze button if required by device)
     - Communicates clearly to all other rescuers to stop touching victim
   - Clears to safely deliver shock
     - Communicates clearly to all other rescuers to stop touching victim
   - Delivers a shock
     - Resumes chest compressions immediately after shock delivery
     - Does *not* turn off AED during CPR

6. **Resumes compressions**
   - Ensures that high-quality chest compressions are resumed immediately after shock delivery
   - Performs same steps for compressions

Pediatric Advanced Life Support
Infant CPR
Skills Testing Checklist (1 of 2)

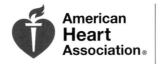

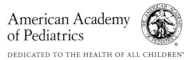

Student Name _____   Date of Test _____

Hospital Scenario: "You are working in a hospital or clinic when a woman runs through the door, carrying an infant. She shouts, 'Help me! My baby's not breathing.' You have gloves and a pocket mask. You send your coworker to activate the emergency response system and to get the emergency equipment."

Prehospital Scenario: "You arrive on the scene for an infant who is not breathing. No bystander CPR has been provided. You approach the scene and ensure that it is safe. Demonstrate what you would do next."

Assessment and Activation

☐ Checks responsiveness   ☐ Shouts for help/Activates emergency response system   ☐ Checks breathing
☐ Checks pulse

Once student shouts for help, instructor says, "Here's the barrier device."

Cycle 1 of CPR (30:2)   *CPR feedback devices preferred for accuracy*

Infant Compressions

☐ Performs high-quality compressions*:
- Placement of 2 fingers in the center of the chest, just below the nipple line
- 30 compressions in no less than 15 and no more than 18 seconds
- Compresses at least one third the depth of the chest, about 1½ inches (4 cm)
- Complete recoil after each compression

Infant Breaths

☐ Gives 2 breaths with a barrier device:
- Each breath given over 1 second
- Visible chest rise with each breath
- Resumes compressions in less than 10 seconds

Cycle 2 of CPR (repeats steps in Cycle 1)   *Only check box if step is successfully performed*

☐ Compressions   ☐ Breaths   ☐ Resumes compressions in less than 10 seconds

Rescuer 2 arrives with bag-mask device and begins ventilation while Rescuer 1 continues compressions with 2 thumb–encircling hands technique.

Cycle 3 of CPR

Rescuer 1: Infant Compressions

☐ Performs high–quality compressions*:
- 15 compressions with 2 thumb–encircling hands technique
- 15 compressions in no less than 7 and no more than 9 seconds
- Compress at least one third the depth of the chest, about 1½ inches (4 cm)
- Complete recoil after each compression

Rescuer 2: Infant Breaths

This rescuer is not evaluated.

(continued)

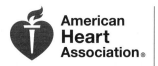

American Academy
of Pediatrics
DEDICATED TO THE HEALTH OF ALL CHILDREN™

Student Name _____   Date of Test _____

Cycle 4 of CPR

Rescuer 2: Infant Compressions

This rescuer is not evaluated.

Rescuer 1: Infant Breaths

☐ Gives 2 breaths with a bag-mask device:
- Each breath given over 1 second
- Visible chest rise with each breath
- Resumes compressions in less than 10 seconds

STOP TEST

Instructor Notes
- Place a ✓ in the box next to each step the student completes successfully.
- If the student does not complete all steps successfully (as indicated by at least 1 blank check box), the student must receive remediation. Make a note here of which skills require remediation (refer to Instructor Manual for information about remediation).

Test Results	Circle **PASS** or **NR** to indicate pass or needs remediation:	**PASS**	**NR**

Instructor Initials _____   Instructor Number _____   Date _____

Infant CPR
Skills Testing Critical Skills Descriptors

1. **Assesses victim and activates emergency response system (this *must* precede starting compressions) within a maximum of 30 seconds. After determining that the scene is safe:**
   - Checks for responsiveness by tapping and shouting
   - Shouts for help/directs someone to call for help *and* get emergency equipment
   - Checks for no breathing or no normal breathing (only gasping)
     - Scans from the head to the chest for a minimum of 5 seconds and no more than 10 seconds
   - Checks brachial pulse
     - Can be done simultaneously with check for breathing
     - Checks for a minimum of 5 seconds and no more than 10 seconds

2. **Performs high-quality chest compressions during 1-rescuer CPR (initiates compressions within 10 seconds of identifying cardiac arrest)**
   - Correct placement of hands/fingers in center of chest
     - 1 rescuer: 2 fingers just below the nipple line
   - Compression rate of 100 to 120/min
     - Delivers 30 compressions in 15 to 18 seconds
   - Adequate depth for age
     - Infant: at least one third the depth of the chest (about 1½ inches [4 cm])
     - Use of a commercial feedback device or high-fidelity manikin is highly recommended
   - Complete chest recoil after each compression
   - Appropriate ratio for age and number of rescuers
     - 1 rescuer: 30 compressions to 2 breaths
   - Minimizes interruptions in compressions
     - Delivers 2 breaths so less than 10 seconds elapses between last compression of one cycle and first compression of next cycle

3. **Provides effective breaths with bag-mask device during 2-rescuer CPR**
   - Opens airway adequately
   - Delivers each breath over 1 second
   - Delivers breaths that produce visible chest rise
   - Avoids excessive ventilation
   - Resumes chest compressions in less than 10 seconds

4. **Switches compression technique at appropriate interval as prompted by the instructor (for purposes of this evaluation). Switch should take no more than 5 seconds.**

5. **Performs high-quality chest compressions during 2-rescuer CPR**
   - Correct placement of hands/fingers in center of chest
     - 2 rescuers: 2 thumb–encircling hands just below the nipple line
   - Compression rate of 100 to 120/min
     - Delivers 15 compressions in 7 to 9 seconds
   - Adequate depth for age
     - Infant: at least one third the depth of the chest (about 1½ inches [4 cm])
   - Complete chest recoil after each compression
   - Appropriate ratio for age and number of rescuers
     - 2 rescuers: 15 compressions to 2 breaths
   - Minimizes interruptions in compressions
   - Delivers 2 breaths so less than 10 seconds elapses between last compression of one cycle and first compression of next cycle

Airway Management Skills Station Competency Checklist

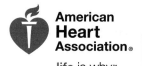 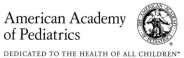

Student Name _____ Date of Test _____

Critical Performance Steps	✓ if done correctly
Verbalizes difference between high-flow and low-flow O₂ delivery systems • High flow: O_2 flow exceeds patient inspiratory flow, preventing entrainment of room air if system is tight-fitting; delivers nearly 1.00 FIO_2, eg, nonrebreathing mask with reservoir, high-flow nasal cannula • Low flow (≤10 L/min): patient inspiratory flow exceeds O_2 flow, allowing entrainment of room air; delivers 0.23 to 0.80 FIO_2, eg, standard nasal cannula, simple O_2 mask	
Verbalizes maximum nasal cannula flow rate for standard nasal cannula (4 L/min)	
Opens airway by using head tilt–chin lift maneuver while keeping mouth open (jaw thrust for trauma victim)	
Verbalizes different indications for OPA and NPA • OPA only for unconscious victim without a gag reflex • NPA for conscious or semiconscious victim	
Selects correctly sized airway by measuring • OPA from corner of mouth to angle of mandible	
Inserts OPA correctly	
Verbalizes assessment for adequate breathing after insertion of OPA	
Suctions with OPA in place; states suctioning not to exceed 10 seconds	
Selects correct mask size for ventilation	
Assembles bag-mask device, opens airway, and creates seal by using E-C clamp technique	
With bag-mask device, gives 1 breath every 3 to 5 seconds for about 30 seconds. Gives each breath in approximately 1 second; each breath should cause chest rise	
Endotracheal Intubation • States equipment needed for endotracheal (ET) tube intubation procedure • Demonstrates technique to confirm proper ET tube placement by physical exam and by using an exhaled CO_2 device • Secures ET tube • Suctions with ET tube in place	
The following steps are optional. They are demonstrated and evaluated only when the student's scope of practice involves ET intubation.	
Endotracheal Intubation • Prepares equipment for ET intubation • Inserts ET tube correctly	

STOP TEST

Instructor Notes
- Place a ✓ in the box next to each step the student completes successfully.
- If the student does not complete all steps successfully (as indicated by at least 1 blank check box), the student must receive remediation. Make a note here of which skills require remediation (refer to Instructor Manual for information about remediation).

Test Results	Circle **PASS** or **NR** to indicate pass or needs remediation:	**PASS**	**NR**

Instructor Initials _____ Instructor Number _____ Date _____

© 2016 American Heart Association

106

Rhythm Disturbances/ Electrical Therapy Skills Station Competency Checklist

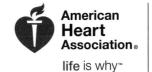

American **Heart** Association®

life is why™

American Academy of Pediatrics

DEDICATED TO THE HEALTH OF ALL CHILDREN™

Student Name _____ Date of Test _____

Critical Performance Steps	✓ if done correctly
Applies 3 ECG leads correctly (or local equipment if >3 leads are used) • Negative (white) lead: to right shoulder • Positive (red) lead: to left lower ribs • Ground (black, green, brown) lead: to left shoulder	
Demonstrates correct operation of monitor • Turns monitor on • Adjusts device to manual mode (not AED mode) to display rhythm in standard limb leads (I, II, III) or paddles/electrode pads	
Verbalizes correct electrical therapy for appropriate core rhythms • Synchronized cardioversion for unstable SVT, VT with pulses • Defibrillation for pulseless VT, VF	
Selects correct paddle/electrode pad for infant or child; places paddles/electrode pads in correct position	
Demonstrates correct and safe synchronized cardioversion • Places device in synchronized mode • Selects appropriate energy (0.5 to 1 J/kg for initial shock) • Charges, clears, delivers current	
Demonstrates correct and safe manual defibrillation • Places device in unsynchronized mode • Selects energy (2 to 4 J/kg for initial shock) • Charges, clears, delivers current	

STOP TEST

Instructor Notes
- Place a ✓ in the box next to each step the student completes successfully.
- If the student does not complete all steps successfully (as indicated by at least 1 blank check box), the student must receive remediation. Make a note here of which skills require remediation (refer to Instructor Manual for information about remediation).

Test Results Circle **PASS** or **NR** to indicate pass or needs remediation:	**PASS**　　　**NR**

Instructor Initials _____ Instructor Number _____ Date _____

Vascular Access
Skills Station
Competency Checklist

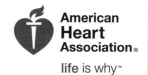 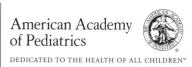

Student Name _____ Date of Test _____

Critical Performance Steps	✓ if done correctly
Verbalizes indications for IO insertion	
Verbalizes sites for IO insertion (anterior tibia, distal femur, medial malleolus, anterior-superior iliac spine)	
Verbalizes contraindications for IO placement • Fracture in extremity • Previous insertion attempt in the same bone • Infection overlying bone	
Inserts IO catheter safely	
Verbalizes how to confirm IO catheter is in correct position; verbalizes how to secure IO catheter	
Attaches IV line to IO catheter; demonstrates giving IO fluid bolus by using 3-way stopcock and syringe	
Shows how to determine correct drug doses by using a color-coded length-based tape or other resource	
The following is optional:	
Verbalizes correct procedure for establishing IV access	

STOP TEST

Instructor Notes
- Place a ✓ in the box next to each step the student completes successfully.
- If the student does not complete all steps successfully (as indicated by at least 1 blank check box), the student must receive remediation. Make a note here of which skills require remediation (refer to Instructor Manual for information about remediation).

Test Results	Circle **PASS** or **NR** to indicate pass or needs remediation:	**PASS**	**NR**

Instructor Initials _____ Instructor Number _____ Date _____

PALS Case Scenario
Testing Checklist
Respiratory Case Scenario
Upper Airway Obstruction

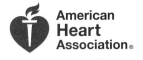 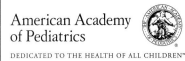

Student Name _____   Date of Test _____

Critical Performance Steps	✓ if done correctly
Team Leader	
Assigns team member roles	
Uses effective communication throughout	
Patient Management	
Directs assessment of airway, breathing, circulation, disability, and exposure, including vital signs	
Directs administration of 100% oxygen or supplementary oxygen as needed to support oxygenation	
Directs application of cardiac monitor and pulse oximetry	
Identifies signs and symptoms of upper airway obstruction	
Categorizes as respiratory distress or failure	
Directs administration of nebulized epinephrine and corticosteroid (for croup), or IM epinephrine and IV corticosteroid (for anaphylaxis)	
States indications for bag-mask ventilation and/or other airway or ventilation support	
If the student does not verbalize the above, prompt the student with the following question: "What are the indications for bag-mask ventilation and/or other airway or ventilation support?"	
Directs establishment of IV or IO access, if indicated	
Directs reassessment of patient in response to treatment	
Case Conclusion/Debriefing	
The following step is evaluated only if the student's scope of practice applies	
Describes how to estimate correct endotracheal tube size for this patient	
If the student does not verbalize the above, prompt the student with the following question: "How would you estimate the endotracheal tube size for this infant with upper airway obstruction?"	

STOP TEST

Instructor Notes
- Place a ✓ in the box next to each step the student completes successfully.
- If the student does not complete all steps successfully (as indicated by at least 1 blank check box), the student must receive remediation. Make a note here of which skills require remediation (refer to Instructor Manual for information about remediation).

Test Results Circle **PASS** or **NR** to indicate pass or needs remediation:	**PASS**　　**NR**

Instructor Initials _____   Instructor Number _____   Date _____

PALS Case Scenario
Testing Checklist
Respiratory Case Scenario
Lower Airway Obstruction

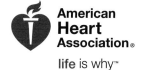

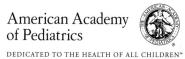

DEDICATED TO THE HEALTH OF ALL CHILDREN™

Student Name _____ Date of Test _____

Critical Performance Steps	✓ if done correctly
Team Leader	
Assigns team member roles	
Uses effective communication throughout	
Patient Management	
Directs assessment of airway, breathing, circulation, disability, and exposure, including vital signs	
Directs administration of 100% oxygen or supplementary oxygen as needed to support oxygenation	
Directs application of cardiac monitor and pulse oximetry	
Identifies signs and symptoms of lower airway obstruction	
Categorizes as respiratory distress or failure	
Directs administration of albuterol and corticosteroids (for asthma) or suctioning or possible additional laboratory studies (for bronchiolitis)	
States indications for bag-mask ventilation and/or other airway or ventilation support	
If the student does not verbalize the above, prompt the student with the following question: *"What are the indications for bag-mask ventilation and/or other airway or ventilation support?"*	
Directs establishment of IV or IO access, if appropriate	
Directs reassessment of patient in response to treatment	
Case Conclusion/Debriefing	
The following step is evaluated only if the student's scope of practice applies	
States indications for endotracheal intubation	
If the student does not verbalize the above, prompt the student with the following question: *"What are the indications for endotracheal intubation?"*	

STOP TEST

Instructor Notes
- Place a ✓ in the box next to each step the student completes successfully.
- If the student does not complete all steps successfully (as indicated by at least 1 blank check box), the student must receive remediation. Make a note here of which skills require remediation (refer to Instructor Manual for information about remediation).

Test Results Circle **PASS** or **NR** to indicate pass or needs remediation:	**PASS** NR

Instructor Initials _____ Instructor Number _____ Date _____

PALS Case Scenario
Testing Checklist
Respiratory Case Scenario
Lung Tissue Disease

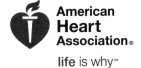 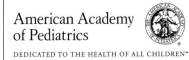

Student Name _____   Date of Test _____

Critical Performance Steps	✓ if done correctly
Team Leader	
Assigns team member roles	
Uses effective communication throughout	
Patient Management	
Directs assessment of airway, breathing, circulation, disability, and exposure, including vital signs	
Directs administration of 100% oxygen (or supplementary oxygen as needed to support oxygenation) and evaluates response	
Identifies indications for bag-mask ventilation and/or additional airway or ventilation support	
Describes methods to verify that bag-mask ventilation is effective	
Directs application of cardiac monitor and pulse oximetry	
Identifies signs and symptoms of lung tissue disease	
Categorizes as respiratory distress or failure	
Directs establishment of IV or IO access	
Directs reassessment of patient in response to treatment	
Identifies need for involvement of advanced provider with expertise in pediatric intubation and mechanical ventilation	
Case Conclusion/Debriefing	
The following step is evaluated only if the student's scope of practice applies	
States indications for endotracheal intubation	
If the student does not verbalize the above, prompt the student with the following question: "What are the indications for endotracheal intubation?"	

STOP TEST

Instructor Notes
- Place a ✓ in the box next to each step the student completes successfully.
- If the student does not complete all steps successfully (as indicated by at least 1 blank check box), the student must receive remediation. Make a note here of which skills require remediation (refer to Instructor Manual for information about remediation).

Test Results Circle **PASS** or **NR** to indicate pass or needs remediation:	**PASS** **NR**

Instructor Initials _____ Instructor Number _____ Date _____

PALS Case Scenario
Testing Checklist
Respiratory Case Scenario
Disordered Control of Breathing

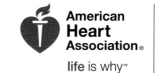 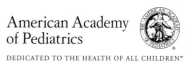

Student Name _____ Date of Test _____

Critical Performance Steps	✓ if done correctly
Team Leader	
Assigns team member roles	
Uses effective communication throughout	
Patient Management	
Directs assessment of airway, breathing, circulation, disability, and exposure, including vital signs	
Directs administration of 100% oxygen (or supplementary oxygen as needed to support oxygenation) and evaluates response	
Identifies indications for bag-mask ventilation and/or additional airway or ventilation support	
Describes methods to verify that bag-mask ventilation is effective	
Directs application of cardiac monitor and pulse oximetry	
Identifies signs of disordered control of breathing	
Categorizes as respiratory distress or failure	
Directs establishment of IV or IO access	
Directs reassessment of patient in response to treatment	
Identifies need for involvement of advanced provider with expertise in pediatric intubation and mechanical ventilation	
Case Conclusion/Debriefing	
The following step is evaluated only if the student's scope of practice applies	
States indications for endotracheal intubation	
If the student does not verbalize the above, prompt the student with the following question: *"What are the indications for endotracheal intubation?"*	

STOP TEST

Instructor Notes
- Place a ✓ in the box next to each step the student completes successfully.
- If the student does not complete all steps successfully (as indicated by at least 1 blank check box), the student must receive remediation. Make a note here of which skills require remediation (refer to Instructor Manual for information about remediation).

Test Results	Circle **PASS** or **NR** to indicate pass or needs remediation:	**PASS**	**NR**

Instructor Initials _____ Instructor Number _____ Date _____

PALS Case Scenario
Testing Checklist
Shock Case Scenario
Hypovolemic Shock

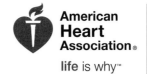 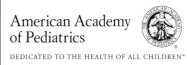

Student Name _____ Date of Test _____

Critical Performance Steps	✓ if done correctly
Team Leader	
Assigns team member roles	
Uses effective communication throughout	
Patient Management	
Directs assessment of airway, breathing, circulation, disability, and exposure, including vital signs	
Directs administration of 100% oxygen	
Directs application of cardiac monitor and pulse oximetry	
Identifies signs and symptoms of hypovolemic shock	
Categorizes as compensated or hypotensive shock	
Directs establishment of IV or IO access	
Directs rapid administration of a 20 mL/kg fluid bolus of isotonic crystalloid; repeats as needed to treat signs of shock	
Reassesses patient during and after each fluid bolus. Stops fluid bolus if signs of heart failure (worsening respiratory distress, development of hepatomegaly or rales/crackles) develop	
Directs reassessment of patient in response to each treatment	
Case Conclusion/Debriefing	
States therapeutic end points during shock management	
If the student does not verbalize the above, prompt the student with the following question: *"What are the therapeutic end points during shock management?"*	

STOP TEST

Instructor Notes
- Place a ✓ in the box next to each step the student completes successfully.
- If the student does not complete all steps successfully (as indicated by at least 1 blank check box), the student must receive remediation. Make a note here of which skills require remediation (refer to Instructor Manual for information about remediation).

Test Results	Circle **PASS** or **NR** to indicate pass or needs remediation:	**PASS**	**NR**

Instructor Initials _____ Instructor Number _____ Date _____

PALS Case Scenario
Testing Checklist
Shock Case Scenario
Obstructive Shock

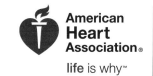 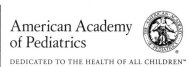

Student Name _____ Date of Test _____

Critical Performance Steps	✓ if done correctly
Team Leader	
Assigns team member roles	
Uses effective communication throughout	
Patient Management	
Directs assessment of airway, breathing, circulation, disability, and exposure, including vital signs	
Directs application of cardiac monitor and pulse oximetry	
Verbalizes DOPE mnemonic for intubated patient who deteriorates	
If the student does not verbalize the above, prompt the student with the following questions: "What mnemonic is helpful to recall when the intubated patient deteriorates? What does this mnemonic mean?"	
Identifies signs and symptoms of obstructive shock	
States at least 2 causes of obstructive shock	
If the student does not state the above, prompt the student with the following statement: "Tell me at least 2 causes of obstructive shock."	
Categorizes as compensated or hypotensive shock	
Directs establishment of IV or IO access, if needed	
Directs rapid administration of a fluid bolus of isotonic crystalloid, if needed (ie, for cardiac tamponade, massive pulmonary embolus)	
Directs appropriate treatment for obstructive shock (needle decompression for tension pneumothorax; fluid bolus, and pericardiocentesis for cardiac tamponade; oxygen, ventilatory support, fluid bolus, and expert consultation for massive pulmonary embolus; prostaglandin infusion and expert consultation for neonate with ductal-dependent congenital heart disease and constriction/closure of the ductus arteriosus)	
Directs reassessment of patient in response to treatment	
Case Conclusion/Debriefing	
States therapeutic end points during shock management	
If the student does not verbalize the above, prompt the student with the following question: "What are the therapeutic end points during shock management?"	

STOP TEST

Instructor Notes
- Place a ✓ in the box next to each step the student completes successfully.
- If the student does not complete all steps successfully (as indicated by at least 1 blank check box), the student must receive remediation. Make a note here of which skills require remediation (refer to Instructor Manual for information about remediation).

Test Results	Circle **PASS** or **NR** to indicate pass or needs remediation:	**PASS**	**NR**

Instructor Initials _____ Instructor Number _____ Date _____

PALS Case Scenario
Testing Checklist
Shock Case Scenario
Distributive Shock

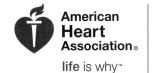 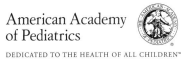

Student Name _____   Date of Test _____

Critical Performance Steps	✓ if done correctly
Team Leader	
Assigns team member roles	
Uses effective communication throughout	
Patient Management	
Directs assessment of airway, breathing, circulation, disability, and exposure, including vital signs	
Directs administration of 100% oxygen	
Directs application of cardiac monitor and pulse oximetry	
Identifies signs and symptoms of distributive (septic) shock	
Categorizes as compensated or hypotensive shock	
Directs establishment of IV or IO access	
Directs rapid administration of a 20 mL/kg fluid bolus of isotonic crystalloid; repeats as needed (with careful reassessment) to treat shock	
Reassesses patient during and after each fluid bolus. Stops fluid bolus if signs of heart failure (worsening respiratory distress, development of hepatomegaly or rales/crackles) develop	
Directs initiation of vasoactive drug therapy within first hour of care for fluid-refractory shock	
Directs reassessment of patient in response to treatment	
Directs early administration of antibiotics (within first hour after shock is identified)	
Case Conclusion/Debriefing	
States therapeutic end points during shock management	
If the student does not verbalize the above, prompt the student with the following question: *"What are the therapeutic end points during shock management?"*	

STOP TEST

Instructor Notes
- Place a ✓ in the box next to each step the student completes successfully.
- If the student does not complete all steps successfully (as indicated by at least 1 blank check box), the student must receive remediation. Make a note here of which skills require remediation (refer to Instructor Manual for information about remediation).

Test Results Circle **PASS** or **NR** to indicate pass or needs remediation:	**PASS** **NR**
Instructor Initials _____ Instructor Number _____ Date _____	

PALS Case Scenario Testing Checklist
Shock Case Scenario
Cardiogenic Shock

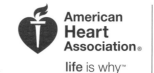 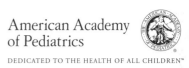

Student Name _____ Date of Test _____

Critical Performance Steps	✓ if done correctly
Team Leader	
Assigns team member roles	
Uses effective communication throughout	
Patient Management	
Directs assessment of airway, breathing, circulation, disability, and exposure, including vital signs	
Directs administration of 100% oxygen	
Directs application of cardiac monitor and pulse oximetry	
Identifies signs and symptoms of cardiogenic shock	
Categorizes as compensated or hypotensive shock	
Directs establishment of IV or IO access	
Directs slow administration of a 5 to 10 mL/kg fluid bolus of isotonic crystalloid over 10 to 20 minutes and reassesses patient during and after fluid bolus. Stops fluid bolus if signs of heart failure worsen	
Directs reassessment of patient in response to treatment	
Recognizes the need to obtain expert consultation from pediatric cardiologist	
Identifies need for inotropic/vasoactive drugs during treatment of cardiogenic shock	
If the student does not indicate the above, prompt the student with the following question: "What are the indications for inotropic/vasoactive drugs during cardiogenic shock?"	
Case Conclusion/Debriefing	
States therapeutic end points during shock management	
If the student does not verbalize the above, prompt the student with the following question: "What are the therapeutic end points during shock management?"	

STOP TEST

Instructor Notes
- Place a ✓ in the box next to each step the student completes successfully.
- If the student does not complete all steps successfully (as indicated by at least 1 blank check box), the student must receive remediation. Make a note here of which skills require remediation (refer to Instructor Manual for information about remediation).

Test Results	Circle **PASS** or **NR** to indicate pass or needs remediation:	**PASS**	**NR**

Instructor Initials _____ Instructor Number _____ Date _____

PALS Case Scenario Testing Checklist
Cardiac Case Scenario
Supraventricular Tachycardia

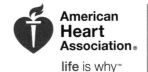 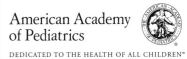

Student Name _____ Date of Test _____

Critical Performance Steps	✓ if done correctly
Team Leader	
Assigns team member roles	
Uses effective communication throughout	
Patient Management	
Directs assessment of airway, breathing, circulation, disability, and exposure, including vital signs	
Directs application of cardiac monitor and pulse oximetry	
Directs administration of supplementary oxygen	
Identifies narrow-complex tachycardia (ie, SVT with adequate perfusion) and verbalizes how to distinguish between ST and SVT	
If the student does not verbalize the above, prompt the student with the following question: "How do you distinguish between ST and SVT?"	
Directs performance of appropriate vagal maneuvers	
Directs establishment of IV or IO access	
Directs preparation and administration of appropriate doses (first and, if needed, second) of adenosine	
States the rationale for the strong recommendation for expert consultation before providing synchronized cardioversion if the stable child with SVT fails to respond to vagal maneuvers and adenosine	
Directs or describes appropriate indications for and safe delivery of attempted cardioversion at 0.5 to 1 J/kg (subsequent doses increased by 0.5 to 1 J/kg, not to exceed 2 J/kg)	
Performs reassessment of patient in response to treatment	
Case Conclusion/Debriefing	
Discusses indications and appropriate energy doses for synchronized cardioversion	
If the student does not verbalize the above, prompt the student with the following question: "What are the indications and appropriate energy doses for synchronized cardioversion?"	

STOP TEST

Instructor Notes
- Place a ✓ in the box next to each step the student completes successfully.
- If the student does not complete all steps successfully (as indicated by at least 1 blank check box), the student must receive remediation. Make a note here of which skills require remediation (refer to Instructor Manual for information about remediation).

Test Results Circle **PASS** or **NR** to indicate pass or needs remediation:	**PASS** NR

Instructor Initials _____ Instructor Number _____ Date _____

PALS Case Scenario
Testing Checklist
Cardiac Case Scenario
Bradycardia

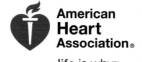 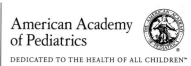

Student Name _____ Date of Test _____

Critical Performance Steps	✓ if done correctly
Team Leader	
Assigns team member roles	
Uses effective communication throughout	
Patient Management	
Directs assessment of airway, breathing, circulation, disability, and exposure, including vital signs	
Identifies bradycardia associated with cardiopulmonary compromise/failure	
Directs initiation of bag-mask ventilation with 100% oxygen	
Directs application of cardiac monitor and pulse oximetry	
Reassesses heart rate and systemic perfusion after initiation of bag-mask ventilation	
Recognizes indications for high-quality CPR (chest compressions plus ventilation) in a bradycardic patient	
If the student does not indicate the above, prompt the student with the following question: *"What are the indications for high-quality CPR in a bradycardic patient?"*	
Directs establishment of IV or IO access	
Directs or discusses preparation for and appropriate administration and dose (0.01 mg/kg) of epinephrine	
Performs reassessment of patient in response to treatment	
Case Conclusion/Debriefing	
Verbalizes consideration of 3 potential causes of bradycardia in infants and children	
If the student does not verbalize the above, prompt the student with the following statement: *"Tell me 3 potential causes of bradycardia in infants and children."*	

STOP TEST

Instructor Notes
- Place a ✓ in the box next to each step the student completes successfully.
- If the student does not complete all steps successfully (as indicated by at least 1 blank check box), the student must receive remediation. Make a note here of which skills require remediation (refer to Instructor Manual for information about remediation).

Test Results	Circle **PASS** or **NR** to indicate pass or needs remediation:	**PASS**	**NR**

Instructor Initials _____ Instructor Number _____ Date _____

PALS Case Scenario
Testing Checklist
Cardiac Case Scenario
Asystole/PEA

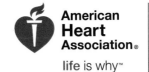 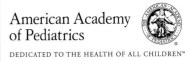

Student Name _____ Date of Test _____

Critical Performance Steps	✓ if done correctly
Team Leader	
Assigns team member roles	
Uses effective communication throughout	
Patient Management	
Identifies cardiac arrest	
Directs immediate initiation of high-quality CPR, and ensures performance of high-quality CPR at all times	
Directs placement of pads/leads and activation of monitor/defibrillator	
Identifies asystole or PEA	
Directs establishment of IO or IV access	
Directs preparation and administration of appropriate dose of epinephrine at appropriate intervals	
Directs checking rhythm approximately every 2 minutes while minimizing interruptions in chest compressions	
Case Conclusion/Debriefing	
Verbalizes at least 3 reversible causes of PEA or asystole	
If the student does not verbalize the above, prompt the student with the following statement: *"Tell me at least 3 reversible causes of PEA or asystole."*	

STOP TEST

Instructor Notes
- Place a ✓ in the box next to each step the student completes successfully.
- If the student does not complete all steps successfully (as indicated by at least 1 blank check box), the student must receive remediation. Make a note here of which skills require remediation (refer to Instructor Manual for information about remediation).

Test Results Circle **PASS** or **NR** to indicate pass or needs remediation:	**PASS** **NR**

Instructor Initials _____ Instructor Number _____ Date _____

PALS Case Scenario
Testing Checklist
Cardiac Case Scenario
VF/Pulseless VT

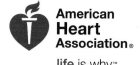 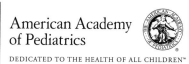

Student Name _____ Date of Test _____

Critical Performance Steps	✓ if done correctly
Team Leader	
Assigns team member roles	
Uses effective communication throughout	
Patient Management	
Identifies cardiac arrest	
Directs immediate initiation of high-quality CPR, and ensures performance of high-quality CPR at all times	
Directs placement of pads/leads and activation of monitor/defibrillator	
Identifies VF or pulseless VT cardiopulmonary arrest	
Directs safe performance of attempted defibrillation at 2 J/kg	
After delivery of every shock, directs immediate resumption of CPR, beginning with chest compressions	
Directs establishment of IO or IV access	
Directs preparation and administration of appropriate dose of epinephrine at appropriate intervals	
Directs safe delivery of second shock at 4 J/kg (subsequent doses 4 to 10 J/kg, not to exceed 10 J/kg or standard adult dose for that defibrillator)	
Directs preparation and administration of appropriate dose of antiarrhythmic (amiodarone or lidocaine) at appropriate time	
Case Conclusion/Debriefing	
Verbalizes possible need for additional doses of epinephrine and antiarrhythmic (amiodarone or lidocaine), and consideration of reversible causes of arrest (H's and T's)	

If the student does not verbalize the above, prompt the student with the following question:
"If VF persists despite the therapies provided, what else should you administer or consider?"

STOP TEST

Instructor Notes
- Place a ✓ in the box next to each step the student completes successfully.
- If the student does not complete all steps successfully (as indicated by at least 1 blank check box), the student must receive remediation. Make a note here of which skills require remediation (refer to Instructor Manual for information about remediation).

Test Results   Circle **PASS** or **NR** to indicate pass or needs remediation: **PASS**   **NR**

Instructor Initials _____   Instructor Number _____   Date _____

© 2016 American Heart Association

120

Appendix B

Instructor Case Scenarios and Debriefing Tools

Hypovolemic Shock
(Child; Uncompensated Shock)

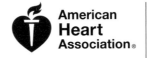
American Heart Association. life is why™

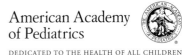
American Academy of Pediatrics
DEDICATED TO THE HEALTH OF ALL CHILDREN™

Scenario Lead-in

Prehospital: You are dispatched to transport a 12 year old with abdominal injuries caused by flipping over bicycle handlebars. Mother reports that this happened about 4 hours ago. There was no loss of consciousness and the child was wearing a helmet. You observe the patient in obvious discomfort, and he says he has worsening abdominal pain. There are no indications of spinal injury.

ED: Parents arrive with their 12 year old with abdominal injuries caused by flipping over bicycle handlebars. Mother reports this happened about 4 hours ago. There was no loss of consciousness and the child was wearing a helmet. Patient appears in obvious discomfort, and he says he has worsening abdominal pain. Spinal injury has been ruled out.

General Inpatient Unit: As a member of the rapid response team, you respond to a 12 year old admitted with abdominal injuries caused by flipping over bicycle handlebars. History and physical exam are consistent with no loss of consciousness at scene, and patient was wearing a helmet. Patient is in obvious discomfort, and he says he has worsening abdominal pain. Spinal injury has been ruled out.

ICU: You are called to the bedside of a 12 year old who has been admitted to the intensive care unit with abdominal injuries caused by flipping over bicycle handlebars. History and physical are consistent with no loss of consciousness at scene and patient was wearing a helmet. Patient is in obvious discomfort, and he says he has worsening abdominal pain. Spinal injury has been ruled out.

Vital Signs	
Heart rate	130/min
Blood pressure	110/50 mm Hg
Respiratory rate	30/min
SpO₂	92% on room air
Temperature	37.5°C (99.5°F)
Weight	46 kg
Age	12 years

Scenario Overview and Learning Objectives

Scenario Overview

Emphasis should be on identification of compensated traumatic hypovolemic shock progressing to hypotensive shock despite bolus fluid administration. Priorities include immediate establishment of intravenous (IV)/intraosseous (IO) access and administration of fluid bolus of isotonic crystalloid, repeated as needed to treat shock signs. Reassessment of cardiorespiratory status is needed during and after each fluid bolus. Glucose concentration should be checked with point-of-care (POC) testing. When this child's shock does not respond to 2-3 fluid boluses of isotonic crystalloid, bolus administration of packed red blood cells is indicated. Providers must recognize the need for expert consultation (eg, pediatric trauma surgeon) and further diagnostic studies.

Scenario-Specific Objectives

- **Recognizes initial compensated shock and hypotensive shock;** this scenario begins with a child in compensated shock who progresses to hypotensive shock despite bolus fluid administration
- **Summarizes signs and symptoms of hypovolemic shock;** key indicators in this scenario include abdominal trauma, tachycardia, mottled skin, weak pulses, and decreased level of consciousness
- **Demonstrates correct interventions for hypovolemic shock;** this patient requires oxygen administration, administration of one or more boluses of isotonic crystalloid with careful reassessment during and after each fluid bolus, administration of packed red blood cells, and surgical consult
- **Summarizes how to evaluate systemic (end-organ) perfusion;** indicators appropriate for this scenario include skin temperature/color, level of consciousness, and urine output

Evaluate—*Initial Impression* (Pediatric Assessment Triangle)	Identify	Intervene
Appearance • Awake, in obvious discomfort **Breathing** • Increased work of breathing, mild tachypnea **Circulation** • Pale, with mottled hands and feet	• Immediate intervention needed	• Activate emergency response system. • Administer 100% oxygen by nonrebreathing mask. • Apply cardiac monitor. • Apply pulse oximeter.

Evaluate—*Primary Assessment* *Focused on Assessment Needed to Support Airway, Oxygenation, Ventilation, and Perfusion*	**Identify**	**Intervene**
• **A**irway: Clear • **B**reathing: Respiratory rate about 30/min; mild subcostal and intercostal retractions; mild nasal flaring; SpO₂ 92% on room air, increases to 95% with 100% oxygen administered via nonrebreathing mask; lungs clear to auscultation • **C**irculation: Heart rate 130/min; central pulses weak, peripheral pulses barely felt; capillary refill about 4 seconds; cool and mottled hands and feet; blood pressure 110/50 mm Hg *Remainder of Primary Assessment performed if airway, ventilation, and perfusion are adequately supported* • **D**isability: Alert • **E**xposure: Rectal temperature 37.5°C (99.5°F); weight 46 kg	• Respiratory distress • Compensated shock • Sinus tachycardia	• Obtain vascular access (IV/IO); send blood sample for stat type and cross match. • Administer a fluid bolus 20 mL/kg of isotonic crystalloid; repeat boluses rapidly IV/IO; assess perfusion; and monitor cardiorespiratory status closely during and immediately after each fluid bolus. – Stop fluid bolus if signs of heart failure develop (eg, increased respiratory distress or development of rales or hepatomegaly). • Check POC glucose concentration and treat hypoglycemia if needed. • Assess response to oxygen.

Evaluate—*Secondary Assessment* *Identify Reversible Causes, but Defer Remainder of Secondary Assessment Until After Initial Shock Therapy*	**Identify**	**Intervene**
SAMPLE history (only to extent needed to evaluate reversible causes) • **S**igns and symptoms: Mechanism of injury, abdominal pain, distended abdomen • **A**llergies: None known • **M**edications: Albuterol inhaler • **P**ast medical history: Mild asthma • **L**ast meal: 6 hours ago • **E**vents (onset): Thrown from bicycle, abdomen caught on handlebars 4 hours ago; initial pain, now worse; increased work of breathing **Physical examination** • *Repeat vital signs after oxygen and 2 boluses of 20 mL/kg fluids:* Heart rate 90-100/min; respiratory rate 15/min; SpO₂ 96% with 100% oxygen via nonrebreathing mask; blood pressure 90/50 mm Hg; capillary refill 4 seconds • *Head, eyes, ears, nose, and throat/neck:* Mucous membranes moist • *Heart and lungs:* No extra heart sounds or murmurs • *Abdomen:* Distended, tender; hypoactive bowel sounds • *Extremities:* Superficial abrasions; central pulses readily palpable, weak peripheral pulses; capillary refill 4 seconds • *Back:* Normal • *Neurologic:* Responds appropriately to questions, but clearly in pain; pupils 4 mm, equal, briskly reactive to light	• Hypotensive shock (likely hypovolemia related to blood loss)	• Repeat bolus of 20 mL/kg of isotonic crystalloid IV/IO push; repeat boluses needed for persistent shock symptoms. • Perform careful and frequent cardiorespiratory assessment during and after each fluid bolus. – Stop fluid bolus if signs of heart failure (increased respiratory distress or development of rales or hepatomegaly). • Consider administration of 10 mL/kg of packed red blood cells if signs of shock and hemodynamic instability persist despite 2-3 boluses of isotonic crystalloids. • Arrange for transfer to surgery if patient cannot achieve hemodynamic stability. • Obtain expert consultation (eg, from trauma surgeon or pediatric surgeon); additional diagnostic studies will be necessary. • Arrange transfer to intensive care unit (ICU) for closer monitoring if child is not already in ICU.

Evaluate—*Diagnostic Assessments* *Perform Throughout the Evaluation of the Patient as Appropriate*	**Identify/Intervene**
Lab data • *Capillary gas:* pH 7.30, PCO₂ 25 mm Hg, PO₂ 30 mm Hg, Hemoglobin 7 g/dL • Glucose (POC) 135 mg/dL (7.5 mmol/L) • *Pending:* Electrolytes, blood urea nitrogen/creatinine, calcium, complete blood count with differential, prothrombin time/international normalized ratio/partial thromboplastin time *Imaging* • *Chest x-ray:* Small heart, clear lung fields • *Abdominal computed tomography:* Moderate liver laceration	• A blood glucose level should be performed as soon as reasonably possible in all critically ill children. Hypoglycemia should be treated immediately. • Child is anemic as the result of blood loss and isotonic crystalloid therapy. • Metabolic acidosis with respiratory compensation. The metabolic acidosis should correct if the child's abdominal injury has stabilized and effective shock resuscitation is provided. • Additional studies will be needed to evaluate abdominal injury.

Re–evaluate-identify-intervene after each intervention.

Debriefing Tool
Practice Case Scenario 1
Hypovolemic Shock (Child; Uncompensated Shock)

General Debriefing Principles

- Use the table below to guide your debriefing; also refer to the **Team Dynamics Debriefing Tool.**
- Debriefings are 10 minutes long.
- Address all learning objectives.
- Summarize take-home messages at the end of the debriefing.
- *Encourage:* Students to self-reflect
  Engagement of all participants
- *Avoid:* Mini-lectures and closed-ended questions
  Dominating the discussion

General Management Objectives

- Uses the PALS Systematic Approach Algorithm to assess and appropriately classify a patient
- Provides oxygen appropriately
- Directs delivery of high-quality CPR (including the use of a feedback device) when indicated
- Demonstrates basic airway maneuvers and use of relevant airway device as appropriate
- Demonstrates application of cardiac and respiratory monitors

- Identifies the cardiac rhythm
- Applies appropriate PBLS or PALS algorithms
- Summarizes general indications, contraindications, and doses of relevant drugs
- Discusses principles of family-centered care in pediatric cardiac arrest
- Applies the 8 elements of effective team dynamics
- Performs frequent reassessment

Action	Gather	Analyze	Summarize
	Student Observations	**Done Well**	**Student-Led Summary**
• Assesses ABCDE, including vital signs • Administers 100% oxygen • Applies cardiac monitor and pulse oximeter • Recognizes signs and symptoms of hypovolemic shock • Categorizes shock as compensated and then hypotensive • Establishes IV or IO access • Directs rapid bolus administration of isotonic crystalloid; monitors for signs of heart failure during and after fluid bolus of isotonic crystalloid • Reassesses patient during and in response to interventions, particularly during and after each fluid bolus • Repeats fluid bolus and administers packed red blood cells as needed to treat shock • Checks glucose with POC testing • Consults pediatric trauma surgeon	• Can you describe the events from your perspective? • How well do you think your treatments worked? • Can you review the events of the scenario (*directed to the Timer/Recorder*)? • What could you have improved? • What did the team do well?	• How were you able to [*insert action here*]? • Why do you think you were able to [*insert action here*]? • Tell me a little more about how you [*insert action here*].	• What are the main things you learned? • Can someone summarize the key points made? • What are the main take-home messages?
	Instructor Observations	**Needs Improvement**	**Instructor-Led Summary**
	• I noticed that [*insert action here*]. • I observed that [*insert action here*]. • I saw that [*insert action here*].	• Why do you think [*insert action here*] occurred? • How do you think [*insert action here*] could have been improved? • What was your thinking while [*insert action here*]? • What prevented you from [*insert action here*]?	• Let's summarize what we learned… • Here is what I think we learned… • The main take-home messages are… • What are the therapeutic end points during shock management? (Answer: Normalized heart rate; improved peripheral perfusion, mental status, and urine output; maintenance of blood pressure) • Which are the indirect signs of improved end-organ function? (Answer: Improved skin blood flow, increased responsiveness/improved level of consciousness, increased urine output, correction of lactic acidosis)

Practice Case Scenario 2
Hypovolemic Shock
(Infant; Nonaccidental Trauma With Increased Intracranial Pressure)

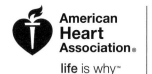

American Academy of Pediatrics

DEDICATED TO THE HEALTH OF ALL CHILDREN™

Scenario Lead-in

Prehospital: You are dispatched to transport a 6 month old with altered level of consciousness. The infant was picked up from day care earlier today and reportedly slept during the car ride home. Her father reports that he was unable to get the infant to eat dinner. She lies listless in father's arms.

ED: Emergency medical services providers arrive with a 6 month old with altered level of consciousness. The infant was reportedly picked up from day care and slept during the car ride home. Her father reports that he was unable to get her to eat dinner. The infant lies listless in her father's arms. The emergency medical services providers were unable to establish peripheral intravenous access.

General Inpatient Unit: As a member of the rapid response team, you respond to a 6-month-old infant with altered level of consciousness who was admitted directly from her physician's office. The father reported that he picked up the infant from day care and she slept during the car ride home. The father reports that he was unable to get the infant to eat dinner. The infant lies listless in the crib. The ward team has been unable to establish peripheral intravenous access.

ICU: You are asked to assess and manage a 6 month old with altered level of consciousness. The infant was picked up from day care by her father, who reports that the infant slept during the car ride home. The father reports that he was unable to get the infant to eat dinner. The infant lies listless in the crib. The infant's peripheral intravenous access has infiltrated.

Vital Signs	
Heart rate	160/min
Blood pressure	84/30 mm Hg
Respiratory rate	10-18/min
SpO$_2$	93% on room air
Temperature	37.0°C (98.6°F)
Weight	8.6 kg
Age	6 months

Scenario Overview and Learning Objectives

Scenario Overview

Emphasis should be on identification of compensated hypovolemic shock. Priorities include immediate establishment of intravenous (IV)/intraosseous (IO) access and administration of fluid bolus of isotonic crystalloid, repeated as needed to treat shock signs. Reassessment of cardiorespiratory status is needed during and after each fluid bolus. Glucose concentration should be checked with point-of-care (POC) testing. This infant's shock is complicated by signs of increased intracranial pressure, probably associated with intracranial injury. Providers must recognize the need for expert consultation and further diagnostic studies.

Scenario-Specific Objectives

- **Recognizes signs of compensated and hypotensive shock;** this scenario illustrates decompensated hypovolemic shock, complicated by increased intracranial pressure (key indicators include decreased level of consciousness, tachycardia, cool and mottled skin, delayed capillary refill, and hypotension)
- **Summarizes signs and symptoms of hypovolemic shock;** key indicators in this case include signs of shock with signs of trauma
- **Demonstrates correct interventions for hypovolemic shock;** this case requires administration of oxygen, administration of an isotonic fluid bolus with careful reassessment during and after the fluid bolus, and consulting someone with surgical expertise (eg, pediatric or neurosurgeon)
- **Summarizes how to evaluate systemic (end-organ) perfusion;** indicators appropriate for this include skin temperature/color, level of consciousness, and urine output
- **Recognizes need for reporting and intervention for possible abuse**

Evaluate—*Initial Impression* *(Pediatric Assessment Triangle)*	Identify	Intervene
Appearance • Lethargic **Breathing** • Irregular and shallow breaths **Circulation** • Pale with significant mottling in extremities	• Immediate intervention needed	• Activate the emergency response system. Emergency medical services requests additional assistance if needed. • Provide bag-mask ventilation with 100% oxygen. • Attach cardiac monitor. • Apply pulse oximeter.

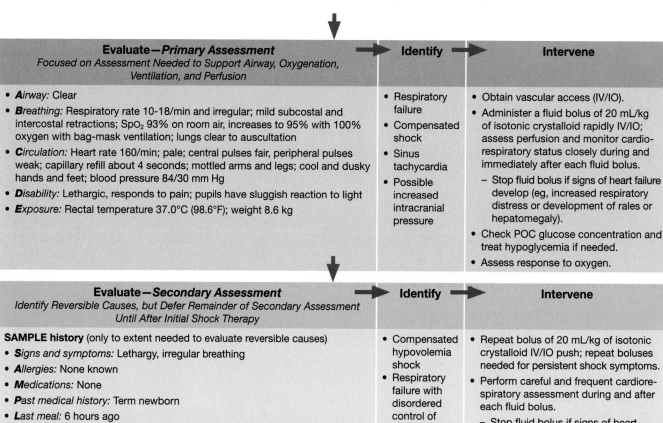

Evaluate—*Primary Assessment*
Focused on Assessment Needed to Support Airway, Oxygenation, Ventilation, and Perfusion

- *Airway:* Clear
- *Breathing:* Respiratory rate 10-18/min and irregular; mild subcostal and intercostal retractions; SpO₂ 93% on room air, increases to 95% with 100% oxygen with bag-mask ventilation; lungs clear to auscultation
- *Circulation:* Heart rate 160/min; pale; central pulses fair, peripheral pulses weak; capillary refill about 4 seconds; mottled arms and legs; cool and dusky hands and feet; blood pressure 84/30 mm Hg
- *Disability:* Lethargic, responds to pain; pupils have sluggish reaction to light
- *Exposure:* Rectal temperature 37.0°C (98.6°F); weight 8.6 kg

Identify
- Respiratory failure
- Compensated shock
- Sinus tachycardia
- Possible increased intracranial pressure

Intervene
- Obtain vascular access (IV/IO).
- Administer a fluid bolus of 20 mL/kg of isotonic crystalloid rapidly IV/IO; assess perfusion and monitor cardio-respiratory status closely during and immediately after each fluid bolus.
  - Stop fluid bolus if signs of heart failure develop (eg, increased respiratory distress or development of rales or hepatomegaly).
- Check POC glucose concentration and treat hypoglycemia if needed.
- Assess response to oxygen.

Evaluate—*Secondary Assessment*
Identify Reversible Causes, but Defer Remainder of Secondary Assessment Until After Initial Shock Therapy

SAMPLE history (only to extent needed to evaluate reversible causes)
- *Signs and symptoms:* Lethargy, irregular breathing
- *Allergies:* None known
- *Medications:* None
- *Past medical history:* Term newborn
- *Last meal:* 6 hours ago
- *Events (onset):* Patient reportedly was "normal self" before being dropped off at day care. Day care told dad that the infant took second nap before being picked up. Infant has demonstrated increasing lethargy, decreased work of breathing, and irregular respiratory rate.

Physical examination
- *Repeat vital signs after oxygen and fluids:* Heart rate 140/min; respiratory rate 30/min bag-mask ventilation; SpO₂ 95% during bag-mask ventilation with 100% oxygen; blood pressure 80/50 mm Hg
- *Head, eyes, nose, and throat/neck:* Bruising to ears
- *Heart and lungs:* Rapid rate, no extra heart sounds or murmurs; lungs sound clear
- *Abdomen:* No palpable liver edge; nondistended; nontender; hypoactive bowel sounds
- *Extremities:* Normal skin turgor
- *Back:* Normal
- *Neurologic:* Lethargic; pupils 4 mm, equal, sluggish reaction to light

Identify
- Compensated hypovolemia shock
- Respiratory failure with disordered control of breathing (decreased level of consciousness)
- Possible intracranial injury with increased intracranial pressure

Intervene
- Repeat bolus of 20 mL/kg of isotonic crystalloid IV/IO push; repeat boluses needed for persistent shock symptoms.
- Perform careful and frequent cardiore-spiratory assessment during and after each fluid bolus.
  - Stop fluid bolus if signs of heart failure (increased respiratory distress or development of rales or hepato-megaly).
- Continue to provide bag-mask ventila-tion; prepare for insertion of advanced airway.
- Identify possible signs of increased intracranial pressure associated with intracranial injury.
- Obtain expert consultation (eg, from trauma surgeon, pediatric surgeon, or neurosurgeon).
  - Additional diagnostic studies will be necessary.
- Arrange transfer to intensive care unit (ICU) for closer monitoring if infant is not already in ICU.

Evaluate—*Diagnostic Assessments*
Perform Throughout the Evaluation of the Patient as Appropriate

Lab data
- *Capillary gas:* pH 7.20, PCO₂ 55 mm Hg, PO₂ 34 mm Hg, base excess –9, hemoglobin 10 g/dL
- *Glucose (POC)* 80 mg/dL (10.3 mmol/L)
- *Pending:* Electrolytes, blood urea nitrogen/creatinine, calcium, complete blood count with differential, prothrombin time/international normalized ratio/partial thromboplastin time
- *Cultures:* Blood, urine

Imaging: Computed tomography (CT)/magnetic resonance imaging (MRI)/ultrasound stat
- *Chest x-ray:* Small heart, clear lung fields
- Head CT/MRI

Identify/Intervene
- A blood glucose concentration should be checked as soon as reasonably possible in all critically ill infants and children. Hypoglycemia should be treated immediately.
- Mixed respiratory and metabolic acidosis should improve with support of ventilation and oxygenation and treatment of possible hypovolemic shock.
- Additional studies will be needed to evaluate the cause of poorly reactive pupils and bruising to ears (eg, CT scan/MRI).

Re–evaluate-identify-intervene after each intervention.

Debriefing Tool
Practice Case Scenario 2
Hypovolemic Shock (Infant; Nonaccidental Trauma With Increased Intracranial Pressure)

General Management Objectives

- Uses the PALS Systematic Approach Algorithm to assess and appropriately classify a patient
- Provides oxygen appropriately
- Directs delivery of high-quality CPR (including the use of a feedback device) when indicated
- Demonstrates basic airway maneuvers and use of relevant airway device as appropriate
- Demonstrates application of cardiac and respiratory monitors
- Identifies the cardiac rhythm
- Applies appropriate PBLS or PALS algorithms
- Summarizes general indications, contraindications, and doses of relevant drugs
- Discusses principles of family-centered care in pediatric cardiac arrest
- Applies the 8 elements of effective team dynamics
- Performs frequent reassessment

Action	Gather	Analyze	Summarize
• Assesses ABCDE, including vital signs • Administers 100% oxygen • Applies cardiac monitor and pulse oximeter • Recognizes signs and symptoms of hypovolemic shock • Categorizes shock as compensated then hypovolemic • Establishes IV or IO access • Directs rapid administration of fluid bolus of isotonic crystalloid; monitors for signs of heart failure during and after fluid bolus • Reassesses patient in response to interventions, particularly during and after each fluid bolus • Repeats fluid bolus as needed to treat shock • Checks glucose with point-of-care testing	*Student Observations* • Can you describe the events from your perspective? • How well do you think your treatments worked? • Can you review the events of the scenario (*directed to the Timer/Recorder*)? • What could you have improved? • What did the team do well? *Instructor Observations* • I noticed that [*insert action here*]. • I observed that [*insert action here*]. • I saw that [*insert action here*].	*Done Well* • How were you able to [*insert action here*]? • Why do you think you were able to [*insert action here*]? • Tell me a little more about how you [*insert action here*]. *Needs Improvement* • Why do you think [*insert action here*] occurred? • How do you think [*insert action here*] could have been improved? • What was your thinking while [*insert action here*]? • What prevented you from [*insert action here*]?	*Student-Led Summary* • What are the main things you learned? • Can someone summarize the key points made? • What are the main take-home messages? *Instructor-Led Summary* • Let's summarize what we learned… • Here is what I think we learned… • The main take-home messages are… • What are the therapeutic end points during shock management? (Answer: Normalized heart rate; improved peripheral perfusion, mental status, and urine output; maintenance of blood pressure) • Which are the indirect signs of improved end-organ function? (Answer: Improved skin blood flow, increased responsiveness/improved level of consciousness, increased urine output, correction of lactic acidosis)

Lower Airway Obstruction
(Child; More Severely Ill)

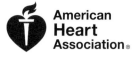

American Heart Association®
life is why™

American Academy of Pediatrics
DEDICATED TO THE HEALTH OF ALL CHILDREN™

Scenario Lead-in

Prehospital: You are responding to a 9-1-1 call for a 10 year old with breathing difficulty.

ED: A 10-year-old girl is brought in by first responders from her home after her mother called 9-1-1 saying that her daughter had difficulty breathing.

General Inpatient Unit: You are called to the room of a 10-year-old girl who is being admitted from the emergency department for respiratory distress.

PICU: You are called to the room of a 10-year-old girl who is being admitted from the emergency department for respiratory distress.

Vital Signs	
Heart rate	140/min
Blood pressure	106/68 mm Hg
Respiratory rate	40/min
SpO₂	86% on room air
Temperature	Afebrile
Weight	35 kg
Age	10 years

Scenario Overview and Learning Objectives

Scenario Overview

Emphasis in this scenario is on rapid identification and management of respiratory distress/potential respiratory failure caused by lower airway obstruction/asthma. The provider must quickly recognize signs of distress (severe tachypnea and hypoxemia on room air) and provide initial therapy, including administration of 100% oxygen, nebulized albuterol, and ipratropium and oral corticosteroids. Continuous nebulized albuterol may also be needed. Early consultation with an expert in the care of children with status asthmaticus is required because this child has a history of status asthmaticus requiring multiple intensive care unit (ICU) admissions. The child improves, so acceleration of care is not required. During the debriefing, the student is asked the indications for endotracheal intubation.

Scenario-Specific Objectives

- **Recognizes signs and symptoms of respiratory distress caused by lower airway obstruction;** in this scenario, they include increased respiratory rate and effort, prolonged expiratory time, and wheezing
- **Performs correct initial interventions for lower airway obstruction;** in this scenario, they include administration of oxygen, nebulized albuterol, and ipratropium bromide and corticosteroids
- **Discusses importance of obtaining expert consultation if child with asthma has a history of ICU admissions and/or fails to respond to initial interventions**

Evaluate—*Initial Impression* (Pediatric Assessment Triangle)	Identify	Intervene
Appearance • Anxious; moderate distress; sitting upright **Breathing** • Increased work of breathing; retractions **Circulation** • Pale skin	• Immediate intervention needed	• Activate the emergency response system. Emergency medical services requests additional assistance if needed. • Administer 100% oxygen by nonrebreathing face mask. • Apply cardiac monitor. • Apply pulse oximeter.

Evaluate—*Primary Assessment* Focused on Assessment Needed to Support Airway, Oxygenation, Ventilation, and Perfusion	Identify	Intervene
• **A**irway: Unobstructed; no abnormal breath sounds are audible • **B**reathing: Moderate suprasternal and intercostal retractions; prolonged expiratory time; expiratory wheezes in the lower lobes; respiratory rate 40/min; SpO₂ 86% on room air, just before 100% oxygen administration • **C**irculation: Heart rate 140/min; pale skin; strong radial pulse; capillary refill 2 seconds; blood pressure 106/68 mm Hg • **D**isability: Awake; speaks in 2- to 3-word sentences • **E**xposure: Afebrile; no rashes; weight 35 kg	• Respiratory distress, possible respiratory failure • Lower airway obstruction	• Allow child to maintain position of comfort. • Assess response to oxygen. • Administer nebulized albuterol and nebulized ipratropium. • Administer oral corticosteroids.

Evaluate—*Secondary Assessment* *Identify Reversible Causes, but Defer Remainder of Secondary Assessment* *Until After Stabilization of Airway, Oxygenation, and Ventilation*		**Identify**	**Intervene**
SAMPLE history • ***S****igns and symptoms:* Cough; respiratory distress • ***A****llergies:* Molds and grass • ***M****edications:* Inhaler that has not been refilled for several weeks • ***P****ast medical history:* Known asthmatic, poorly controlled due to poor compliance with medical care; 3 ICU admissions for respiratory failure; family members smoke in the house • ***L****ast meal:* 3 hours ago • ***E****vents (onset):* Cold symptoms for the last 3 days; increased cough and distress for past 24 hours **Physical examination** • *Repeat vital signs after oxygen and fluids:* Heart rate 140/min; respiratory rate 32/min; SpO$_2$ 94% when receiving 100% oxygen via nonrebreathing face mask; blood pressure 112/71 mm Hg • *Head, eyes, ears, nose, and throat/neck:* Normal • *Heart and lungs:* Wheezing on expiration in lower lobes; poor air movement; persistent moderate suprasternal and intercostal retractions • *Abdomen:* Normal • *Extremities:* Normal • *Back:* Normal • *Neurologic:* Anxious; no other abnormalities; now speaking in 3- to 4-word sentences		• Respiratory distress • Lower airway obstruction	• Assess response to albuterol and ipratropium. • If wheezing and aeration are not improved, consider provision of continuous nebulized albuterol. • Obtain vascular access. • Check glucose with point-of-care (POC) testing. • Consider obtaining expert consultation regarding the management of pediatric status asthmaticus. • If no improvement in signs of lower airway obstruction despite continuous albuterol and administration of ipratropium bromide, consider additional interventions (eg, magnesium sulfate) and diagnostic testing (arterial blood gas, chest x-ray), and consult an expert in the management of pediatric status asthmaticus (if not already done). • Arrange for transfer of child to the ICU (if the child is not already in the ICU) so that child may receive additional monitoring and therapy. • If child's condition does improve, be prepared to titrate inspired oxygen concentration, as tolerated, to keep SpO$_2$ 94% or greater.

Evaluate—*Diagnostic Assessments* *Perform Throughout the Evaluation of the Patient as Appropriate*	**Identify/Intervene**
Lab data • Glucose (POC testing) 126 mg/dL (7.0 mmol/L)	• Although laboratory tests are generally not appropriate during the immediate management, a blood glucose concentration should be checked as soon as reasonably possible in all critically ill infants and children. Hypoglycemia should be treated immediately. • Additional testing (eg, chest x-ray) may be performed if child demonstrates any additional respiratory signs or symptoms.

Re–evaluate-identify-intervene after each intervention.

Debriefing Tool

Practice Case Scenario 3
Lower Airway Obstruction (Child; More Severely Ill)

General Debriefing Principles

- Use the table below to guide your debriefing; also refer to the **Team Dynamics Debriefing Tool.**
- Debriefings are 10 minutes long.
- Address all learning objectives.
- Summarize take-home messages at the end of the debriefing.
- *Encourage:* Students to self-reflect
  Engagement of all participants
- *Avoid:* Mini-lectures and closed-ended questions
  Dominating the discussion

General Management Objectives

- Uses the PALS Systematic Approach Algorithm to assess and appropriately classify a patient
- Provides oxygen appropriately
- Directs delivery of high-quality CPR (including the use of a feedback device) when indicated
- Demonstrates basic airway maneuvers and use of relevant airway device as appropriate
- Demonstrates application of cardiac and respiratory monitors
- Identifies the cardiac rhythm
- Applies appropriate PBLS or PALS algorithms
- Summarizes general indications, contraindications, and doses of relevant drugs
- Discusses principles of family-centered care in pediatric cardiac arrest
- Applies the 8 elements of effective team dynamics
- Performs frequent reassessment

Action	Gather	Analyze	Summarize
• Directs assessment of ABCDE and vital signs • Directs administration of 100% oxygen • Applies cardiac monitor and pulse oximeter • Recognizes signs and symptoms of lower airway obstruction • Initiates therapy for asthma, including continued oxygen administration, nebulized albuterol, and corticosteroids • Directs establishment of intravenous or intraosseous access • Directs reassessment of patient in response to each intervention • Summarizes additional therapy to provide if indicated (ie, give nebulized albuterol continuously, administer nebulized ipratropium bromide, consider magnesium sulfate) • States the importance of early consultation with expert in the care of children with status asthmaticus	***Student Observations*** • Can you describe the events from your perspective? • How well do you think your treatments worked? • Can you review the events of the scenario (*directed to the Timer/Recorder*)? • What could you have improved? • What did the team do well? ***Instructor Observations*** • I noticed that [*insert action here*]. • I observed that [*insert action here*]. • I saw that [*insert action here*].	***Done Well*** • How were you able to [*insert action here*]? • Why do you think you were able to [*insert action here*]? • Tell me a little more about how you [*insert action here*]. ***Needs Improvement*** • Why do you think [*insert action here*] occurred? • How do you think [*insert action here*] could have been improved? • What was your thinking while [*insert action here*]? • What prevented you from [*insert action here*]?	***Student-Led Summary*** • What are the main things you learned? • Can someone summarize the key points made? • What are the main take-home messages? ***Instructor-Led Summary*** • Let's summarize what we learned… • Here is what I think we learned… • The main take-home messages are… • In this scenario, the child gradually improved. If this child continued to deteriorate despite the care provided, and expert consultation was available, what would be the indications for bag-mask ventilation or other airway or ventilation support? (Answer includes decreased level of consciousness; decreased air movement; and decreased wheezing, bradycardia, and pulsus paradoxus.)

Practice Case Scenario 4
Upper Airway Obstruction
(Child; Moderate to Severe)

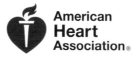

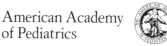

DEDICATED TO THE HEALTH OF ALL CHILDREN™

Scenario Lead-in

Prehospital: You are responding to a 9-1-1 call for a 1 year old with breathing difficulty.

ED: A 1-year-old girl is brought in by first responders from her home after mother called 9-1-1 because the child was having difficulty breathing.

General Inpatient Unit: You are called to the room of a 1-year-old girl who is being admitted from the emergency department for respiratory distress and croup-like symptoms.

ICU: You are called to the room of a 1-year-old girl who is being admitted from the emergency department for respiratory distress and croup-like symptoms.

Vital Signs	
Heart rate	154/min
Blood pressure	75/43 mm Hg
Respiratory rate	64/min
SpO$_2$	84% on room air
Temperature	36.3°C (97.4°F)
Weight	10 kg
Age	1 year

Scenario Overview and Learning Objectives

Scenario Overview

Emphasis in this scenario is on rapid recognition and management of respiratory distress associated with significant upper airway obstruction. The child's lethargy, signs of increased respiratory effort, and stridor at rest all indicate the need to remove the child from the parents, position the child to open the airway and suction the nares, administer nebulized epinephrine and dexamethasone, and prepare for more-advanced care, including early expert consultation. Discussion during the debriefing addresses estimation of endotracheal tube size.

Scenario-Specific Objectives

- **Identifies the signs and symptoms of significant upper airway obstruction;** in this scenario, they include significant tachypnea and increased work of breathing, inspiratory stridor, fair chest movement, and decreased level of consciousness

- **Recognizes that removing the child from the parent's arms is indicated for this child;** in this scenario, the child is lethargic with only fair chest rise and mild cyanosis

- **Performs correct interventions for significant upper airway obstruction;** in this scenario, these include positioning to open airway, suctioning of nares, oxygen administration, nebulized epinephrine (may be repeated), administration of dexamethasone, and preparation for respiratory support

- **Identifies the need to obtain expert consultation to be available for insertion of advanced airway**

Evaluate—*Initial Impression* (Pediatric Assessment Triangle)	Identify	Intervene
Appearance • Being held by parent; appears lethargic, not moving much **Breathing** • Tachypneic with increased work of breathing; high-pitched inspiratory stridor; only fair chest rise noted **Circulation** • Mild cyanosis of lips	• Immediate intervention needed	• Activate the emergency response system. Emergency medical services requests additional assistance if needed. • Place patient on bed and reposition to open airway using head tilt–chin lift. • Administer 100% oxygen by nonrebreathing face mask. • Apply cardiac monitor. • Apply pulse oximeter.

Evaluate—*Primary Assessment* Focused on Assessment Needed to Support Airway, Oxygenation, Ventilation, and Perfusion	Identify	Intervene
• **A**irway: Patent; no oral obstruction • **B**reathing: High-pitched, faint, inspiratory stridor; respiratory rate 64/min; moderate, suprasternal, intercostal, and subcostal retractions; SpO$_2$ 84% before oxygen administration, then 95% after provision of 100% inspired oxygen; nasal flaring present with copious secretions; improved chest rise with repositioning; transmitted upper airway sounds with overall poor air entry • **C**irculation: Heart rate 154/min; mild cyanosis of lips before oxygen administration (lips now pink); warm skin centrally and peripherally; strong central and peripheral pulses; capillary refill 3 seconds; blood pressure 75/43 mm Hg • **D**isability: Lethargic, but withdraws and whimpers to tactile stimulation; anterior fontanel soft and flat • **E**xposure: Temperature 36.3°C (97.4°F); weight 10 kg	• Respiratory distress or failure • Upper airway obstruction	• Continue positioning/oxygen administration. • Suction nares. • Administer nebulized epinephrine. • Contact expert help to be available if child fails to improve or deteriorates further and to develop plan of care.

Evaluate—*Secondary Assessment* *Identify Reversible Causes, but Defer Remainder of Secondary Assessment Until After Stabilization of Airway, Oxygenation, and Ventilation*	Identify	Intervene
SAMPLE history • **S**igns and symptoms: Awoke yesterday with fever, barking, and seal-like cough; seemed to improve yesterday, but worse overnight • **A**llergies: None known • **M**edications: Acetaminophen for fever given by mother 2 hours ago • **P**ast medical history: Otitis media at 10 and 11 months • **L**ast meal: 8 hours ago; refused bottle and breakfast this morning • **E**vents (onset): Symptoms worse at night; increased work of breathing and more lethargic this morning **Physical examination** • *Repeat vital signs after oxygen and racemic epinephrine:* Heart rate 161/min; respiratory rate 56/min; SpO₂ 99% on supplementary oxygen; blood pressure 77/48 mm Hg • *Head, eyes, ears, nose, and throat/neck:* Nasal flaring persists; less nasal secretions; airway remains patent with support and positioning; moist mucous membranes • *Heart and lungs:* Lungs clear; transmitted upper airway sounds (less pronounced); suprasternal, intercostal, and subcostal retractions improved; improved bilateral chest rise; stridor is louder • *Abdomen:* Normal • *Extremities:* Normal • *Back:* Normal • *Neurologic:* Becoming more alert	• Respiratory distress • Upper airway obstruction	• Evaluate response to nebulized epinephrine. • Repeat nebulized epinephrine and reassess response. • Providers may consider use of heliox, but it can't be used if the child requires a high concentration of inspired oxygen. • Check glucose using point-of-care testing. • Administer oral/intravenous/intramuscular corticosteroids (eg, dexamethasone); administer oral corticosteroids if child is sufficiently alert. • Be prepared to provide initial advanced care, such as immediate bag-mask ventilation, if the child's condition fails to improve or deteriorates further. • Arrange for the child to have careful, close observation as severe symptoms may recur, requiring transfer to intensive care unit (ICU) (if child is not already in ICU).

Evaluate—*Diagnostic Assessments* *Perform Throughout the Evaluation of the Patient as Appropriate*	Identify/Intervene
Lab data • Glucose 72 mg/dL (4.2 mmol/L) • Consider complete blood count and electrolytes **Imaging** • Lateral soft-tissue neck radiographs may be considered but are generally not necessary	• Laboratory tests are generally not appropriate during the immediate management (initially providers should minimize stimulation until child's airway obstruction and work of breathing are more stable). • A blood glucose concentration should be checked as soon as reasonably possible in all critically ill infants and children. – This child has not been eating well, so it will be important to check the glucose. Hypoglycemia should be treated immediately. • Lateral neck radiographs may be considered to identify causes of upper airway obstruction that may not respond to initial interventions.

Re–evaluate–identify–intervene after each intervention.

Debriefing Tool
Practice Case Scenario 4
Upper Airway Obstruction (Child; Moderate to Severe)

General Debriefing Principles

- Use the table below to guide your debriefing; also refer to the **Team Dynamics Debriefing Tool.**
- Debriefings are 10 minutes long.
- Address all learning objectives.
- Summarize take-home messages at the end of the debriefing.
- *Encourage:* Students to self-reflect
    Engagement of all participants
- *Avoid:* Mini-lectures and closed-ended questions
    Dominating the discussion

General Management Objectives

- Uses the PALS Systematic Approach Algorithm to assess and appropriately classify a patient
- Provides oxygen appropriately
- Directs delivery of high-quality CPR (including the use of a feedback device) when indicated
- Demonstrates basic airway maneuvers and use of relevant airway device as appropriate
- Demonstrates application of cardiac and respiratory monitors

- Identifies the cardiac rhythm
- Applies appropriate PBLS or PALS algorithms
- Summarizes general indications, contraindications, and doses of relevant drugs
- Discusses principles of family-centered care in pediatric cardiac arrest
- Applies the 8 elements of effective team dynamics
- Performs frequent reassessment

Action	Gather	Analyze	Summarize
• Directs assessment of ABCDE and vital signs • Administers 100% oxygen • Applies cardiac monitor and pulse oximeter • Recognizes signs of severe upper airway obstruction • Provides appropriate initial management of significant upper airway obstruction, including positioning the child and opening the airway, suctioning the nares, providing oxygen, and giving nebulized epinephrine and dexamethasone • Reassesses the child frequently and evaluates response to interventions, watching closely for signs of deterioration • Identifies the need to obtain early expert consultation to develop plan of care should the child deteriorate further, including possible insertion of an advanced airway and other advanced care and monitoring • Arranges transfer of child to ICU (if child is not already in ICU)	***Student Observations*** • Can you describe the events from your perspective? • How well do you think your treatments worked? • Can you review the events of the scenario (*directed to the Timer/Recorder*)? • What could you have improved? • What did the team do well? ***Instructor Observations*** • I noticed that [*insert action here*]. • I observed that [*insert action here*]. • I saw that [*insert action here*].	***Done Well*** • How were you able to [*insert action here*]? • Why do you think you were able to [*insert action here*]? • Tell me a little more about how you [*insert action here*]. ***Needs Improvement*** • Why do you think [*insert action here*] occurred? • How do you think [*insert action here*] could have been improved? • What was your thinking while [*insert action here*]? • What prevented you from [*insert action here*]?	***Student-Led Summary*** • What are the main things you learned? • Can someone summarize the key points made? • What are the main take-home messages? ***Instructor-Led Summary*** • Let's summarize what we learned… • Here is what I think we learned… • The main take-home messages are… • In this scenario, the child improved somewhat after interventions to relieve upper airway obstruction. What would be the signs of deterioration and possible indications for bag-mask ventilation or other airway or ventilation support? (Answer: Very rapid or inadequate respiratory rate or irregular breathing pattern; signs of increased work of breathing; decreased breath sounds or aeration; deterioration in level of consciousness, hypoxemia, or cyanosis) • How would you estimate the correct uncuffed endotracheal tube size? (Answer: Would estimate a tube size about 0.5 mm smaller than typical for length and age)

137

Asystole
(Infant; Arrest)*

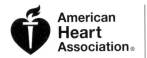

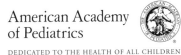

American Academy of Pediatrics

DEDICATED TO THE HEALTH OF ALL CHILDREN™

Vital Signs	
Heart rate	CPR in progress
Blood pressure	CPR in progress
Respiratory rate	Bag-mask ventilation (CPR)
SpO₂	Not obtainable
Temperature	Deferred
Weight	7 kg
Age	6 months

Scenario Lead-in

Prehospital: You are dispatched to a house where a 6-month-old infant has had respiratory distress; she is now unresponsive.

ED: An ambulance is en route to the emergency department with a 6-month-old infant who was found unresponsive in her crib; CPR is ongoing.

General Inpatient Unit: You are called as a member of the rapid response team to see a 6 month old who was admitted with respiratory distress, but she has now become limp and unresponsive.

ICU: You are called to see a 6 month old who became progressively limp and unresponsive. The infant was admitted with respiratory distress with the remainder of the emergency department workup unremarkable.

Scenario Overview and Learning Objectives

Scenario Overview

This scenario focuses on the identification and management of cardiac arrest and a "nonshockable" rhythm. Emphasis is placed on immediate delivery of high-quality CPR and early administration of epinephrine. The student should identify potential reversible causes of asystole (H's and T's); respiratory distress and failure may have caused hypoxia and acidosis in this scenario. Although not required for successful completion of the scenario, the instructor may (if time allows) discuss important elements of post–cardiac arrest care, including titration of inspired oxygen concentration to maintain SpO₂ of 94%-99%; targeted temperature management (especially avoidance or aggressive treatment of fever); hemodynamic support; support of airway, ventilation, and perfusion; and support of neurologic and other end-organ function.

Scenario-Specific Objectives

- **Identifies cardiac arrest with a nonshockable rhythm;** in this scenario, the infant has asystole
- **Describes correct dose and rationale for epinephrine administration**
- **Summarizes potentially reversible causes of asystole;** during the scenario, the student considers possible reversible causes of cardiac arrest (recalled by conditions beginning with H's and T's); in this infant, respiratory distress may have produced hypoxia and acidosis
- **Discusses principles of post–cardiac arrest care;** for this scenario, these include titration of inspired oxygen concentration as tolerated; targeted temperature management (especially prevention of fever); hemodynamic support; support of airway, oxygenation, and ventilation; and support of neurologic and other end-organ function

Evaluate—*Initial Impression* (Pediatric Assessment Triangle)	Identify	Intervene
Appearance • Extremities appear to be limp; no spontaneous movement and no visible reaction to noise **Breathing** • No spontaneous breathing **Circulation** • Cyanotic/pale extremities and lips; severe mottling	• Immediate intervention needed	• Activate the emergency response system. Emergency medical services requests additional assistance if needed. • Check for response (no response), and perform simultaneous check for breathing (none) while checking for brachial pulse (none). • Immediately begin high-quality CPR.

*Could also use as pulseless electrical activity case if needed

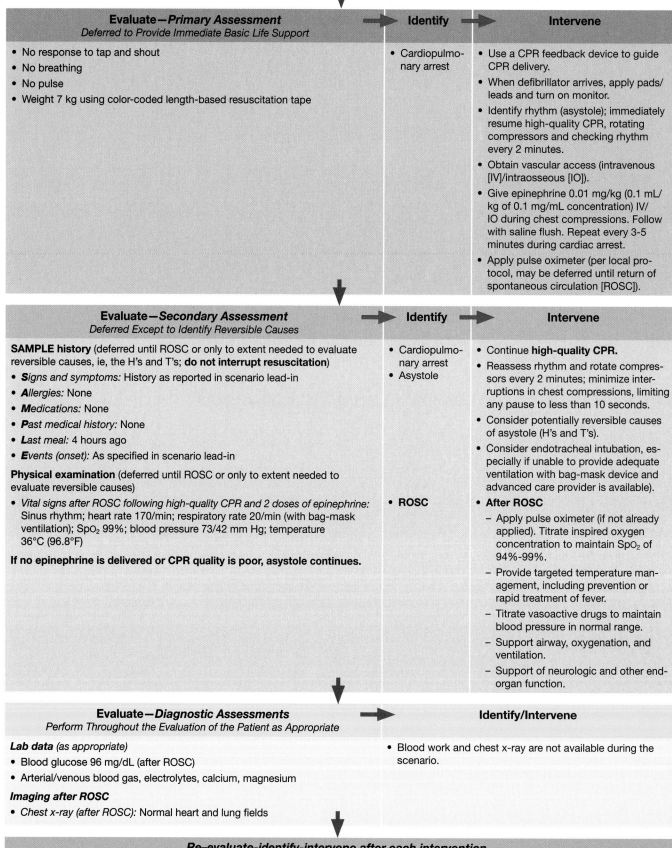

Evaluate—*Primary Assessment* *Deferred to Provide Immediate Basic Life Support*	Identify	Intervene
• No response to tap and shout • No breathing • No pulse • Weight 7 kg using color-coded length-based resuscitation tape	• Cardiopulmonary arrest	• Use a CPR feedback device to guide CPR delivery. • When defibrillator arrives, apply pads/leads and turn on monitor. • Identify rhythm (asystole); immediately resume high-quality CPR, rotating compressors and checking rhythm every 2 minutes. • Obtain vascular access (intravenous [IV]/intraosseous [IO]). • Give epinephrine 0.01 mg/kg (0.1 mL/kg of 0.1 mg/mL concentration) IV/IO during chest compressions. Follow with saline flush. Repeat every 3-5 minutes during cardiac arrest. • Apply pulse oximeter (per local protocol, may be deferred until return of spontaneous circulation [ROSC]).

Evaluate—*Secondary Assessment* *Deferred Except to Identify Reversible Causes*	Identify	Intervene

SAMPLE history (deferred until ROSC or only to extent needed to evaluate reversible causes, ie, the H's and T's; **do not interrupt resuscitation**)
• *Signs and symptoms:* History as reported in scenario lead-in
• *Allergies:* None
• *Medications:* None
• *Past medical history:* None
• *Last meal:* 4 hours ago
• *Events (onset):* As specified in scenario lead-in
 	
Physical examination (deferred until ROSC or only to extent needed to evaluate reversible causes)
• *Vital signs after ROSC following high-quality CPR and 2 doses of epinephrine:* Sinus rhythm; heart rate 170/min; respiratory rate 20/min (with bag-mask ventilation); SpO$_2$ 99%; blood pressure 73/42 mm Hg; temperature 36°C (96.8°F)
 	
If no epinephrine is delivered or CPR quality is poor, asystole continues.
	• Cardiopulmonary arrest
	• Asystole
	
	• ROSC
		• Continue **high-quality CPR.**
		• Reassess rhythm and rotate compressors every 2 minutes; minimize interruptions in chest compressions, limiting any pause to less than 10 seconds.
		• Consider potentially reversible causes of asystole (H's and T's).
		• Consider endotracheal intubation, especially if unable to provide adequate ventilation with bag-mask device and advanced care provider is available).
		• **After ROSC**
		  – Apply pulse oximeter (if not already applied). Titrate inspired oxygen concentration to maintain SpO$_2$ of 94%-99%.
		  – Provide targeted temperature management, including prevention or rapid treatment of fever.
		  – Titrate vasoactive drugs to maintain blood pressure in normal range.
		  – Support airway, oxygenation, and ventilation.
		  – Support of neurologic and other end-organ function.

Evaluate—*Diagnostic Assessments* *Perform Throughout the Evaluation of the Patient as Appropriate*	Identify/Intervene
Lab data (as appropriate) • Blood glucose 96 mg/dL (after ROSC) • Arterial/venous blood gas, electrolytes, calcium, magnesium *Imaging after ROSC* • Chest x-ray (after ROSC): Normal heart and lung fields	• Blood work and chest x-ray are not available during the scenario.

Re–evaluate-identify-intervene after each intervention.

Debriefing Tool
Practice Case Scenario 5
Asystole (Infant; Arrest)

Action	Gather	Analyze	Summarize
- Identifies cardiac arrest - Directs immediate initiation of high-quality CPR with the use of a feedback device (if available) - Applies monitor leads/pads and activation of monitor - Identifies asystole - Directs establishment of IV or IO access - Directs preparation and administration of 0.01 mg/kg epinephrine (0.1 mL/kg of 0.1 mg/mL concentration) IV/IO bolus at appropriate intervals - Directs checking rhythm approximately every 2 minutes while minimizing interruptions in chest compressions - Identifies at least 3 potential reversible causes of pulseless electrical activity (recalled by the H's and T's) - Performs appropriate reassessments	***Student Observations*** - Can you describe the events from your perspective? - How well do you think your treatments worked? - Can you review the events of the scenario (*directed to the Timer/Recorder*)? - What could you have improved? - What did the team do well? ***Instructor Observations*** - I noticed that [*insert action here*]. - I observed that [*insert action here*]. - I saw that [*insert action here*].	***Done Well*** - How were you able to [*insert action here*]? - Why do you think you were able to [*insert action here*]? - Tell me a little more about how you [*insert action here*]. ***Needs Improvement*** - Why do you think [*insert action here*] occurred? - How do you think [*insert action here*] could have been improved? - What was your thinking while [*insert action here*]? - What prevented you from [*insert action here*]?	***Student-Led Summary*** - What are the main things you learned? - Can someone summarize the key points made? - What are the main take-home messages? ***Instructor-Led Summary*** - Let's summarize what we learned… - Here is what I think we learned… - The main take-home messages are… - Of the potential reversible causes of asystole in this patient, which are most likely? (Answer: Hypoxia) - Although not covered in this scenario, what are the key elements of post–cardiac arrest care? (Answer should include titration of oxygen; targeted temperature management; hemodynamic support and support of airway, oxygenation, and ventilation; and support of neurologic and other end-organ function.)

Pulseless Electrical Activity
(Child; Arrest)

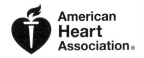

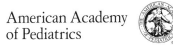

Scenario Lead-in

Prehospital: You are dispatched to a house where a 3-year-old child is now unresponsive. Prescription pills, including his grandmother's oral hypoglycemic agent, are scattered throughout the child's room.

ED: An ambulance is en route to the emergency department with a 3-year-old child who was found unresponsive in his bed. Prescription pills, including his grandmother's oral hypoglycemic agent, were scattered throughout the child's room.

General Inpatient Unit: You are called as a member of the rapid response team to see a 3 year old who was admitted with lethargy; he has now become limp and unresponsive. Emergency medical services had found prescription pills, including his grandmother's oral hypoglycemic agent, scattered throughout the child's room.

ICU: You are called to see a 3 year old who was admitted with lethargy; he now has become progressively limp and unresponsive. Emergency medical services found prescription pills, including his grandmother's oral hypoglycemic agent, scattered throughout the child's room.

Vital Signs	
Heart rate	CPR in progress
Blood pressure	CPR in progress
Respiratory rate	100% bag-mask ventilation (CPR)
SpO₂	Not obtainable
Temperature	Deferred
Weight	17 kg
Age	3 years

Scenario Overview and Learning Objectives

Scenario Overview

This scenario focuses on the identification and management of the child with cardiac arrest and a "nonshockable" rhythm. Emphasis is placed on immediate delivery of high-quality CPR and early administration of epinephrine. The student should identify potential causes of pulseless electrical activity (PEA) (H's and T's). The child has significant hypoglycemia that must be corrected, and other drug toxicities may be present (the team must identify the drugs collected by emergency medical services [EMS] providers). Although not required for successful completion of the scenario, the instructor may (if time allows) discuss important elements of post–cardiac arrest care, including titration of inspired oxygen concentration to maintain SpO₂ of 94%-99%; targeted temperature management (especially avoidance or aggressive treatment of fever); hemodynamic support; support of airway, ventilation, and perfusion; and support of neurologic and other end-organ function.

Scenario-Specific Objectives

- **Identifies cardiac arrest with a nonshockable rhythm;** in this scenario, the child has PEA
- **Describes correct dose and rationale for epinephrine administration**
- **Summarizes potentially reversible causes of PEA;** during the scenario, the student/provider considers possible reversible causes of cardiac arrest (recalled by conditions beginning with H's and T's); in this child, significant hypoglycemia and possible other toxic drugs have contributed to the arrest
- **Discuss principles of post–cardiac arrest care;** these include titration of inspired oxygen concentration as tolerated; targeted temperature management (especially prevention of fever); hemodynamic support; support of airway, oxygenation, and ventilation; and support of neurologic and other end-organ function

Evaluate—*Initial Impression* *(Pediatric Assessment Triangle)*	Identify	Intervene
Appearance • Appears to be limp; no spontaneous movement and no visible reaction to noise **Breathing** • No spontaneous breathing **Circulation** • Cyanotic/pale extremities and lips; severe mottling	• Immediate intervention needed	• Activate the emergency response system. Emergency medical services requests additional assistance if needed. • Check for response (no response), and perform simultaneous check for breathing (none) while checking for carotid pulse (none). • Immediately begin high-quality CPR.

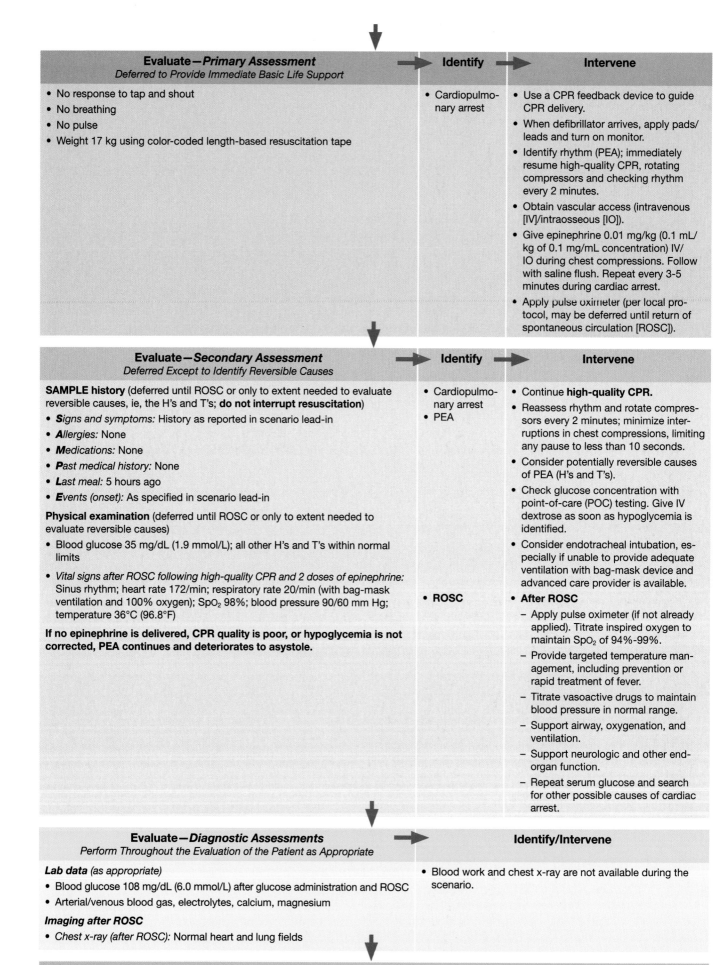

Evaluate—*Primary Assessment*
Deferred to Provide Immediate Basic Life Support

Identify

Intervene

- No response to tap and shout
- No breathing
- No pulse
- Weight 17 kg using color-coded length-based resuscitation tape

- Cardiopulmonary arrest

- Use a CPR feedback device to guide CPR delivery.
- When defibrillator arrives, apply pads/leads and turn on monitor.
- Identify rhythm (PEA); immediately resume high-quality CPR, rotating compressors and checking rhythm every 2 minutes.
- Obtain vascular access (intravenous [IV]/intraosseous [IO]).
- Give epinephrine 0.01 mg/kg (0.1 mL/kg of 0.1 mg/mL concentration) IV/IO during chest compressions. Follow with saline flush. Repeat every 3-5 minutes during cardiac arrest.
- Apply pulse oximeter (per local protocol, may be deferred until return of spontaneous circulation [ROSC]).

Evaluate—*Secondary Assessment*
Deferred Except to Identify Reversible Causes

Identify

Intervene

SAMPLE history (deferred until ROSC or only to extent needed to evaluate reversible causes, ie, the H's and T's; **do not interrupt resuscitation**)
- *Signs and symptoms:* History as reported in scenario lead-in
- *Allergies:* None
- *Medications:* None
- *Past medical history:* None
- *Last meal:* 5 hours ago
- *Events (onset):* As specified in scenario lead-in

Physical examination (deferred until ROSC or only to extent needed to evaluate reversible causes)
- Blood glucose 35 mg/dL (1.9 mmol/L); all other H's and T's within normal limits
- *Vital signs after ROSC following high-quality CPR and 2 doses of epinephrine:* Sinus rhythm; heart rate 172/min; respiratory rate 20/min (with bag-mask ventilation and 100% oxygen); SpO₂ 98%; blood pressure 90/60 mm Hg; temperature 36°C (96.8°F)

If no epinephrine is delivered, CPR quality is poor, or hypoglycemia is not corrected, PEA continues and deteriorates to asystole.

- Cardiopulmonary arrest
- PEA

- ROSC

- Continue **high-quality CPR.**
- Reassess rhythm and rotate compressors every 2 minutes; minimize interruptions in chest compressions, limiting any pause to less than 10 seconds.
- Consider potentially reversible causes of PEA (H's and T's).
- Check glucose concentration with point-of-care (POC) testing. Give IV dextrose as soon as hypoglycemia is identified.
- Consider endotracheal intubation, especially if unable to provide adequate ventilation with bag-mask device and advanced care provider is available.
- **After ROSC**
  - Apply pulse oximeter (if not already applied). Titrate inspired oxygen to maintain SpO₂ of 94%-99%.
  - Provide targeted temperature management, including prevention or rapid treatment of fever.
  - Titrate vasoactive drugs to maintain blood pressure in normal range.
  - Support airway, oxygenation, and ventilation.
  - Support neurologic and other end-organ function.
  - Repeat serum glucose and search for other possible causes of cardiac arrest.

Evaluate—*Diagnostic Assessments*
Perform Throughout the Evaluation of the Patient as Appropriate

Identify/Intervene

Lab data *(as appropriate)*
- Blood glucose 108 mg/dL (6.0 mmol/L) after glucose administration and ROSC
- Arterial/venous blood gas, electrolytes, calcium, magnesium

Imaging after ROSC
- *Chest x-ray (after ROSC):* Normal heart and lung fields

- Blood work and chest x-ray are not available during the scenario.

Re–evaluate-identify-intervene after each intervention.

Debriefing Tool
Practice Case Scenario 6
PEA (Child; Arrest)

General Debriefing Principles

- Use the table below to guide your debriefing; also refer to the **Team Dynamics Debriefing Tool.**
- Debriefings are 10 minutes long.
- Address all learning objectives.
- Summarize take-home messages at the end of the debriefing.
- *Encourage:* Students to self-reflect
    - Engagement of all participants
- *Avoid:* Mini-lectures and closed-ended questions
    - Dominating the discussion

General Management Objectives

- Uses the PALS Systematic Approach Algorithm to assess and appropriately classify a patient
- Provides oxygen appropriately
- Directs delivery of high-quality CPR (including the use of a feedback device) when indicated
- Demonstrates basic airway maneuvers and use of relevant airway device as appropriate
- Demonstrates application of cardiac and respiratory monitors
- Identifies the cardiac rhythm
- Applies appropriate PBLS or PALS algorithms
- Summarizes general indications, contraindications, and doses of relevant drugs
- Discusses principles of family-centered care in pediatric cardiac arrest
- Applies the 8 elements of effective team dynamics
- Performs frequent reassessment

Action	Gather	Analyze	Summarize
	Student Observations	*Done Well*	*Student-Led Summary*
- Identifies cardiac arrest - Directs immediate initiation of high-quality CPR with the use of a feedback device (if available) - Applies cardiac monitor and pulse oximeter - Identifies PEA - Directs establishment of IV or IO access - Directs preparation and administration of 0.01 mg/kg (0.1 mL/kg of 0.1 mg/mL concentration) epinephrine IV/IO bolus at appropriate intervals - Directs checking rhythm on monitor approximately every 2 minutes while minimizing interruptions in chest compressions - Identifies at least 3 potential reversible causes of PEA (recalled by the H's and T's) - Checks glucose early with POC testing because child likely ingested hypoglycemic agent - Performs appropriate reassessments	- Can you describe the events from your perspective? - How well do you think your treatments worked? - Can you review the events of the scenario (*directed to the Timer/Recorder*)? - What could you have improved? - What did the team do well?	- How were you able to [*insert action here*]? - Why do you think you were able to [*insert action here*]? - Tell me a little more about how you [*insert action here*].	- What are the main things you learned? - Can someone summarize the key points made? - What are the main take-home messages?
	Instructor Observations	*Needs Improvement*	*Instructor-Led Summary*
	- I noticed that [*insert action here*]. - I observed that [*insert action here*]. - I saw that [*insert action here*].	- Why do you think [*insert action here*] occurred? - How do you think [*insert action here*] could have been improved? - What was your thinking while [*insert action here*]? - What prevented you from [*insert action here*]?	- Let's summarize what we learned… - Here is what I think we learned… - The main take-home messages are… - Of the potential reversible causes of PEA in this patient, which are most likely? (Answer: Hypoglycemia, perhaps other electrolyte imbalances) - Although not covered in this scenario, what are the key elements of post–cardiac arrest care? (Answer should include titration of oxygen; targeted temperature management; hemodynamic support and support of airway, oxygenation, and ventilation; and support of neurologic and other end-organ function.)

Lung Tissue (Parenchymal) Disease (Infant)

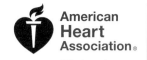

American Heart Association®
life is why™

American Academy of Pediatrics
DEDICATED TO THE HEALTH OF ALL CHILDREN™

Scenario Lead-in

Prehospital: You respond to a 6 month old in respiratory distress.

ED: Emergency medical services providers arrive with a 6-month-old boy brought from home with respiratory distress.

General Inpatient Unit: You are called to the room of a 6-month-old boy being directly admitted for respiratory distress.

PICU: You are called to the room of a 6-month-old boy just admitted to the intensive care unit for respiratory distress.

Vital Signs	
Heart rate	160/min
Blood pressure	90/60 mm Hg
Respiratory rate	80/min
SpO_2	82% on room air
Temperature	39.2°C (102.5°F)
Weight	6 kg
Age	6 months

Scenario Overview and Learning Objectives

Scenario Overview

Emphasis in this scenario is on rapid recognition of respiratory failure associated with lung tissue (parenchymal) disease. Recognition of signs of respiratory failure (including significant respiratory effort, hypoxemia despite high-flow supplementary oxygen, decreased level of consciousness, and cyanosis) should prompt immediate initiation of appropriate therapy, starting with administration of 100% oxygen and bag-mask ventilation. The provider should quickly consult a provider with advanced expertise when the infant fails to improve. This infant needs intubation and mechanical ventilation by an expert in the care of children with respiratory failure. Pediatric intensive care unit (PICU) care is required. During debriefing, the method to estimate endo-tracheal tube size (cuffed and uncuffed) is discussed. Although not required for successful completion of the scenario, the possible use of continuous positive airway pressure (CPAP) or noninvasive ventilation can be addressed with emphasis that such therapy must be provided in appropriate settings where continuous monitoring is provided and intubation equipment and appropriate provider expertise are readily available.

Scenario-Specific Objectives

- **Distinguishes between respiratory distress and respiratory failure;** in this scenario, the infant's clinical signs are consistent with respiratory failure

- **Identifies signs and symptoms of lung tissue disease in a pediatric patient;** in this scenario, the signs of lung tissue disease include tachypnea, increased respiratory effort, grunting, crackles (rales), tachycardia, and hypoxemia despite oxygen administration

- **Implements correct interventions for lung tissue disease;** in this scenario, those interventions include administration of a high concentration of oxygen, appropriate monitoring, reassessing the infant, and advancing to more support of oxygenation and ventilation when the infant fails to improve

- **Recalls the common causes of lung tissue disease;** common causes include pneumonia and aspiration

Evaluate—*Initial Impression* (Pediatric Assessment Triangle)	Identify	Intervene
Appearance • Lethargic **Breathing** • Shallow, rapid respirations; grunting **Circulation** • Pale skin; cyanosis	• Immediate intervention needed	• Administer 100% oxygen by nonre-breathing face mask. • Apply cardiac monitor. • Apply pulse oximeter.

Evaluate—*Primary Assessment* Focused on Assessment Needed to Support Airway, Oxygenation, Ventilation, and Perfusion	Identify	Intervene
• **A**irway: Unobstructed but noisy; grunting • **B**reathing: Shallow, rapid respirations; mild intercostal and subcostal retractions; bilateral crackles; no stridor or wheezing; expiratory phase is not prolonged; respiratory rate 80/min; SpO_2 82% on room air and increased to 88% on 100% oxygen via a nonrebreathing face mask • **C**irculation: Heart rate 160/min; pale skin; cyanosis; strong central and peripheral pulses; capillary refill 2 seconds; blood pressure 90/60 mm Hg • **D**isability: Lethargic; arousable by voice • **E**xposure: Temperature 39.2°C (102.5°F); weight 6 kg	• Respiratory failure • Lung tissue disease	• Assess response to oxygen. • Provide bag-mask ventilation with 100% oxygen.

Evaluate—*Secondary Assessment*	**Identify**	**Intervene**
Identify Reversible Causes, but Defer Remainder of Secondary Assessment Until After Stabilization of Airway, Oxygenation, and Ventilation		

SAMPLE history

- **S**igns and symptoms: Sudden onset of respiratory distress after an episode of vomiting; no previous cold symptoms or cough
- **A**llergies: None known
- **M**edications: Metoclopramide
- **P**ast medical history: None
- **L**ast meal: 2 hours ago
- **E**vents (onset): Previously well other than history of severe gastroesophageal reflux

Physical examination

- *Repeat vital signs after bag-mask ventilation with 100% oxygen:* Respiratory rate 24/min; heart rate 160/min; SpO_2 96% with bag-mask ventilation; blood pressure 100/70 mm Hg
- *Head, eyes, ears, nose, and throat/neck:* Normal
- *Heart and lungs:* Diminished breath sounds; bilateral diffuse crepitations
- *Abdomen:* Normal
- *Extremities:* Normal
- *Back:* Normal
- *Neurologic:* Lethargic; becoming less responsive and more difficult to arouse

Identify

- Respiratory distress
- Lung tissue disease

Intervene

- Continue bag-mask ventilation.
- Contact a more-advanced provider with appropriate expertise.
  - *Note:* If the child's level of consciousness improves and continuous monitoring is provided, critical care providers may consider use of noninvasive ventilation support (CPAP or noninvasive positive-pressure ventilation) *if* there is equipment and appropriate expertise for rapid intubation immediately available.
- Obtain vascular access.
- Obtain arterial/venous blood gas.
- Check glucose with point-of-care (POC) testing.
- Prepare equipment and skilled personnel for endotracheal intubation using a cuffed tracheal tube.
- Treat fever with antipyretics.
- Arrange transfer of the child to an intensive care unit (ICU) (unless the child is already in the ICU).
- Consider specific interventions for lung tissue disease (eg, antibiotics for suspected pneumonia).

Evaluate—*Diagnostic Assessments*	**Identify/Intervene**
Perform Throughout the Evaluation of the Patient as Appropriate	

Lab data

- Glucose (POC testing) 136 mg/dL (7.5 mmol/L)
- Complete blood count, blood culture, arterial/venous blood gas pending

Imaging

- Chest x-ray

Identify/Intervene

- Laboratory tests generally are not appropriate during the first 5-10 minutes when attempting to stabilize a hypoxemic child with severe respiratory distress/respiratory failure.
- A blood glucose concentration should be checked as soon as reasonably possible in all critically ill infants and children. Hypoglycemia should be treated immediately.
- Chest x-ray shows diffuse bilateral airspace disease.

Re–evaluate-identify-intervene after each intervention.

Debriefing Tool
Practice Case Scenario 7
Lung Tissue (Parenchymal) Disease (Infant)

General Debriefing Principles

- Use the table below to guide your debriefing; also refer to the **Team Dynamics Debriefing Tool.**
- Debriefings are 10 minutes long.
- Address all learning objectives.
- Summarize take-home messages at the end of the debriefing.
- *Encourage:* Students to self-reflect
  Engagement of all participants
- *Avoid:* Mini-lectures and closed-ended questions
  Dominating the discussion

General Management Objectives

- Uses the PALS Systematic Approach Algorithm to assess and appropriately classify a patient
- Provides oxygen appropriately
- Directs delivery of high-quality CPR (including the use of a feedback device) when indicated
- Demonstrates basic airway maneuvers and use of relevant airway device as appropriate
- Demonstrates application of cardiac and respiratory monitors

- Identifies the cardiac rhythm
- Applies appropriate PBLS or PALS algorithms
- Summarizes general indications, contraindications, and doses of relevant drugs
- Discusses principles of family-centered care in pediatric cardiac arrest
- Applies the 8 elements of effective team dynamics
- Performs frequent reassessment

Action	Gather	Analyze	Summarize
• Directs assessment of ABCDE and vital signs • Directs administration of 100% oxygen via nonrebreathing face mask and evaluates response • Establishes cardiac monitoring and pulse oximeter • Identifies respiratory failure • Identifies signs of lung tissue disease • Reassesses child and identifies need for additional intervention (beyond administration of 100% oxygen via nonrebreathing face mask) • Provides or directs bag-mask ventilation • Directs establishment of intravenous or intraosseous access • Performs frequent reassessment of patient • Identifies need for involvement of advanced provider with expertise in pediatric intubation and mechanical ventilation • Summarizes specific interventions for lung tissue disease • Identifies indications for endotracheal intubation	***Student Observations*** • Can you describe the events from your perspective? • How well do you think your treatments worked? • Can you review the events of the scenario (*directed to the Timer/Recorder*)? • What could you have improved? • What did the team do well? ***Instructor Observations*** • I noticed that [*insert action here*]. • I observed that [*insert action here*]. • I saw that [*insert action here*].	***Done Well*** • How were you able to [*insert action here*]? • Why do you think you were able to [*insert action here*]? • Tell me a little more about how you [*insert action here*]. ***Needs Improvement*** • Why do you think [*insert action here*] occurred? • How do you think [*insert action here*] could have been improved? • What was your thinking while [*insert action here*]? • What prevented you from [*insert action here*]?	***Student-Led Summary*** • What are the main things you learned? • Can someone summarize the key points made? • What are the main take-home messages? ***Instructor-Led Summary*** • Let's summarize what we learned… • Here is what I think we learned… • The main take-home messages are… • This infant requires intubation. How will you estimate the appropriate cuffed endotracheal tube size? • Can you explain why CPAP or noninvasive positive-pressure ventilation might improve this child's oxygenation? (Answer: It will increase alveolar ventilation and ventilation-perfusion match.) Discuss why it is important that such care be provided in a setting where continuous monitoring of the child is possible and appropriate expertise is immediately available.

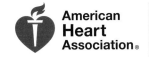

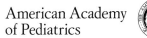

DEDICATED TO THE HEALTH OF ALL CHILDREN™

Vital Signs	
Heart rate	130/min
Blood pressure	80/30 mm Hg
Respiratory rate	35/min
SpO$_2$	93% on room air
Temperature	39.0°C (102.2°F)
Weight	41 kg
Age	12 years

Scenario Lead-in

Prehospital: You are dispatched to transport a 12-year-old girl with a 24-hour history of high fever and lethargy. She has become progressively more confused in the last hour.

ED: Parents arrive with their 12-year-old girl who has a 24-hour history of high fever and lethargy. She has become progressively more confused in the last hour.

General Inpatient Unit: You have just received a 12-year-old girl directly admitted to the ward from her physician's office. She has a 24-hour history of high fever and lethargy. She has become progressively more confused in the last hour. You are unable to establish intravenous access.

ICU: You are called to the bedside of a 12-year-old girl who has been admitted to the intensive care unit with a 24-hour history of high fever and lethargy. She has become progressively more confused in the last hour. The intravenous access placed at the time of admission has infiltrated.

Scenario Overview and Learning Objectives

Scenario Overview

Emphasis should be on identification of hypotensive distributive/septic shock. Priorities include immediate establishment of intravenous (IV)/ intraosseous (IO) access and administration of fluid bolus(es) of isotonic crystalloid with careful reassessment of cardiorespiratory function during and after each fluid bolus. The provider should be able to discuss the importance of detection of signs of heart failure and need to stop bolus fluid administration if such signs develop. Within the first hour of identification of signs of septic shock, providers must give bolus fluid therapy, administer antibiotics, and initiate vasoactive drug therapy (if shock persists despite bolus fluids). The provider should also make plans to transfer child to an appropriate setting (unless child is already in the intensive care unit [ICU]).

Scenario-Specific Objectives

- **Recognizes hypotensive vs compensated shock;** in this scenario, the child has hypotensive shock
- **Recognizes need for early/rapid intervention with bolus administration of isotonic crystalloids and vasoactive drug therapy within the first hour if shock signs/symptoms persist despite bolus fluid administration**
- **Recognizes the need for careful and frequent cardiorespiratory reassessment during and after each fluid bolus;** the provider looks for signs of heart failure (increased respiratory distress or development of rales or hepatomegaly) and the need to stop bolus fluid administration if signs of heart failure develop
- **Recognizes need for early/rapid administration of antibiotics (during the first hour after identification of shock symptoms)**

Evaluate—*Initial Impression* *(Pediatric Assessment Triangle)*	Identify	Intervene
Appearance • Lethargic; irritable; mumbling **Breathing** • Increased rate, but no distress **Circulation** • Pale and mottled	• Immediate intervention needed	• Activate the emergency response system. Emergency medical services requests additional assistance if needed. • Administer 100% oxygen by nonrebreathing face mask. • Apply cardiac monitor. • Apply pulse oximeter.

Evaluate—*Primary Assessment* *Focused on Assessment Needed to Support Airway, Oxygenation, Ventilation, and Perfusion*	Identify	Intervene

• **A**irway: Clear
• **B**reathing: Respiratory rate about 35/min; SpO$_2$ 93% on room air, increased to 97% with administration of 100% oxygen; lungs clear to auscultation
• **C**irculation: Heart rate 130/min; central pulses good, peripheral pulses bounding; flash capillary refill (less than 1 second); warm, but mottled hands and feet; blood pressure 80/30 mm Hg
• **D**isability: Lethargic; mumbling; confused
• **E**xposure: Rectal temperature 39.0°C (102.2°F); petechial-purpuric rash over extremities and torso; weight 41 kg
	• Hypotensive shock (likely septic shock)
	• Sinus tachycardia
		• Obtain vascular access (IV/IO).
		• Administer a 20 mL/kg bolus of isotonic crystalloid IV/IO.
		  – Reassess during and after fluid bolus.
		  – Stop fluid bolus if signs of heart failure develop (eg, development of respiratory distress rales or hepatomegaly).
		• Administer antibiotics (if not already done) within first hour of recognition of shock. If possible, obtain blood culture before antibiotic administration, but don't delay antibiotic or fluid administration.
		• Check point-of-care (POC) glucose and treat hypoglycemia if needed.

Evaluate—Secondary Assessment	**Identify**	**Intervene**
Identify Reversible Causes, but Defer Remainder of Secondary Assessment Until Hypotension Corrected		

SAMPLE history (only to extent needed to evaluate reversible causes)

- **S**igns and symptoms: Fever and lethargy for 24 hours
- **A**llergies: None known
- **M**edications: None
- **P**ast medical history: Previously well
- **L**ast meal: No oral intake for 6 hours
- **E**vents (onset): 24-hour history of fever and increasing lethargy; noted to be confused in last 2 hours

Physical examination

- *Repeat vital signs after oxygen and fluids:* Heart rate 122/min; respiratory rate 35/min; SpO₂ 100% with 100% inspired oxygen; blood pressure 84/32 mm Hg
- *Head, eyes, ears, nose, and throat/neck:* Mucous membranes slightly dry; neck supple
- *Heart and lungs:* Rapid rate; no extra heart sounds or murmurs; lungs sound clear
- *Abdomen:* No palpable liver edge; nondistended; nontender; normal bowel sounds
- *Extremities:* Warm hands and feet; mottled; bounding peripheral pulses
- *Back:* Normal
- *Neurologic:* Lethargic; pupils 4 mm, equal, reactive

Identify:

- Hypotensive distributive/ septic shock

Intervene:

- If signs of shock persist, repeat fluid bolus of 20 mL/kg of isotonic crystalloid IV/IO as needed. Reassess during and after each fluid bolus.
  - Stop fluid bolus if signs of heart failure develop (eg, development of respiratory distress, rales, or hepatomegaly).
- Begin vasoactive drug therapy within first hour of the recognition of shock if systemic perfusion fails to improve after bolus fluid therapy.
  - Consider administration of epinephrine infusion (or dopamine, if epinephrine is not available).
- Ensure that bolus fluid therapy, administration of antibiotics, and initiation of vasoactive therapy (if shock is fluid refractory) are all accomplished within the first hour after the identification of signs of septic shock.
- Assess response to oxygen administration.
- Arrange for transfer to ICU for closer monitoring if child is not already in ICU.

Evaluate—Diagnostic Assessments	**Identify/Intervene**
Perform Throughout the Evaluation of the Patient as Appropriate	

Lab data

- *Capillary gas:* pH 7.16; PCO₂ 20 mm Hg; PO₂ 20 mm Hg; base deficit/excess −10; lactate 5.0 mmol/L; hemoglobin 11 g/dL
- *Glucose (POC)* 185 mg/dL (10.3 mmol/L)
- *Pending:* Electrolytes, blood urea nitrogen/creatinine, calcium, complete blood count with differential, prothrombin time/international normalized ratio/partial thromboplastin time
- *Cultures:* Blood, urine

Imaging

- *Chest x-ray:* Small heart, clear lung fields

Identify/Intervene:

- The blood glucose concentration should be checked with POC testing whenever the infant or child is critically ill. Hypoglycemia should be treated immediately.
- Metabolic acidosis with partial respiratory compensation should correct if shock resuscitation is effective.

Re–evaluate-identify-intervene after each intervention.

Debriefing Tool

Practice Case Scenario 8
Distributive Shock (Adolescent; Septic Shock)

General Debriefing Principles

- Use the table below to guide your debriefing; also refer to the **Team Dynamics Debriefing Tool.**
- Debriefings are 10 minutes long.
- Address all learning objectives.
- Summarize take-home messages at the end of the debriefing.
- *Encourage:* Students to self-reflect
  Engagement of all participants
- *Avoid:* Mini-lectures and closed-ended questions
  Dominating the discussion

General Management Objectives

- Uses the PALS Systematic Approach Algorithm to assess and appropriately classify a patient
- Provides oxygen appropriately
- Directs delivery of high-quality CPR (including the use of a feedback device) when indicated
- Demonstrates basic airway maneuvers and use of relevant airway device as appropriate
- Demonstrates application of cardiac and respiratory monitors

- Identifies the cardiac rhythm
- Applies appropriate PBLS or PALS algorithms
- Summarizes general indications, contraindications, and doses of relevant drugs
- Discusses principles of family-centered care in pediatric cardiac arrest
- Applies the 8 elements of effective team dynamics
- Performs frequent reassessment

Action	Gather	Analyze	Summarize
• Directs assessment of ABCDE and vital signs • Administers 100% oxygen • Applies cardiac monitor and pulse oximeter • Identifies signs and symptoms of distributive (septic) shock in an adolescent • Categorizes shock as hypotensive • Directs establishment of IV or IO access • Directs rapid administration of a 20 mL/kg fluid bolus of isotonic crystalloid • Reassesses the patient during and in response to interventions, particularly during and after each fluid bolus; stops fluid bolus if signs of heart failure develop • Repeats fluid bolus as needed to treat shock with careful reassessment during and after each fluid bolus • Checks glucose with POC testing early in the care of the lethargic infant • Directs early (ie, within first hour after identification of shock signs) administration of antibiotics • Directs initiation of vasoactive drug therapy within the first hour after the recognition of shock if shock fails to respond to fluid boluses • Verbalizes therapeutic end points during shock management (normalization of heart rate and blood pressure; improvement in peripheral perfusion, mental status, and urine output)	***Student Observations*** • Can you describe the events from your perspective? • How well do you think your treatments worked? • Can you review the events of the scenario (*directed to the Timer/Recorder*)? • What could you have improved? • What did the team do well? ***Instructor Observations*** • I noticed that [*insert action here*]. • I observed that [*insert action here*]. • I saw that [*insert action here*].	***Done Well*** • How were you able to [*insert action here*]? • Why do you think you were able to [*insert action here*]? • Tell me a little more about how you [*insert action here*]. ***Needs Improvement*** • Why do you think [*insert action here*] occurred? • How do you think [*insert action here*] could have been improved? • What was your thinking while [*insert action here*]? • What prevented you from [*insert action here*]?	***Student-Led Summary*** • What are the main things you learned? • Can someone summarize the key points made? • What are the main take-home messages? ***Instructor-Led Summary*** • Let's summarize what we learned… • Here is what I think we learned… • The main take-home messages are… • What are the therapeutic end points during shock management? (Answer: Normalized heart rate; improved peripheral perfusion, mental status, and urine output; normalized blood pressure; correction of metabolic/lactic acidosis)

Supraventricular Tachycardia
(Adolescent; Unstable)

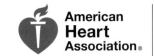
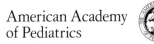

Vital Signs	
Heart rate	235/min
Blood pressure	75/55 mm Hg
Respiratory rate	34/min
SpO$_2$	92% on room air
Temperature	37.6°C (99.7°F)
Weight	50 kg
Age	12 years

Scenario Lead-in

Prehospital: You are dispatched to a house where a 12-year-old boy has lethargy, tachypnea, and a racing heart.

ED: An ambulance is en route to the emergency department with a 12-year-old boy with lethargy, tachypnea, and a racing heart.

General Inpatient Unit: You are called to examine a 12-year-old boy with lethargy, tachypnea, and a racing heart.

ICU: You are called to the bedside of a 12-year-old boy who says he has a racing heart and now has lethargy.

Scenario Overview and Learning Objectives

Scenario Overview

Emphasis should be on diagnosis and management of supraventricular tachycardia (SVT) in an unstable patient, including possible rapid bolus administration of adenosine (only if intravenous [IV]/intraosseous [IO] access is readily available) and the safe delivery of synchronized cardioversion using appropriate doses. Vagal maneuvers may be performed while preparing adenosine or while preparing for synchronized cardioversion but should not delay intervention. If time allows, the instructor may briefly discuss the need for expert consultation before administering a precardioversion sedative to a child with hemodynamic instability.

Scenario-Specific Objectives

- **Differentiates between SVT and sinus tachycardia;** in this scenario, the child has unstable SVT
- **Describes potential vagal maneuvers used for a child with SVT;** potential maneuvers used in children include blowing through an obstructed straw and carotid sinus massage
- **Demonstrates the proper rapid bolus technique to administer adenosine**
- **Discusses indications for synchronized cardioversion;** in this scenario, the child has poor perfusion, including hypotension, acutely altered mental status (new lethargy), and signs of shock
- **Demonstrates safe delivery of synchronized cardioversion with appropriate dose in a patient with SVT and poor perfusion**

Evaluate—*Initial Impression* *(Pediatric Assessment Triangle)*	Identify	Intervene
Appearance • Moaning; minimal response to caregivers **Breathing** • Increased rate and effort, including nasal flaring **Circulation** • Pale and mottled	• Immediate intervention needed	• Activate the emergency response system. Emergency medical services requests additional assistance if needed. • Administer 100% oxygen by nonrebreathing face mask. • Apply cardiac monitor. • Apply pulse oximeter.

Evaluate—*Primary Assessment* *Focused on Assessment Needed to Support Airway, Oxygenation, Ventilation, and Perfusion*	Identify	Intervene

• **A**irway: Clear
• **B**reathing: Respiratory rate 34/min; SpO$_2$ 92% before supplementary oxygen and 100% after; crackles throughout lung fields
• **C**irculation: Heart rate 235/min; weak central pulses, thready peripheral pulses; cool/mottled skin; capillary refill about 6 seconds; blood pressure 75/55 mm Hg
• **D**isability: Deferred until after successful rhythm conversion
• **E**xposure: Temperature 37.6°C (99.7°F); weight 50 kg
	• Altered level of consciousness
	• Narrow-complex tachycardia/SVT with a pulse and poor perfusion
	• Respiratory distress vs respiratory failure
	• *Hypotensive shock*
		• Establish IV/IO access if possible but **do not delay cardioversion if IV/IO access is not readily available.**
		• Guide child to perform vagal maneuvers **if they do not delay adenosine or cardioversion.**
		• If functional IV is in place or is established immediately, administer adenosine.
		  – Begin recording continuous rhythm strip.
		  – Give adenosine 0.1 mg/kg (max 6 mg) IV/IO by rapid bolus followed by rapid saline flush.

Evaluate—*Primary Assessment* *Focused on Assessment Needed to Support Airway, Oxygenation, Ventilation, and Perfusion*	Identify	Intervene
		– If first dose of adenosine is unsuccessful, administer adenosine 0.2 mg/kg rapid bolus (max 12 mg), if it can be given more rapidly than synchronized cardioversion. Ensure that rapid bolus technique is used to administer the drug. – If adenosine is ineffective, provide immediate synchronized cardioversion. • Deliver synchronized cardioversion as soon as it is available, unless other therapies (eg, adenosine) have worked by the time synchronized cardioversion can be delivered. (*Note:* Do not delay cardioversion to attempt other therapies if synchronized cardioversion can be provided immediately.) – If functional IV/IO access and expertise is immediately available, provide sedation before cardioversion *if it won't delay cardioversion*. Use caution; expertise is required to avoid worsening hemodynamic instability. – As soon as a monitor/defibrillator arrives, attach pads and begin recording rhythm strip. – "Clear" and perform synchronized cardioversion (0.5 to 1 J/kg). – If synchronized cardioversion is unsuccessful, "clear" and perform synchronized cardioversion with 2 J/kg. • Prepare to assist ventilation (with bag-mask device) if needed.

Evaluate—*Secondary Assessment* *Deferred Until After Rhythm Conversion*	Identify	Intervene
SAMPLE history • **S**igns and symptoms: Tachycardia; lethargy; hypotension • **A**llergies: None known • **M**edications: None • **P**ast medical history: History of SVT about 4 years ago • **L**ast meal: Ate 6 hours ago • **E**vents (onset): Acute onset 30 minutes ago **Physical examination** • *Repeat vital signs after successful rhythm conversion:* Heart rate 104/min; sinus rhythm; respiratory rate 28/min; SpO$_2$ 100% on 100% oxygen by non-rebreathing mask; blood pressure 100/60 mm Hg • *Head, eyes, ears, nose, and throat/neck:* Clear; no audible breath sounds • *Heart and lungs:* Sinus rhythm; central and peripheral pulses strong; capillary refill 3 seconds; no murmur, gallop, or rub appreciated; fine scattered crackles at bases on auscultation • *Abdomen:* Liver not palpable below the costal margin • *Extremities:* Cool peripherally • *Back:* Unremarkable • *Neurologic:* Cries out in pain with cardioversion; opens eyes and moves spontaneously, answering questions with single words or short phrases • Point-of-care (POC) glucose concentration (see below) **If no rhythm conversion or delay in administering adenosine or cardioversion** • *Vital signs:* Heart rate 235/min; weak central pulses, peripheral pulses barely palpable; cool/mottled skin; capillary refill about 6 seconds; respiratory rate 34/min; SpO$_2$ 93% despite 100% oxygen via nonrebreathing mask; crackles throughout lung fields; blood pressure 72/54 mm Hg	• SVT with poor perfusion converts to sinus rhythm if rapid adenosine or cardioversion is provided.	• **After rhythm conversion** – Reassess and monitor patient's cardiorespiratory status. – Evaluate for signs of heart failure (enlarged liver, extra heart sounds or murmurs, crackles/rales). – Prepare to insert advanced airway if needed. – Wean supplementary oxygen as tolerated if child stabilizes. – Obtain 12-lead electrocardiogram (ECG). – Check glucose with POC testing.

Evaluate—*Diagnostic Assessments*	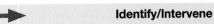 Identify/Intervene
Perform Throughout the Evaluation of the Patient as Appropriate	

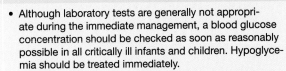

Lab data
- Blood glucose
- Electrolytes

Imaging
- Chest x-ray, 12-lead ECG in SVT and in sinus rhythm

- Although laboratory tests are generally not appropriate during the immediate management, a blood glucose concentration should be checked as soon as reasonably possible in all critically ill infants and children. Hypoglycemia should be treated immediately.

- Laboratory studies (other than POC glucose testing) are deferred until rhythm is converted and systemic perfusion and hemodynamic function are improved.

Re–evaluate-identify-intervene after each intervention.

Debriefing Tool
Practice Case Scenario 9
SVT (Adolescent; Unstable)

General Debriefing Principles

- Use the table below to guide your debriefing; also refer to the **Team Dynamics Debriefing Tool.**
- Debriefings are 10 minutes long.
- Address all learning objectives.
- Summarize take-home messages at the end of the debriefing.
- *Encourage:* Students to self-reflect
  Engagement of all participants
- *Avoid:* Mini-lectures and closed-ended questions
  Dominating the discussion

General Management Objectives

- Uses the PALS Systematic Approach Algorithm to assess and appropriately classify a patient
- Provides oxygen appropriately
- Directs delivery of high-quality CPR (including the use of a feedback device) when indicated
- Demonstrates basic airway maneuvers and use of relevant airway device as appropriate
- Demonstrates application of cardiac and respiratory monitors

- Identifies the cardiac rhythm
- Applies appropriate PBLS or PALS algorithms
- Summarizes general indications, contraindications, and doses of relevant drugs
- Discusses principles of family-centered care in pediatric cardiac arrest
- Applies the 8 elements of effective team dynamics
- Performs frequent reassessment

Action	Gather	Analyze	Summarize
• Directs assessment of ABCDE and vital signs • Applies cardiac monitor and pulse oximeter • Directs administration of supplementary oxygen • Identifies rhythm as SVT with a pulse and poor perfusion and distinguishes it from sinus tachycardia • Describes how to perform appropriate vagal maneuvers for a child • Directs establishment of IV/IO access if it will not delay synchronized cardioversion • Directs preparation and rapid bolus administration of appropriate dose of adenosine • Directs safe delivery of attempted cardioversion at dose of 0.5 J/kg; if ineffective, increases dose to 2 J/kg • Performs frequent reassessments after each intervention	***Student Observations*** • Can you describe the events from your perspective? • How well do you think your treatments worked? • Can you review the events of the scenario (*directed to the Timer/Recorder*)? • What could you have improved? • What did the team do well? ***Instructor Observations*** • I noticed that [*insert action here*]. • I observed that [*insert action here*]. • I saw that [*insert action here*].	***Done Well*** • How were you able to [*insert action here*]? • Why do you think you were able to [*insert action here*]? • Tell me a little more about how you [*insert action here*]. ***Needs Improvement*** • Why do you think [*insert action here*] occurred? • How do you think [*insert action here*] could have been improved? • What was your thinking while [*insert action here*]? • What prevented you from [*insert action here*]?	***Student-Led Summary*** • What are the main things you learned? • Can someone summarize the key points made? • What are the main take-home messages? ***Instructor-Led Summary*** • Let's summarize what we learned… • Here is what I think we learned… • The main take-home messages are… • Ask students to state the indications for synchronized cardioversion. • If time allows, discuss need for expert consultation before administering precardioversion sedative to child with SVT and hemodynamic instability.

Wide-Complex Tachycardia, Possible Ventricular Tachycardia
(Infant; Stable)

American Heart Association
life is why™

American Academy of Pediatrics
DEDICATED TO THE HEALTH OF ALL CHILDREN™

Vital Signs	
Heart rate	220/min
Blood pressure	96/54 mm Hg
Respiratory rate	36/min
SpO$_2$	97% while receiving 30% oxygen by face mask
Temperature	Afebrile
Weight	6 kg
Age	3 months

Scenario Lead-in

Prehospital: You are en route to a call for a 3-month-old infant with irritability and cold-like symptoms.

ED: You are called to the emergency department to help out with a 3-month-old infant with irritability and cold-like symptoms.

General Inpatient Unit: You are called to the bedside of a 3-month-old infant who was admitted with irritability and cold-like symptoms.

ICU: You are called to see a 3-month-old infant who was admitted to the intensive care unit for a respiratory distress episode earlier in the day.

Scenario Overview and Learning Objectives

Scenario Overview

Emphasis should be on the recognition of wide-complex tachycardia in a stable patient and consideration of adenosine (if rhythm regular and QRS is monomorphic). In addition, providers should search for and treat reversible causes (eg, hypokalemia or hyperkalemia). Provision of synchronized cardioversion and administration of antiarrhythmics are beyond the scope of this scenario, but discussion regarding indications for synchronized cardioversion, including appropriate dose and safe delivery, should occur after completing the scenario. Expert consultation with a pediatric cardiologist is strongly recommended before such interventions because expertise is required to minimize potential negative hemodynamic effects.

Scenario-Specific Objectives

- **Differentiates between ventricular tachycardia (VT) and supraventricular tachycardia (SVT) with a pulse and poor perfusion;** in this scenario, the child's wide-complex tachycardia is probably VT
- **Differentiates between pulseless VT and wide-complex tachycardia (possible VT) with a pulse**
- **Describes the indications for synchronized cardioversion in VT;** in this scenario, the infant has respiratory distress but no hypotension, acutely altered mental status or signs of shock, so does not require immediate synchronized cardioversion
- **Discusses possible administration of adenosine;** in this scenario, the wide complexes are in regular rhythm and QRS morphology is monomorphic, so adenosine can be considered
- **Describes safe delivery of synchronized cardioversion (if needed) with appropriate dose in an infant with VT and a pulse**
- **Discusses reason that expert consultation is advised before performing synchronized cardioversion in a stable child with VT**

Evaluate—*Initial Impression* (Pediatric Assessment Triangle) → Identify → Intervene

Appearance
- Awake; crying

Breathing
- Spontaneous; nasal congestion; no increased work of breathing apparent

Circulation
- Pale skin

Identify
- No immediate intervention needed

Intervene
- Proceed to Primary Assessment.

Evaluate—*Primary Assessment* → Identify → Intervene

- **A**irway: Crying
- **B**reathing: Upper airway congestion; bilateral air entry; no use of accessory muscles; no nasal flaring; respiratory rate 36/min; SpO$_2$ 97% when receiving 30% oxygen by face mask
- **C**irculation: Heart rate 220/min; blood pressure 96/54 mm Hg; pale skin; capillary refill 3 seconds; strong central pulses, palpable peripheral pulses; QRS complexes are regular and monomorphic
- **D**isability: Awake; fussy; eyes open
- **E**xposure: Afebrile; weight 6 kg

Identify
- Wide-complex tachycardia (possible VT) with a pulse and adequate perfusion (stable)
- Regular, monomorphic complexes

Intervene
- Activate the emergency response system. Emergency medical services requests additional assistance if needed.
- Administer supplementary oxygen if needed.
- Apply cardiac monitor.
- Apply pulse oximeter.
- Identify rhythm: wide-complex tachycardia (possible VT) with a pulse and adequate perfusion.
- Obtain 12-lead electrocardiogram (ECG).
- Search for and treat reversible causes.
- Obtain vascular access (intravenous [IV]).

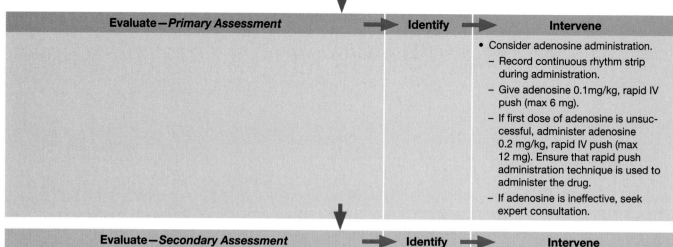

Evaluate—*Primary Assessment*	Identify	Intervene

		• Consider adenosine administration.
		  – Record continuous rhythm strip during administration.
		  – Give adenosine 0.1mg/kg, rapid IV push (max 6 mg).
		  – If first dose of adenosine is unsuccessful, administer adenosine 0.2 mg/kg, rapid IV push (max 12 mg). Ensure that rapid push administration technique is used to administer the drug.
		  – If adenosine is ineffective, seek expert consultation.

Evaluate—*Secondary Assessment*

SAMPLE history

- **S**igns and symptoms: Fussy; agitated since early morning
- **A**llergies: None
- **M**edications: None
- **P**ast medical history: Delivery at 39 weeks; no problems
- **L**ast meal: 1 oz formula 4 hours ago
- **E**vents: Admitted to floor 6 hours ago with fussiness, agitation, and cold-like symptoms

Physical examination

- *Repeat vital signs (adenosine has no effect):* Heart rate 218/min (wide-complex tachycardia persists); blood pressure 96/56 mm Hg; respiratory rate 24/min; SpO$_2$ 97% on room air
- *Head, eyes, ears, nose, and throat/neck:* Normal
- *Heart and lungs:* No murmur, gallop, or rub; lungs clear; capillary refill 3 seconds; peripheral pulses weak
- *Abdomen:* Nondistended; nontender; no masses; normal bowel sounds; no hepatomegaly
- *Extremities:* No edema; no rash; cool hands and feet
- *Back:* Normal
- *Neurologic:* Pupils equal and reactive equal

If sedation and/or cardioversion undertaken without expert consultation

- *Vital signs:* Heart rate 218/min; wide-complex tachycardia persists; blood pressure 64/38 mm Hg; development of signs of heart failure and poor perfusion

Identify

- Persistent stable, wide-complex tachycardia with a pulse and adequate perfusion

Intervene

- Monitor cardiorespiratory function for signs of heart failure (enlarged liver, extra heart sounds or murmurs, crackles/rales).
- Search for and treat reversible causes.
- Obtain 12-lead ECG.
- Wean supplementary oxygen as tolerated.

Evaluate—*Diagnostic Assessments*
Perform Throughout the Evaluation of the Patient as Appropriate

Identify/Intervene

Lab data

- Blood glucose
- Electrolytes
- A blood gas (arterial, venous, or capillary blood gas) not indicated in the immediate management of this infant, but could be considered after stabilization to guide further management

Imaging

- Not indicated

- Although laboratory tests are generally not appropriate during the immediate management, a blood glucose concentration should be checked with point-of-care testing as soon as reasonable in all critically ill children. Hypoglycemia should be treated immediately.
- Serum electrolytes should also be checked as soon as possible. An electrolyte abnormality such hypokalemia or hyperkalemia may cause ventricular arrhythmias.

Re–evaluate-identify-intervene after each intervention.

Debriefing Tool
Practice Case Scenario 10
Wide-Complex Tachycardia, Possible VT (Infant; Stable)

General Management Objectives

- Uses the PALS Systematic Approach Algorithm to assess and appropriately classify a patient
- Provides oxygen appropriately
- Directs delivery of high-quality CPR (including the use of a feedback device) when indicated
- Demonstrates basic airway maneuvers and use of relevant airway device as appropriate
- Demonstrates application of cardiac and respiratory monitors
- Identifies the cardiac rhythm
- Applies appropriate PBLS or PALS algorithms
- Summarizes general indications, contraindications, and doses of relevant drugs
- Discusses principles of family-centered care in pediatric cardiac arrest
- Applies the 8 elements of effective team dynamics
- Performs frequent reassessment

Action	Gather	Analyze	Summarize
• Directs assessment of ABCDE and vital signs • Applies cardiac monitor and pulse oximeter • Directs administration of supplementary oxygen • Identifies VT with a pulse and stable perfusion • Directs establishment of IV access • Identifies when it would be appropriate to obtain expert consultation • Discusses preparation and administration of correct doses of adenosine using rapid bolus technique • Explains the rationale for expert consultation before synchronized cardioversion or antiarrhythmics if stable wide-complex tachycardia fails to respond to adenosine • States the reason it is important to search for and treat reversible causes of wide-complex tachycardias • Performs frequent reassessment	***Student Observations*** • Can you describe the events from your perspective? • How well do you think your treatments worked? • Can you review the events of the scenario (*directed to the Timer/Recorder*)? • What could you have improved? • What did the team do well? ***Instructor Observations*** • I noticed that [*insert action here*]. • I observed that [*insert action here*]. • I saw that [*insert action here*].	***Done Well*** • How were you able to [*insert action here*]? • Why do you think you were able to [*insert action here*]? • Tell me a little more about how you [*insert action here*]. ***Needs Improvement*** • Why do you think [*insert action here*] occurred? • How do you think [*insert action here*] could have been improved? • What was your thinking while [*insert action here*]? • What prevented you from [*insert action here*]?	***Student-Led Summary*** • What are the main things you learned? • Can someone summarize the key points made? • What are the main take-home messages? ***Instructor-Led Summary*** • Let's summarize what we learned… • Here is what I think we learned… • The main take-home messages are… • The patient in this scenario did not require synchronized cardioversion. Please describe the indications for synchronized cardioversion, the appropriate first and second energy doses, and how to safely deliver synchronized cardioversion.

Practice Case Scenario 11
Wide-Complex Tachycardia (Possible Ventricular Tachycardia) With a Pulse and Poor Perfusion
(Child; Unstable)

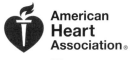

American Heart Association®
life is why™

American Academy of Pediatrics
DEDICATED TO THE HEALTH OF ALL CHILDREN™

Scenario Lead-in

Prehospital: You are en route to a house where a 10-year-old child has acutely developed difficulty breathing.

ED: You are called to the emergency department to help out when a 10-year-old child is brought in after acutely developing difficulty breathing.

General Inpatient Unit: You are called as a member of the rapid response team to see a 10-year-old child who acutely developed difficulty breathing.

ICU: You are called to see a 10-year-old child who was admitted to the intensive care unit for a syncopal episode earlier in the day; he is now having acute difficulty breathing.

Vital Signs	
Heart rate	185/min
Blood pressure	74/35 mm Hg
Respiratory rate	46/min
SpO₂	82% on room air
Temperature	37.6°C (99.7°F)
Weight	30 kg
Age	10 years

Scenario Overview and Learning Objectives

Scenario Overview

*Emphasis should be on diagnosis and management of unstable wide-complex tachycardia to convert the rhythm and improve systemic perfusion and hemodynamic function. This is accomplished immediately with synchronized cardioversion. If functional intravenous (IV)/intraosseous (IO) access has been established or can be established **immediately** and expertise is available, sedation may be provided. However, synchronized cardioversion should not be delayed. Providers should also search for and treat reversible causes. Expert consultation is advised. Administration of adenosine or other antiarrhythmics is beyond the scope of this scenario, but discussion regarding indications for adenosine and vagal maneuvers will verify student familiarity with treatment of other tachycardias with a pulse (eg, supraventricular tachycardia [SVT] with a pulse and adequate perfusion).*

Scenario-Specific Objectives

- Differentiates between narrow-complex (likely SVT) and wide-complex tachycardia/possible ventricular tachycardia (VT) with a pulse and poor perfusion
- Differentiates between pulseless VT and wide-complex tachycardia (possible VT) with a pulse
- Describes the indications for synchronized cardioversion for wide-complex tachycardia with a pulse and poor perfusion; in this scenario, the child demonstrates hypotension, acutely altered mental status, and signs of shock—these are indications for immediate synchronized cardioversion
- Demonstrates safe delivery of synchronized cardioversion with appropriate shock dose in a patient with wide-complex tachycardia with a pulse
- Describes the reason for caution and need for expertise when considering giving sedative before cardioversion for a child who has tachycardia with a pulse and poor perfusion

---

Evaluate—*Initial Impression* (Pediatric Assessment Triangle)	Identify	Intervene
Appearance • Lethargic; opens eyes to voice but not talking spontaneously **Breathing** • Spontaneous, rapid rate; significant retractions; grunting **Circulation** • Pale; mottled	• Immediate intervention needed	• Activate the emergency response system. Emergency medical services requests additional assistance if needed. • Administer 100% oxygen by nonrebreathing face mask. • Apply cardiac monitor or monitor/defibrillator. • Apply pulse oximeter.

Evaluate—*Primary Assessment* Focused on Assessment Needed to Support Airway, Oxygenation, Ventilation, and Perfusion	Identify	Intervene
• **A**irway: Clear • **B**reathing: Respiratory rate 46/min; SpO₂ 82% (improves to 94% with 100% oxygen via nonrebreathing mask); subcostal and intercostal retractions; nasal flaring • **C**irculation: Heart rate 185/min; blood pressure 74/35 mm Hg; central pulses weak, peripheral pulses very weak; cool peripherally; capillary refill 4-5 seconds • **D**isability: Opens eyes to voice; intermittently moaning • **E**xposure: Temperature 37.6°C (99.7°F); weight 30 kg	• Altered level of consciousness • Wide-complex tachycardia, possible VT, with a pulse and poor perfusion	• Obtain vascular access (IV/IO), but **do not delay cardioversion.** • Deliver synchronized cardioversion as soon as monitor/defibrillator arrives: – *If functional IV/IO access and expertise is immediately available, provide sedation if it won't delay cardioversion. Use caution; expertise is required to avoid worsening hemodynamic instability.*

Evaluate—*Primary Assessment*	**Identify**	**Intervene**

Focused on Assessment Needed to Support Airway, Oxygenation, Ventilation, and Perfusion	• Participant may also note
	  – Respiratory distress vs respiratory failure
	  – Hypotensive shock
		– Attach pads and begin recording rhythm strip.
		– "Clear" and perform synchronized cardioversion (0.5-1 J/kg).
		– If initial synchronized cardioversion is unsuccessful, immediately "clear" and perform synchronized cardioversion with 2 J/kg.

Evaluate—*Secondary Assessment*	**Identify**	**Intervene**

Identify Reversible Causes, but Defer Remainder of Secondary Assessment Until Rhythm Conversion	• Altered level of consciousness
	• Wide-complex tachycardia (possible VT) with a pulse and poor perfusion converts to sinus rhythm if synchronized cardioversion provided correctly
	• Respiratory distress vs respiratory failure
		• Obtain expert consultation.
		• Search for and treat reversible causes.
		• **After rhythm conversion**
		  – Reassess and monitor cardiorespiratory status.
		  – Evaluate for signs of heart failure (enlarged liver, extra heart sounds or murmurs, crackles).
		  – Assist ventilation with bag-mask device if needed.
		  – Prepare to insert advanced airway if needed.
		  – Wean supplementary oxygen as tolerated if child remains stable after cardioversion.
		  – Obtain 12-lead electrocardiogram (ECG).
		  – Check glucose with point-of-care testing.

SAMPLE history (review with parent/primary caretaker only to identify reversible causes)

- **S**igns and symptoms: Developed acute shortness of breath and difficulty breathing; no chest pain; no recent illnesses
- **A**llergies: None
- **M**edications: None
- **P**ast medical history: Fractured clavicle at age 6
- **L**ast meal: Supper with family
- **E**vents: Sudden shortness of breath and difficulty breathing

Physical examination if cardioversion correctly performed

- *Repeat vital signs postcardioversion:* Heart rate 124/min; sinus rhythm; respiratory rate 28/min; SpO$_2$ 97% with 100% oxygen via nonrebreathing mask; blood pressure 105/78 mm Hg
- *Head, eyes, ears, nose, and throat/neck:* Clear; no abnormal audible breath sounds
- *Heart and lungs:* No murmur, gallop, or rub; subcostal and intercostal retractions less pronounced; breath sounds equal bilaterally; no wheezes or crackles; central pulses now strong; peripheral pulses; capillary refill 3 seconds
- *Abdomen:* Nondistended; nontender; no masses; normal bowel sounds
- *Extremities:* Warming
- *Back:* Normal
- *Neurologic:* Pupils equal and reactive; now opens eyes and moves all extremities spontaneously; answers healthcare providers' questions
- *Point-of-care glucose:* 88 mg/dL

If no cardioversion

- *Vital signs:* Heart rate 185/min; blood pressure 68/33 mm Hg; worsening perfusion (weak central and very faint peripheral pulses); capillary refill 6-7 seconds

Evaluate—*Diagnostic Assessments*	**Identify/Intervene**
Perform Throughout the Evaluation of the Patient as Appropriate	

Lab data

- *Blood glucose:* 88 mg/dL
- Electrolytes
- A blood gas (arterial, venous, or capillary blood gas) and electrolytes not indicated in the immediate management of this child, but could be considered after stabilization to guide further management

Imaging

- Chest x-ray (evaluate for cardiomegaly, pulmonary edema, or effusions)
- Repeat ECG

- Although laboratory tests are generally not appropriate during the immediate management, a blood glucose concentration should be checked as soon as reasonably possible in all critically ill infants and children. Hypoglycemia should be treated immediately.
- Serum electrolytes should also be checked as soon as possible. An electrolyte abnormality such hypokalemia or hyperkalemia may cause ventricular arrhythmias.

Re–evaluate-identify-intervene after each intervention.

Debriefing Tool
Practice Case Scenario 11
Wide-Complex Tachycardia (Possible VT) With a Pulse and Poor Perfusion
(Child; Unstable)

General Management Objectives

- Uses the PALS Systematic Approach Algorithm to assess and appropriately classify a patient
- Provides oxygen appropriately
- Directs delivery of high-quality CPR (including the use of a feedback device) when indicated
- Demonstrates basic airway maneuvers and use of relevant airway device as appropriate
- Demonstrates application of cardiac and respiratory monitors
- Identifies the cardiac rhythm
- Applies appropriate PBLS or PALS algorithms
- Summarizes general indications, contraindications, and doses of relevant drugs
- Discusses principles of family-centered care in pediatric cardiac arrest
- Applies the 8 elements of effective team dynamics
- Performs frequent reassessment

Action	Gather	Analyze	Summarize
• Directs assessment of ABCDE and vital signs • Applies cardiac monitor and pulse oximeter • Directs administration of supplementary (100%) oxygen • Identifies wide-complex tachycardia with a pulse and poor perfusion • Identifies the need for prompt synchronized cardioversion and is able to deliver it or help others do so • Directs establishment of IV or IO access provided it does not delay cardioversion • Identifies the need and rational for obtaining expert consultation to provide sedation before cardioversion attempt • Directs safe delivery of attempted cardioversion at dose of 0.5 J/kg; if ineffective, increases dose to 2 J/kg • States the reason it is important to search for and treat reversible causes of wide-complex tachycardias • Performs frequent reassessments after each intervention	***Student Observations*** • Can you describe the events from your perspective? • How well do you think your treatments worked? • Can you review the events of the scenario (*directed to the Timer/Recorder*)? • What could you have improved? • What did the team do well? ***Instructor Observations*** • I noticed that [*insert action here*]. • I observed that [*insert action here*]. • I saw that [*insert action here*].	***Done Well*** • How were you able to [*insert action here*]? • Why do you think you were able to [*insert action here*]? • Tell me a little more about how you [*insert action here*]. ***Needs Improvement*** • Why do you think [*insert action here*] occurred? • How do you think [*insert action here*] could have been improved? • What was your thinking while [*insert action here*]? • What prevented you from [*insert action here*]?	***Student-Led Summary*** • What are the main things you learned? • Can someone summarize the key points made? • What are the main take-home messages? ***Instructor-Led Summary*** • Let's summarize what we learned… • Here is what I think we learned… • The main take-home messages are… • What are the indications for synchronized cardioversion in a child with tachycardia and a pulse and poor perfusion? (Answer: Hypotension, acutely altered mental status, signs of shock) • Although this patient had unstable wide-complex tachycardia, what interventions would be appropriate if this child demonstrated stable, narrow-complex tachycardia? (Answers: Vagal maneuvers, adenosine [first dose 0.1 mg/kg rapid bolus, maximum 6 mg; second dose 0.2 mg/kg rapid bolus) • If this child had no central pulses, how would you treat the child? (Answer: As cardiac arrest with shockable rhythm)

Pulseless Arrest, Pulseless Ventricular Tachycardia
(Infant; Arrest)

American Heart Association®
life is why™

American Academy of Pediatrics
DEDICATED TO THE HEALTH OF ALL CHILDREN™

Scenario Lead-in

Prehospital: You are dispatched to a home where a 6 month old suddenly became gray and apneic. Babysitter called 9-1-1 and initiated CPR.

ED: An ambulance is en route with a 6-month-old infant who suddenly became limp and gray. CPR is in progress.

General Inpatient Unit: You are called as a member of the rapid response team to see a 6 month old who suddenly became limp and gray. The infant was admitted for observation following a period of apnea. CPR is in progress.

ICU: You are called to see a 6 month old who suddenly became limp and gray. Patient was admitted following a period of apnea. CPR is in progress.

Vital Signs	
Heart rate	CPR in progress
Blood pressure	CPR in progress
Respiratory rate	Bag-mask ventilation (CPR)
SpO₂	Not obtainable
Temperature	Deferred
Weight	8 kg
Age	6 months

Scenario Overview and Learning Objectives

Scenario Overview

This scenario focuses on the identification and management of cardiac arrest and a "shockable" rhythm. Emphasis is placed on immediate delivery of high-quality CPR and integration of shock delivery while minimizing interruptions in CPR. One shock followed by CPR, and then (when pulseless ventricular tachycardia [VT] persists) a second shock followed by CPR + epinephrine, and then (when pulseless VT persists) a third shock followed by CPR + antiarrhythmic (amiodarone or lidocaine) are administered before return of spontaneous circulation (ROSC). Identification of potential causes (H's and T's) should be discussed during debriefing.

Insertion of advanced airway and post-ROSC care are beyond the scope this scenario. Post-ROSC care is addressed with the asystole scenario.

Scenario-Specific Objectives

- **Identifies cardiac arrest with a shockable rhythm;** in this scenario, the infant has pulseless VT
- **Demonstrates safe shock delivery with appropriate dose and minimal interruption of chest compressions;** the correct initial dose is 2 J/kg, second shock is 4 J/kg, and subsequent doses are at least 4 J/kg (maximum 10 J/kg or adult dose for the defibrillator)
- **Describes correct dose and rationale for epinephrine administration**
- **Uses appropriate antiarrhythmic in ventricular fibrillation (VF)/ pulseless VT;** the 2015 AHA Guidelines Update for CPR and ECC noted that either amiodarone or lidocaine is equally acceptable
- **Identifies reversible causes of persistent pulseless VT;** during the debriefing, the student should be asked to recall possible reversible causes of cardiac arrest (recalled by conditions beginning with H's and T's)

Evaluate—*Initial Impression* (Pediatric Assessment Triangle)	Identify	Intervene
Appearance • Extremities appear to be limp; no spontaneous movement and no visible reaction to noise **Breathing** • No spontaneous breathing **Circulation** • Cyanotic/pale extremities and lips; overall gray color	• Immediate intervention needed	• Activate the emergency response system. Emergency medical services requests additional assistance if needed. • Check for response (no response) and perform simultaneous check for breathing (none) and brachial pulse (none). • Immediately begin high-quality CPR.

Evaluate—*Primary Assessment* Deferred to Initiate Immediate Basic Life Support, and Then Focused on Assessment Needed to Support Airway, Oxygenation, Ventilation, and Perfusion	Identify	Intervene
• Should verify airway, breathing, and circulation support • Monitor reveals pulseless VT • Weight 8 kg per color-coded length-based resuscitation tape	• Cardiopulmonary arrest • Pulseless VT cardiac arrest	• Use a CPR feedback device, if available, to guide CPR delivery. • When defibrillator arrives, apply pads/leads and turn on monitor. • Identify rhythm (pulseless VT, shockable). • Attempt defibrillation with 2 J/kg as soon as possible. • Resume high-quality CPR immediately after shock delivery. • Obtain vascular access (intravenous [IV]/intraosseous [IO]). • Apply pulse oximeter (per local protocol, may be deferred until return of spontaneous circulation [ROSC]).

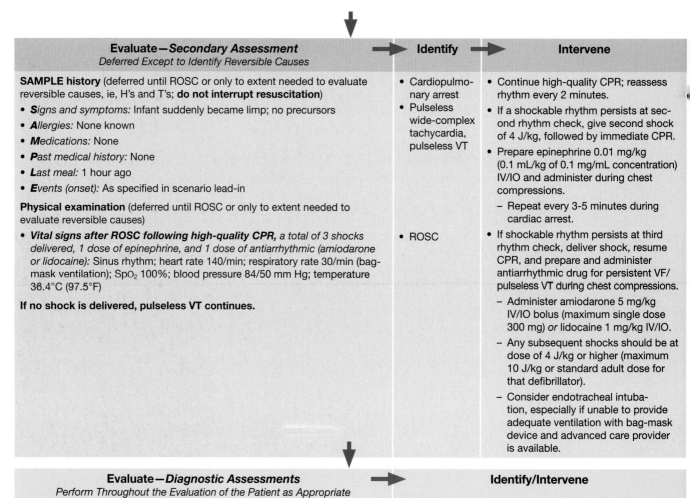

Evaluate—*Secondary Assessment* *Deferred Except to Identify Reversible Causes*	Identify	Intervene

SAMPLE history (deferred until ROSC or only to extent needed to evaluate reversible causes, ie, H's and T's; **do not interrupt resuscitation**)
 	
 • *Signs and symptoms:* Infant suddenly became limp; no precursors
 • *Allergies:* None known
 • *Medications:* None
 • *Past medical history:* None
 • *Last meal:* 1 hour ago
 • *Events (onset):* As specified in scenario lead-in
 	
 Physical examination (deferred until ROSC or only to extent needed to evaluate reversible causes)
 	
 • *Vital signs after ROSC following high-quality CPR, a total of 3 shocks delivered, 1 dose of epinephrine, and 1 dose of antiarrhythmic (amiodarone or lidocaine):* Sinus rhythm; heart rate 140/min; respiratory rate 30/min (bag-mask ventilation); SpO$_2$ 100%; blood pressure 84/50 mm Hg; temperature 36.4°C (97.5°F)
 	
 If no shock is delivered, pulseless VT continues.
	• Cardiopulmonary arrest
	 • Pulseless wide-complex tachycardia, pulseless VT
	
	 • ROSC
		• Continue high-quality CPR; reassess rhythm every 2 minutes.
		 • If a shockable rhythm persists at second rhythm check, give second shock of 4 J/kg, followed by immediate CPR.
		 • Prepare epinephrine 0.01 mg/kg (0.1 mL/kg of 0.1 mg/mL concentration) IV/IO and administer during chest compressions.
		  – Repeat every 3-5 minutes during cardiac arrest.
		 • If shockable rhythm persists at third rhythm check, deliver shock, resume CPR, and prepare and administer antiarrhythmic drug for persistent VF/pulseless VT during chest compressions.
		  – Administer amiodarone 5 mg/kg IV/IO bolus (maximum single dose 300 mg) *or* lidocaine 1 mg/kg IV/IO.
		  – Any subsequent shocks should be at dose of 4 J/kg or higher (maximum 10 J/kg or standard adult dose for that defibrillator).
		  – Consider endotracheal intubation, especially if unable to provide adequate ventilation with bag-mask device and advanced care provider is available.

Evaluate—*Diagnostic Assessments* *Perform Throughout the Evaluation of the Patient as Appropriate*	Identify/Intervene
Lab data *(as appropriate)* • Blood glucose 112 mg/dL (6.2 mmol/L) (after ROSC) • Arterial/venous blood gas, electrolytes, calcium, magnesium **Imaging** • *Chest x-ray (after ROSC):* Normal heart and lung fields	• Blood work and chest x-ray are not available during the scenario.

Re–evaluate-identify-intervene after each intervention.

Debriefing Tool
Practice Case Scenario 12
Pulseless Arrest, Pulseless VT (Infant; Arrest)

General Management Objectives

- Uses the PALS Systematic Approach Algorithm to assess and appropriately classify a patient
- Provides oxygen appropriately
- Directs delivery of high-quality CPR (including the use of a feedback device) when indicated
- Demonstrates basic airway maneuvers and use of relevant airway device as appropriate
- Demonstrates application of cardiac and respiratory monitors

- Identifies the cardiac rhythm
- Applies appropriate PBLS or PALS algorithms
- Summarizes general indications, contraindications, and doses of relevant drugs
- Discusses principles of family-centered care in pediatric cardiac arrest
- Applies the 8 elements of effective team dynamics
- Performs frequent reassessment

Action	Gather	Analyze	Summarize
	Student Observations	***Done Well***	***Student-Led Summary***
- Identifies cardiac arrest - Directs immediate initiation of high-quality CPR with the use of a feedback device (if available) and monitors quality throughout resuscitation - Directs placement of monitor leads/pads and activation of monitor - Identifies pulseless VT cardiopulmonary arrest - Directs safe performance of first shock of 2 J/kg	- Can you describe the events from your perspective? - How well do you think your treatments worked? - Can you review the events of the scenario (*directed to the Timer/Recorder*)? - What could you have improved? - What did the team do well?	- How were you able to [*insert action here*]? - Why do you think you were able to [*insert action here*]? - Tell me a little more about how you [*insert action here*].	- What are the main things you learned? - Can someone summarize the key points made? - What are the main take-home messages?
- After each shock, directs immediate resumption of high-quality CPR, beginning with chest compressions - Directs establishment of IV or IO access - If pulseless VT persists at second rhythm check, directs safe delivery of a second shock, using a dose of 4 J/kg; any subsequent shocks should use a dose of 4 J/kg or higher (maximum 10 J/kg or standard adult dose) - Directs preparation and administration of appropriate IV/IO dose (0.01 mg/kg [0.1 mL/kg of the 0.1 mg/mL concentration]) of epinephrine at appropriate intervals - If VF persists at third rhythm check, directs that antiarrhythmic with appropriate dose (amiodarone 5 mg/kg or lidocaine 1 mg/kg) be administered when compressions resume - Performs appropriate reassessments	***Instructor Observations*** - I noticed that [*insert action here*]. - I observed that [*insert action here*]. - I saw that [*insert action here*].	***Needs Improvement*** - Why do you think [*insert action here*] occurred? - How do you think [*insert action here*] could have been improved? - What was your thinking while [*insert action here*]? - What prevented you from [*insert action here*]?	***Instructor-Led Summary*** - Let's summarize what we learned… - Here is what I think we learned… - The main take-home messages are… - If the infant's VF failed to respond to the therapies given, what else should you consider? (Answer: H's and T's—ie, reversible causes) - If a third shock is needed, what dose is used? (Answer: 4 J/kg or higher; maximum 10 J/kg or standard adult dose for that defibrillator)

Obstructive Shock
(Child; Hypotensive; Tension Pneumothorax)

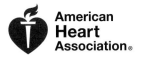
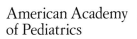

Scenario Lead-in

Prehospital: You are on scene with an 8-year-old boy. He was intubated with an oral-tracheal tube because of depressed mental status, and then he suddenly deteriorated and is being manually ventilated by another care provider. An intravenous catheter is in place.

ED: An 8-year-old boy is being transported by emergency medical services. He has been intubated with an oral-tracheal tube for decreased level of consciousness (a Glasgow Coma Scale Score of 4). He suddenly deteriorated and is being manually ventilated through the endotracheal tube. An intravenous catheter is in place.

General Inpatient Unit: You are called to the room of an 8-year-old boy who was just intubated by the rapid response team for pneumonia and hypoxemia. An oral-tracheal tube was placed. As the team was preparing to transport him to the intensive care unit, the child suddenly deteriorated and is being manually ventilated through the endotracheal tube. An intravenous catheter is in place.

ICU: You are called to the room of an 8-year-old boy who is intubated and mechanically ventilated. He has suddenly deteriorated and is being manually ventilated through the endotracheal tube. An intravenous catheter is in place.

Vital Signs	
Heart rate	140/min
Blood pressure	80/54 mm Hg
Respiratory rate	Manual ventilation
SpO$_2$	68% on 100% oxygen
Temperature	37.2°C (99.0°F)
Weight	20 kg
Age	8 years

Scenario Overview and Learning Objectives

Scenario Overview

*Emphasis is placed on immediate recognition of respiratory failure and signs of obstructive shock. The provider should use the DOPE (**D**isplacement of the tube, **O**bstruction of the tube, **P**neumothorax, **E**quipment failure) mnemonic to quickly identify a tension pneumothorax as the cause and then must perform immediate needle decompression followed by chest tube insertion. Emphasize the importance of performing the needle decompression before obtaining a chest x-ray.*

Scenario-Specific Objectives

- **Recognizes compensated vs hypotensive shock;** this case illustrates hypotensive shock (key indicators in this case include hypotension, tachycardia, and decreased level of consciousness)
- **Summarizes signs and symptoms of obstructive shock;** key indicators in this case include signs of shock combined with evidence of tension pneumothorax
- **Summarizes the elements of the DOPE mnemonic for an intubated patient with sudden deterioration;** in this scenario, displacement of tube, obstruction of tube, and equipment failure should be ruled out before needle decompression
- **Demonstrates correct interventions for tension pneumothorax;** in this scenario, interventions include needle decompression, a chest x-ray, and chest tube insertion
- **Discusses conditions under which fluid bolus administration would be appropriate for treatment of obstructive shock;** although fluid resuscitation is not needed in this scenario, bolus fluid administration may be helpful for cardiac tamponade, until pericardiocentesis can be performed and in massive pulmonary embolus

Evaluate—*Initial Impression* *(Pediatric Assessment Triangle)*	Identify	Intervene
Appearance • No spontaneous movement; flaccid extremities; no visible reaction to noise **Breathing** • Orally intubated; poor chest wall movement with manual ventilation using a resuscitation bag **Circulation** • Pale skin; dusky mucous membranes	• Immediate intervention needed	• Activate the emergency response system. Emergency medical services requests additional assistance if needed. • Continue manual ventilation with 100% oxygen. • Apply cardiac monitor. • Apply pulse oximeter.

Evaluate—*Primary Assessment* *Focused on Assessment Needed to Restore Patent Airway, Oxygenation, Ventilation, and Perfusion*	Identify	Intervene
• **A**irway: Orally intubated with a 6.0 cuffed endotracheal tube (ETT); secured at 18 cm at the lip • **B**reathing: Manually ventilated; asymmetric chest rise, absent breath sounds on the right; increasing inspiratory pressure needed to produce chest expansion; SpO$_2$ 68% despite receiving 100% inspired oxygen. As student evaluates using DOPE mnemonic, provide the following responses to student queries and actions:	• Respiratory failure and hypotensive shock	• Analyze rhythm (sinus tachycardia). • Assess response to oxygen and manual ventilation (no change). • Check waveform capnography (if applicable).

Evaluate—*Primary Assessment* *Focused on Assessment Needed to Support Airway, Oxygenation, Ventilation, and Perfusion*	**Identify**	**Intervene**
– Displacement: Depth of insertion unchanged; breath sounds present on left; exhaled CO_2 still detectable – Obstruction: Normal breath sounds on left; *if ETT is withdrawn slightly to detect and treat possible left main stem intubation, there is no change in the breath sounds, chest rise, or resistance to manual ventilation* – Pneumothorax (consistent with current clinical picture) – Equipment failure: Ruled out by switching to manual ventilation with bag • *Circulation:* Heart rate 140/min; weak pulses; capillary refill 5 seconds; blood pressure 80/54 mm Hg • *Disability:* Unconscious; pupils equal and reactive to light • *Exposure:* Temperature 37.2°C (99.0°F); weight 20 kg	• Probable tension pneumothorax and obstructive shock	• Rule out endotracheal tube displacement and obstruction and equipment failure. • Perform needle decompression on right side (inserting an 18- to 20-gauge over-the-needle catheter over the top of the child's third rib, second intercostal space in the midclavicular line). • Obtain chest x-ray and insert chest tube.

Evaluate—*Secondary Assessment* *Identify Reversible Causes, but Defer Remainder of Secondary Assessment Until Effective Ventilation Established (After Needle Thoracostomy)*	**Identify**	**Intervene**
SAMPLE history (only to extent needed to evaluate reversible causes) • *Signs and symptoms:* Orally intubated for respiratory failure; sudden deterioration • *Allergies:* None known • *Medications:* None • *Past medical history:* None • *Last meal:* Nothing by mouth • *Events (onset):* Sudden deterioration in intubated patient **Physical examination** • *Repeat vital signs after oxygen:* Heart rate 175/min; manual ventilation at 24 breaths/min – If needle decompression performed: SpO_2 85% and rising; blood pressure increases to 110/65 mm Hg; capillary refill 3 seconds – If needle decompression *not* performed: SpO_2 58% and falling; blood pressure becomes undetectable and cardiac arrest develops; capillary refill extremely prolonged • *Head, eyes, ears, nose, and throat/neck* – If needle decompression performed: Normal – If needle decompression *not* performed: Jugular vein distention • *Heart and lungs* – If needle decompression performed: Breath sounds equal bilaterally and there is decreased resistance to manual ventilation – If needle decompression *not* performed: Breath sounds absent on right • *Abdomen:* Normal • *Extremities* – If needle decompression performed: 2+ central and peripheral pulses, capillary refill 3 seconds – If needle decompression *not* performed: No palpable pulses, capillary refill extremely prolonged • *Back:* Normal • *Neurologic:* Unconscious	• Respiratory failure • Hypotensive obstructive shock (corrects when needle decompression performed; if needle decompression is *not* performed, pulseless arrest develops) • Tension pneumothorax	• Reassess cardiorespiratory function (particularly ventilation and perfusion); immediate improvement should be noted following needle decompression. • Verify that intravenous catheter remains patent. • Check glucose with point-of-care (POC) testing. • Arrange for transfer to intensive care unit (ICU) (if child is not already in ICU) for closer monitoring and treatment of underlying conditions.

Evaluate—*Diagnostic Assessments* *Perform Throughout the Evaluation of the Patient as Appropriate*	**Identify/Intervene**
Lab data • *Pending:* Arterial blood gas or venous blood gas **Imaging** • Chest radiograph (should not delay intervention until chest x-ray performed)	• Laboratory diagnostic testing is deferred until treatment of the tension pneumothorax. • A blood glucose concentration should be checked as soon as reasonably possible in all critically ill children, particularly neonates and infants. Hypoglycemia should be treated immediately. • *Note:* Needle decompression is performed before obtaining chest x-ray (ie, the chest x-ray should follow needle decompression but can precede chest tube insertion).

Re–evaluate-identify-intervene after each intervention.

Debriefing Tool
Practice Case Scenario 13
Obstructive Shock (Child; Hypotensive; Tension Pneumothorax)

General Management Objectives

- Uses the PALS Systematic Approach Algorithm to assess and appropriately classify a patient
- Provides oxygen appropriately
- Directs delivery of high-quality CPR (including the use of a feedback device) when indicated
- Demonstrates basic airway maneuvers and use of relevant airway device as appropriate
- Demonstrates application of cardiac and respiratory monitors
- Identifies the cardiac rhythm
- Applies appropriate PBLS or PALS algorithms
- Summarizes general indications, contraindications, and doses of relevant drugs
- Discusses principles of family-centered care in pediatric cardiac arrest
- Applies the 8 elements of effective team dynamics
- Performs frequent reassessment

Action	Gather	Analyze	Summarize
• Assesses ABCDE, including vital signs • Applies cardiac monitor and pulse oximeter • Identifies signs and symptoms of obstructive shock • Categorizes as hypotensive shock • Verbalizes DOPE mnemonic for intubated patient who deteriorates • Identifies tension pneumothorax • Describes performance of needle decompression for tension pneumothorax • Reassesses patient's response to needle decompression	***Student Observations*** • Can you describe the events from your perspective? • How well do you think your treatments worked? • Can you review the events of the scenario (*directed to the Timer/Recorder*)? • What could you have improved? • What did the team do well? ***Instructor Observations*** • I noticed that [*insert action here*]. • I observed that [*insert action here*]. • I saw that [*insert action here*].	***Done Well*** • How were you able to [*insert action here*]? • Why do you think you were able to [*insert action here*]? • Tell me a little more about how you [*insert action here*]. ***Needs Improvement*** • Why do you think [*insert action here*] occurred? • How do you think [*insert action here*] could have been improved? • What was your thinking while [*insert action here*]? • What prevented you from [*insert action here*]?	***Student-Led Summary*** • What are the main things you learned? • Can someone summarize the key points made? • What are the main take-home messages? ***Instructor-Led Summary*** • Let's summarize what we learned… • Here is what I think we learned… • The main take-home messages are… • Name 2 additional causes of obstructive shock. (Answer: Cardiac tamponade, massive pulmonary embolism, and closure of the ductus arteriosus in infants with ductal-dependent congenital heart lesions) • Please highlight key aspects of the management of cardiac tamponade (fluid bolus and pericardiocentesis), massive pulmonary embolus (oxygen, ventilatory support, fluid bolus, and expert consultation) and ductal closure in neonates with ductal-dependent congenital heart disease (prostaglandin infusion and expert consultation).

(continued)

(continued)

Action	Gather	Analyze	Summarize
			• What are the therapeutic end points during shock management? (Answer: Normalized heart rate; improved peripheral perfusion, mental status, and urine output; normalized blood pressure; correction of metabolic/lactic acidosis)

Practice Case Scenario 14

Cardiogenic Shock
(Infant; Cardiomyopathy)

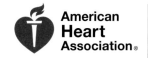

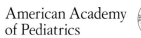

Vital Signs	
Heart rate	180/min
Blood pressure	60/30 mm Hg
Respiratory rate	60/min
SpO$_2$	89% on room air
Temperature	35.7°C (96.2°F)
Weight	7 kg
Age	4 months

Scenario Lead-in

Prehospital: You have been dispatched to transport a 4-month-old female infant with a 48-hour history of respiratory distress.

ED: You are asked to assess and manage a 4-month-old female infant who has increased work of breathing with substernal and intercostal retractions, a breathless cry, and wheezing. She has a 3-day history of respiratory distress and increased lethargy. The infant was seen by her pediatrician 2 days ago for wheezing and respiratory distress and was given steroids and nebulizer treatments with no improvement.

General Inpatient Unit: You are called to assess a 4-month-old female infant who has been admitted to the ward with a 24-hour history of increased work of breathing and increased oxygen requirement.

ICU: You are called to the bedside of a 4-month-old female infant who has been admitted to the intensive care unit with a 24-hour history of increased respiratory distress. She has crackles and wheezing and an increased oxygen requirement. Her occasional cry sounds "breathless." The infant now appears mottled and lethargic. Her intravenous access is no longer functioning.

Scenario Overview and Learning Objectives

Scenario Overview

Emphasis should be on identification and rapid treatment of hypotensive cardiogenic shock. Priorities include immediate establishment of intravenous (IV) access and careful administration of a small bolus of isotonic crystalloid over 10-20 minutes, with careful reassessment of cardiorespiratory function during and after the fluid bolus. The provider should recognize the development of signs of worsening heart failure during the administration of the fluid bolus and stop bolus fluid administration. The infant requires inotropic therapy to improve cardiac function and vasoactive drug therapy to improve blood pressure and systemic perfusion. The infant may need additional support with continuous positive airway pressure (CPAP), noninvasive bilevel positive-pressure ventilation, or other positive-pressure ventilation support to improve oxygenation. Expert consultation from a pediatric cardiologist and further diagnostic studies (including echocardiography) are needed.

Scenario-Specific Objectives

- **Differentiates compensated vs hypotensive shock;** in this scenario, the child is hypotensive, so has hypotensive shock
- **Differentiates the signs and symptoms of cardiogenic shock from other types of shock;** in this scenario, the combination of signs of hypotensive shock with signs of heart failure (labored breathing, crackles, and hepatomegaly) and evidence of decreased perfusion (mottling, cyanosis, lethargy) point to likely cardiogenic shock
- **Provides correct interventions for cardiogenic shock;** in this scenario, these interventions include establishment of cardiac monitoring and pulse oximetry, careful bolus administration of isotonic crystalloids, careful reassessment during and after each fluid bolus, and initiation and titration of inotropic/vasoactive drugs
- **Describes correct volume and duration of bolus fluid administration for cardiogenic shock and describes possible negative effects of excessive bolus fluid administration;** in this scenario, signs of intolerance of bolus fluid administration include worsening of signs of heart failure with no improvement in shock signs

Evaluate—*Initial Impression* (Pediatric Assessment Triangle)	Identify	Intervene
Appearance • Lethargic; minimal reaction to noises in room **Breathing** • Labored breathing with moderate to severe intercostal and subcostal retractions **Circulation** • Pale; significant mottling with peripheral cyanosis noted	• Immediate intervention needed	• Activate emergency response system, if appropriate. • Administer 100% oxygen by nonrebreathing face mask. • Apply cardiac monitor. • Apply pulse oximeter.

Evaluate—*Primary Assessment* Focused on Assessment Needed to Support Airway, Oxygenation, Ventilation, and Perfusion	Identify	Intervene
• **A**irway: Patent • **B**reathing: Respiratory rate about 60/min; mild intercostal retractions; nasal flaring and intermittent grunting; SpO$_2$ 89% on room air, 100% with 100% oxygen • **C**irculation: Heart rate 180/min; central pulses present (not strong) and peripheral pulses weak and thready; capillary refill about 4 seconds; cool, mottled hands and feet; blood pressure 60/30 mm Hg • **D**isability: Lethargic; responds to painful stimuli • **E**xposure: Temperature 35.7°C (96.2°F); weight 7 kg	• Respiratory distress • Hypotensive shock, probably cardiogenic • Sinus tachycardia	• Obtain vascular (IV/intraosseous [IO]) access. • Administer a fluid bolus of 5-10 mL/kg of isotonic crystalloid IV/IO over 10-20 minutes. • Perform careful and frequent reassessment during and after fluid bolus. Stop fluid bolus if respiratory distress worsens or rales or hepatomegaly develop/worsen. • Check glucose using point-of-care (POC) testing.

Evaluate—*Secondary Assessment* *Identify Reversible Causes, but Defer Remainder of Secondary Assessment Until After Initial Shock Therapy*	Identify	Intervene
SAMPLE history (only to extent needed to evaluate reversible causes) • **S**igns and symptoms: Increased work of breathing and lethargy • **A**llergies: No known allergies • **M**edications: None • **P**ast medical history: No past history of illness • **L**ast meal: Poor intake for last 12 hours • **E**vents (onset): 24 hours of increased respiratory distress and difficulty breathing, no improvement with steroids or nebulizer treatments **Physical examination** • *Repeat vital signs after oxygen and first fluid bolus:* Heart rate 180/min; respiratory rate 75/min; SpO₂ 89% while receiving 100% oxygen by nonrebreather face mask; blood pressure 56/30 mm Hg • *Head, eyes, ears, nose, and throat/neck:* Mucous membranes slightly dry • *Heart and lungs:* Rapid rate; systolic murmur now detected; crackles and retractions worsening • *Abdomen:* Liver edge palpable at 3 cm below costal margin; nondistended abdomen; hypoactive bowel sounds • *Extremities:* Cold upper and lower extremities; mottled; weak peripheral pulses • *Back:* Normal • *Neurologic:* Lethargic; pupils 4 mm, equal, reactive	• Cardiogenic shock • Hypotensive shock • Worsening respiratory distress after fluid bolus • Possible respiratory failure	• Stop bolus fluid administration (signs of heart failure worsening). • Begin appropriate inotropic/vasoactive support if hypotension and assess response. • Assess response to oxygen administration. • Identify persistent hypoxemia despite oxygen administration. – Administer CPAP or noninvasive bilevel positive-pressure ventilation or other support if hypoxemia and respiratory distress continue. • Obtain 12-lead electrocardiogram (ECG). • Obtain a pediatric cardiology consultation and an echocardiogram, if available. • Arrange for transfer to the intensive care unit (ICU) for closer monitoring, if infant is not already in ICU.

Evaluate—*Diagnostic Assessments* *Perform Throughout the Evaluation of the Patient as Appropriate*	Identify/Intervene
Lab data • *Arterial blood gas (after initiation of CPAP or positive-pressure ventilation):* pH 7.25; PCO₂ 20 mm Hg; PO₂ 170 mm Hg; lactate 4.9 mmol/L • Glucose (POC testing) 80 mg/dL (4.4 mmol/L) • *Pending:* Electrolytes, blood urea nitrogen/creatinine, calcium, complete blood count with differential, prothrombin time/international normalized ratio/partial thromboplastin time • *Cultures:* Blood, urine **Imaging** • *Chest x-ray:* Cardiomegaly; increased pulmonary vascular markings	• A blood glucose concentration should be checked as soon as reasonably possible in all critically ill infants and children. Hypoglycemia should be treated immediately. • Arterial blood gas confirms metabolic acidosis associated with inadequate cardiac output. • Chest x-ray shows cardiomegaly and pulmonary edema consistent with heart failure/cardiogenic shock. • Obtain echocardiogram when available.

Re–evaluate-identify-intervene after each intervention.

Debriefing Tool
Practice Case Scenario 14
Cardiogenic Shock (Infant; Cardiomyopathy)

General Debriefing Principles

- Use the table below to guide your debriefing; also refer to the **Team Dynamics Debriefing Tool.**
- Debriefings are 10 minutes long.
- Address all learning objectives.
- Summarize take-home messages at the end of the debriefing.
- *Encourage:* Students to self-reflect
  Engagement of all participants
- *Avoid:* Mini-lectures and closed-ended questions
  Dominating the discussion

General Management Objectives

- Uses the PALS Systematic Approach Algorithm to assess and appropriately classify a patient
- Provides oxygen appropriately
- Directs delivery of high-quality CPR (including the use of a feedback device) when indicated
- Demonstrates basic airway maneuvers and use of relevant airway device as appropriate
- Demonstrates application of cardiac and respiratory monitors

- Identifies the cardiac rhythm
- Applies appropriate PBLS or PALS algorithms
- Summarizes general indications, contraindications, and doses of relevant drugs
- Discusses principles of family-centered care in pediatric cardiac arrest
- Applies the 8 elements of effective team dynamics
- Performs frequent reassessment

Action	Gather	Analyze	Summarize
• Directs assessment of ABCDE and vital signs • Applies cardiac monitor and pulse oximeter • Administers 100% oxygen • Recognizes signs and symptoms of cardiogenic shock • Categorizes shock as hypotensive • Directs establishment of IV or IO access • Directs administration of a 5-10 mL/kg bolus of isotonic crystalloid IV/IO over 10-20 minutes • Reassesses patient during and in response to interventions, particularly during and after each fluid bolus • Identifies signs of worsening heart failure and stops bolus fluid administration • Identifies need for inotropic/vasoactive support; titrates to improve cardiac output and systemic perfusion • Obtains expert consultation from a pediatric cardiologist and obtains an echocardiogram or other diagnostic studies as recommended by cardiologist	***Student Observations*** • Can you describe the events from your perspective? • How well do you think your treatments worked? • Can you review the events of the scenario (*directed to the Timer/Recorder*)? • What could you have improved? • What did the team do well? ***Instructor Observations*** • I noticed that [*insert action here*]. • I observed that [*insert action here*]. • I saw that [*insert action here*].	***Done Well*** • How were you able to [*insert action here*]? • Why do you think you were able to [*insert action here*]? • Tell me a little more about how you [*insert action here*]. ***Needs Improvement*** • Why do you think [*insert action here*] occurred? • How do you think [*insert action here*] could have been improved? • What was your thinking while [*insert action here*]? • What prevented you from [*insert action here*]?	***Student-Led Summary*** • What are the main things you learned? • Can someone summarize the key points made? • What are the main take-home messages? ***Instructor-Led Summary*** • Let's summarize what we learned… • Here is what I think we learned… • The main take-home messages are… • What are the therapeutic end points during shock management? (Answer: Normalized heart rate; improved peripheral perfusion, mental status, and urine output; normalized blood pressure; correction of metabolic/lactic acidosis)

Practice Case Scenario 15
Disordered Control of Breathing Disease (Infant)

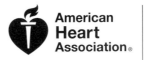 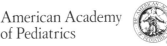

Vital Signs	
Heart rate	146/min
Blood pressure	88/56 mm Hg
Respiratory rate	12/min
SpO₂	80% on room air
Temperature	39.7°C (103.5°F)
Weight	7 kg
Age	6 months

Scenario Lead-in

Prehospital: You respond to a 9-1-1 call for a 6 month old having a seizure.

ED: Emergency medical services arrives with a 6-month-old boy brought from his home after mother called 9-1-1 because her child had a seizure.

General Inpatient Unit: You are called to the room of a 6-month-old boy who is being admitted after having a seizure.

Scenario Overview and Learning Objectives

Scenario Overview

Emphasis of this scenario is on recognition and immediate management of an infant with respiratory failure and disordered control of breathing (inadequate respiratory rate and effort and decreased level of consciousness after a seizure that likely complicates an episode of meningitis). This infant requires immediate opening of the airway and bag-mask ventilation with 100% oxygen. During debriefing, discuss indications for intubation in this patient and methods to estimate appropriate cuffed and uncuffed endotracheal tube sizes.

Scenario-Specific Objectives

- **Identifies respiratory distress vs respiratory failure;** in this scenario, respiratory failure is present
- **Summarizes signs of disordered control of breathing;** in this scenario, the infant demonstrated inadequate spontaneous respiratory effort with very slow and shallow breaths, although they were regular
- **Recalls causes of disordered control of breathing;** cues to the instructor: common causes include drugs, increased intracranial pressure, and seizures
- **Discusses correct interventions for disordered control of breathing;** in this scenario, interventions include opening the airway and bag-mask ventilation with 100% oxygen

Evaluate—*Initial Impression* *(Pediatric Assessment Triangle)*	Identify	Intervene
Appearance • Lethargic; eyes closed; no visible reaction to his mother's voice or noises in environment **Breathing** • Very slow respiratory rate with minimal chest rise **Circulation** • Pink skin	• Immediate intervention needed	• Activate the emergency response system. Emergency medical services requests additional assistance if needed. • Position the infant to open airway. • Begin bag-mask ventilation with 100% oxygen. • Apply cardiac monitor. • Apply pulse oximeter.

Evaluate—*Primary Assessment* *Focused on Assessment Needed to Support Airway, Oxygenation, Ventilation, and Perfusion*	Identify	Intervene
• **A**irway: Paradoxical movement of chest and abdomen when breathing, relieved when airway opened • **B**reathing: Spontaneous respiratory rate 12/min; shallow and regular; SpO₂ 80% on room air and 99% with bag-mask ventilation with 100% oxygen at a rate of 30/min • **C**irculation: Heart rate 146/min; dusky (before bag-mask ventilation with 100% oxygen); strong central and peripheral pulses; capillary refill 2 seconds; blood pressure 88/56 mm Hg • **D**isability: Lethargic; responsive to painful stimuli • **E**xposure: Temperature 39.7°C (103.5°F); weight 7 kg	• Respiratory failure (inadequate respiratory rate and effort)	• Verify chest rise with bag-mask ventilation and monitor response to bag-mask ventilation with oxygen. • Continue bag-mask ventilation with 100% oxygen and monitor for increase in infant's spontaneous respiratory effort—match ventilation with infant's effort if possible. • Consider insertion of oropharyngeal airway if infant is unresponsive with no cough or gag reflex. • Establish vascular access (intravenous). • Treat fever with antipyretic.

Evaluate—Secondary Assessment *Identify Reversible Causes, but Defer Remainder of Secondary Assessment Until After Stabilization of Airway, Oxygenation, and Ventilation*	**Identify**	**Intervene**
SAMPLE history • *Signs and symptoms:* Fever, irritable for the last 3 days • *Allergies:* None known • *Medications:* Acetaminophen given by mother 2 hours ago • *Past medical history:* None—no history of previous seizure disorder • *Last meal:* Ate 3 hours ago • *Events (onset):* Abrupt onset of tonic-clonic seizure lasting approximately 5 minutes **Physical examination** • *Repeat vital signs with assisted ventilation with 100% oxygen:* Respiratory rate 30/min with bag-mask ventilation now assisting the infant's spontaneous respiratory effort; heart rate 136/min; SpO$_2$ 99% with inspired oxygen concentration of 100%; blood pressure 94/58 mm Hg • *Head, eyes, ears, nose, and throat/neck:* Airway clear; pupils 3 mm bilateral and reactive; tense anterior fontanelle • *Heart and lungs:* Clear breath sounds; good chest rise with assisted ventilation; rate and depth of spontaneous breaths increasing • *Abdomen:* Normal • *Extremities:* No edema; no rash • *Back:* Normal • *Neurologic:* Level of consciousness unchanged; moves all 4 extremities with painful stimulus but in nonpurposeful fashion	• Respiratory failure (inadequate respiratory rate and depth) • Disordered control of breathing	• Closely monitor infant's level of consciousness, spontaneous respiratory effort, and airway protective mechanisms (ability to cough to protect airway). Remove oral airway if responsiveness improves or cough or gag reflex returns. • If infant's spontaneous respiratory effort improves, provide bag-mask ventilation that assists the infant's respiratory effort. • As patient will continue to be bradypneic with a reduced level of consciousness, continue bag-mask ventilation with 100% oxygen, and obtain expert consultation to plan for advanced airway insertion and support of ventilation. • Check glucose using point-of-care testing. • Arrange for transfer to higher level of care for evaluation, observation, and care.

Evaluate—Diagnostic Assessments *Perform Throughout the Evaluation of the Patient as Appropriate*	**Identify/Intervene**
Lab data • Glucose (bedside) 166 mg/dL (9.2 mmol/L) • Electrolytes; blood urea nitrogen/creatinine; complete blood count with differential; blood culture **Imaging** • Chest x-ray: Ordered	• A blood glucose concentration should be checked as soon as reasonably possible in all critically ill infants and children. This infant had a seizure and still has decreased level of consciousness, so it will be important to check the glucose. • It is not always possible to obtain an arterial blood gas.

Re–evaluate-identify-intervene after each intervention.

Debriefing Tool
Practice Case Scenario 15
Disordered Control of Breathing Disease (Infant)

General Debriefing Principles

- Use the table below to guide your debriefing; also refer to the **Team Dynamics Debriefing Tool.**
- Debriefings are 10 minutes long.
- Address all learning objectives.
- Summarize take-home messages at the end of the debriefing.
- *Encourage:* Students to self-reflect
  Engagement of all participants
- *Avoid:* Mini-lectures and closed-ended questions
  Dominating the discussion

General Management Objectives

- Uses the PALS Systematic Approach Algorithm to assess and appropriately classify a patient
- Provides oxygen appropriately
- Directs delivery of high-quality CPR (including the use of a feedback device) when indicated
- Demonstrates basic airway maneuvers and use of relevant airway device as appropriate
- Demonstrates application of cardiac and respiratory monitors
- Identifies the cardiac rhythm
- Applies appropriate PBLS or PALS algorithms
- Summarizes general indications, contraindications, and doses of relevant drugs
- Discusses principles of family-centered care in pediatric cardiac arrest
- Applies the 8 elements of effective team dynamics
- Performs frequent reassessment

Action	Gather	Analyze	Summarize
• Directs assessment of ABCDE and vital signs • Provides or directs bag-mask ventilation with 100% oxygen • Applies cardiac monitor and pulse oximeter • Identifies respiratory failure • Identifies signs of disordered control of breathing • Directs establishment of intravenous access • Performs frequent reassessment of patient • Describes methods to verify that bag-mask ventilation is effective • Identifies need for involvement of advanced provider with expertise in pediatric intubation and mechanical ventilation • Summarizes specific interventions for disordered control of breathing	***Student Observations*** • Can you describe the events from your perspective? • How well do you think your treatments worked? • Can you review the events of the scenario (*directed to the Timer/Recorder*)? • What could you have improved? • What did the team do well? ***Instructor Observations*** • I noticed that [*insert action here*]. • I observed that [*insert action here*]. • I saw that [*insert action here*].	***Done Well*** • How were you able to [*insert action here*]? • Why do you think you were able to [*insert action here*]? • Tell me a little more about how you [*insert action here*]. ***Needs Improvement*** • Why do you think [*insert action here*] occurred? • How do you think [*insert action here*] could have been improved? • What was your thinking while [*insert action here*]? • What prevented you from [*insert action here*]?	***Student-Led Summary*** • What are the main things you learned? • Can someone summarize the key points made? • What are the main take-home messages? ***Instructor-Led Summary*** • Let's summarize what we learned… • Here is what I think we learned… • The main take-home messages are… • What were the indications for endotracheal intubation in an infant with disordered control of breathing? (Answers: Inadequate spontaneous respiratory effort and/or failure to maintain a patent airway, signs of possible increased intracranial pressure) • If the infant requires intubation, how would you estimate the size of cuffed and uncuffed endotracheal tube to use?

Bradycardia
(Child; Seizure)

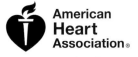

American Heart Association.

life is why™

American Academy
of Pediatrics

DEDICATED TO THE HEALTH OF ALL CHILDREN™

Vital Signs	
Heart rate	45/min
Blood pressure	85/54 mm Hg
Respiratory rate	6/min
SpO$_2$	62% before bag-mask ventilation with oxygen
Temperature	39.3°C (102.7°F)
Weight	27 kg
Age	8 years

Scenario Lead-in

Prehospital: You are dispatched to the home of an 8-year-old child who was having a generalized seizure and received rectal diazepam; he now has decreased respiratory effort.

ED: Paramedics arrive with an 8-year-old child who was having a generalized seizure and received rectal diazepam; he now has decreased respiratory effort.

General Inpatient Unit: You are a member of the rapid response team called to evaluate an 8 year old who had a generalized seizure on the floor and received intravenous lorazepam; he now has decreased respiratory effort.

ICU: You are asked to evaluate an 8 year old who just had a seizure and received intravenous lorazepam; he now has decreased respiratory effort.

Scenario Overview and Learning Objectives

Scenario Overview

Emphasis should be placed on identification and treatment of hypoxic bradycardia associated with disordered control of breathing/respiratory depression and upper airway obstruction. Priorities include immediate establishment of a patent airway and effective bag-mask ventilation with 100% oxygen. Provider may need to reopen airway and reattempt bag-mask ventilation before it produces effective chest rise. Chest compressions are not required because the heart rate, oxygenation, and perfusion rise quickly once effective bag-mask ventilation is provided. If the patient cannot maintain a patent airway and does not recover adequate spontaneous ventilation, providers should prepare for advanced airway insertion. The student should describe how to estimate the child's endotracheal tube size. Discussion of flumazenil as a receptor antagonist is beyond the scope of the scenario and the drug is contraindicated for this patient (it can lower seizure threshold).

Scenario-Specific Objectives

- **Demonstrates support of oxygenation and ventilation in a patient with hypoxic bradycardia**
- **Recognizes indications for CPR in bradycardic patient;** in this scenario, compressions are not needed because the child's heart rate and oxygenation quickly improve once effective bag-mask ventilation with oxygen is provided
- **States 3 causes of bradycardia;** these include hypoxia (most common), vagal stimulation, heart block, and drug overdose
- **Describes appropriate indications for and dose of epinephrine for bradycardia**

Evaluate—*Initial Impression*
(Pediatric Assessment Triangle)

Appearance
- No visible reaction to noise

Breathing
- Very slow respiratory rate

Circulation
- Pale; lips slightly dusky

Identify

- Immediate intervention needed

Intervene

- Activate the emergency response system. Emergency medical services requests additional assistance if needed.
- Check for response (no response) and perform simultaneous check for breathing (still very slow) and carotid pulse (slow pulse detected).
- Begin bag-mask ventilation with 100% oxygen.
- Apply cardiac monitor.
- Apply pulse oximeter.

Evaluate—*Primary Assessment*	**Identify**	**Intervene**
Focused on Assessment Needed to Support Airway, Oxygenation, Ventilation, and Perfusion		

- **A**irway: Snoring respirations
- **B**reathing: Spontaneous respiratory rate 6/min; SpO₂ 62% on room air; initially bag-mask ventilation with 100% oxygen produces no chest rise and poor air entry bilaterally; if provider reopens airway and reattempts bag-mask ventilation, significant improvement in ease of ventilation and chest rise is apparent, and SpO₂ rises rapidly
- **C**irculation: Initial heart rate 45/min (sinus bradycardia); weak peripheral pulses; 2+ central pulses; capillary refill 3-4 seconds; blood pressure 85/54 mm Hg; heart rate increases to 95/min with effective bag-mask ventilation with 100% oxygen
- **D**isability: Unresponsive
- **E**xposure: Temperature 39.3°C (102.7°F); weight 27 kg; no rashes

Identify
- Respiratory failure due to upper airway obstruction and disordered control of breathing
- Sinus bradycardia *(rate 45/min increases to 95/min with bag-mask ventilation)*
- Decreased level of consciousness

Intervene
- Insert oral airway.
- Reopen airway, reposition face mask, ensure adequate seal to face, and provide bag-mask ventilation that produces chest rise.
- Assess heart rate response to ventilation and oxygen administration to determine the need for additional intervention.
- Obtain vascular access (intravenous [IV]/intraosseous [IO]).

Evaluate—*Secondary Assessment*	**Identify**	**Intervene**
Identify Reversible Causes, but Defer Remainder of Secondary Assessment Until Heart Rate 60/min or Greater With Adequate Perfusion		

SAMPLE history
- **S**igns and symptoms: Had generalized tonic-clonic seizure and received benzodiazepine as noted
- **A**llergies: None
- **M**edications: Levetiracetam
- **P**ast medical history: Known seizure disorder; last seizure was 6 months ago
- **L**ast meal: Ate normally 2 hours ago
- **E**vents (onset): Upper respiratory infection symptoms for 2 days; generalized tonic-clonic seizure lasting 12 minutes; seizure activity stopped 5 minutes before team's arrival

Physical examination
- *Repeat vital signs after effective bag-mask ventilation:* Heart rate increases to 95/min; SpO₂ 95% with bag-mask ventilation at a rate of 16-20/min with 100% oxygen; blood pressure 95/54 mm Hg
- *Head, eyes, ears, nose, and throat/neck:* Continues to be ventilated with bag-mask device with oropharyngeal airway in place; pupils 3 mm, equal, and reactive to light
- *Heart and lungs:* No murmur; good air entry with positive-pressure ventilation; 2+ central and peripheral pulses; capillary refill 3 seconds
- *Abdomen:* Soft; no organomegaly
- *Extremities:* Unremarkable
- *Back:* Unremarkable
- *Neurologic:* Remains unresponsive to painful stimulation; pupils 3 mm, equal, and reactive to light
- Point-of-care (POC) glucose (see below)

Identify
- Altered level of consciousness
- Sinus rhythm with correction of bradycardia
- Respiratory failure due to upper airway obstruction and disordered control of breathing

Intervene
- Continue bag-mask ventilation as needed. If SpO₂ is greater than 94% and perfusion is improving with bag-mask ventilation, do the following:
  - Wean supplementary oxygen as tolerated.
  - Evaluate spontaneous respiratory effort and provide assisted ventilation to support spontaneous respiratory efforts.
  - Remove oral airway if child begins to respond at all or develops cough or gag reflex.
  - Stop bag-mask ventilation if child's spontaneous ventilation effort becomes adequate.
- If child does not recover effective spontaneous ventilation and airway protective mechanisms, consider placement of advanced airway. Obtain expert consultation.
- Check POC glucose concentration.

Evaluate—*Diagnostic Assessments*	**Identify/Intervene**
Perform Throughout the Evaluation of the Patient as Appropriate	

Lab data
- Blood glucose 107 mg/dL
- A blood gas (arterial, venous, or capillary) not indicated in the immediate management of this child

Imaging
- Head computed tomography if there is a history or physical findings to suggest trauma

Identify/Intervene
- A blood glucose concentration should be checked as soon as reasonably possible in all critically ill infants and children. Hypoglycemia should be promptly treated.
- Laboratory studies (other than POC glucose testing) are deferred until effective airway, oxygenation, ventilation, and heart rate/perfusion are established.

Re–evaluate-identify-intervene after each intervention.

Debriefing Tool
Practice Case Scenario 16
Bradycardia (Child; Seizure)

- Use the table below to guide your debriefing; also refer to the **Team Dynamics Debriefing Tool.**
- Debriefings are 10 minutes long.
- Address all learning objectives.
- Summarize take-home messages at the end of the debriefing.
- *Encourage:* Students to self-reflect
  Engagement of all participants
- *Avoid:* Mini-lectures and closed-ended questions
  Dominating the discussion

General Management Objectives

- Uses the PALS Systematic Approach Algorithm to assess and appropriately classify a patient
- Provides oxygen appropriately
- Directs delivery of high-quality CPR (including the use of a feedback device) when indicated
- Demonstrates basic airway maneuvers and use of relevant airway device as appropriate
- Demonstrates application of cardiac and respiratory monitors

- Identifies the cardiac rhythm
- Applies appropriate PBLS or PALS algorithms
- Summarizes general indications, contraindications, and doses of relevant drugs
- Discusses principles of family-centered care in pediatric cardiac arrest
- Applies the 8 elements of effective team dynamics
- Performs frequent reassessment

Action	Gather	Analyze	Summarize
• Directs assessment of ABCDE and vital signs • Identifies bradycardia associated with hypoxia that is caused by upper airway obstruction and disordered control of breathing (ie, hypoventilation) • Directs insertion of oral airway and bag-mask ventilation with 100% oxygen • Applies cardiac monitor and pulse oximeter • Reassesses heart rate and perfusion after initiation of bag-mask ventilation with oxygen • Determines that chest compressions and epinephrine administration are not needed because heart rate increases adequately with establishment of patent airway, adequate oxygenation, and ventilation • Directs establishment of IV or IO access • Checks glucose with POC testing in this unresponsive patient • Discusses preparation for advanced airway placement • Performs frequent reassessment	***Student Observations*** • Can you describe the events from your perspective? • How well do you think your treatments worked? • Can you review the events of the scenario (*directed to the Timer/Recorder*)? • What could you have improved? • What did the team do well? ***Instructor Observations*** • I noticed that [*insert action here*]. • I observed that [*insert action here*]. • I saw that [*insert action here*].	***Done Well*** • How were you able to [*insert action here*]? • Why do you think you were able to [*insert action here*]? • Tell me a little more about how you [*insert action here*]. ***Needs Improvement*** • Why do you think [*insert action here*] occurred? • How do you think [*insert action here*] could have been improved? • What was your thinking while [*insert action here*]? • What prevented you from [*insert action here*]?	***Student-Led Summary*** • What are the main things you learned? • Can someone summarize the key points made? • What are the main take-home messages? ***Instructor-Led Summary*** • Let's summarize what we learned… • Here is what I think we learned… • The main take-home messages are… • The child in this scenario did not require chest compressions. What would have been the indications for the addition of chest compressions to ventilation (CPR)? (Answer: Heart rate is less than 60/min with signs of poor perfusion despite adequate oxygenation and ventilation.) • The child in this scenario did not require epinephrine administration. If it had been necessary, what dose would be appropriate? (Answer: 0.01 mg/kg [0.1 mL/kg of the 0.1 mg/mL concentration]) • In addition to hypoxia, what are 3 other causes of bradycardia in infants and children?

(continued)

(continued)

Action	Gather	Analyze	Summarize
			• This scenario did not include advanced airway insertion. In preparing for intubation, how would you estimate the correct cuffed and uncuffed endotracheal tube size for this infant?

Hypovolemic Shock
(Child)

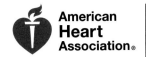

American Heart Association®

life is why™

American Academy of Pediatrics

DEDICATED TO THE HEALTH OF ALL CHILDREN™

Scenario Lead-in

Prehospital: You have been dispatched to transport a 5 year old with a 3-day history of fever and diarrhea. She has been increasingly lethargic in the last 2 hours.

ED: You are asked to assess and manage a 5 year old with a 3-day history of fever and diarrhea. She has been increasingly lethargic in the last 2 hours. Efforts for a peripheral intravenous access have been unsuccessful.

General Inpatient Unit: You are called to assess a 5 year old who has been admitted to the ward with a 3-day history of fever and diarrhea. She has been increasingly lethargic in the last hour and has had severe ongoing diarrhea. Her intravenous access is no longer functioning.

ICU: You are called to the bedside of a 5 year old who has been admitted to the intensive care unit with a 3-day history of fever and diarrhea. She has been increasingly lethargic in the last 2 hours and has had severe ongoing diarrhea. Her intravenous access is no longer functioning.

Vital Signs	
Heart rate	140/min
Blood pressure	100/80 mm Hg
Respiratory rate	36/min
SpO₂	92% on room air
Temperature	38.0°C (100.4°F)
Weight	21 kg
Age	5 years

Scenario Overview and Learning Objectives

Scenario Overview

Emphasis in this scenario should be on identification of compensated hypovolemic shock. Priorities include oxygen, immediate establishment of intravenous (IV) access, and administration of fluid bolus of isotonic crystalloid, repeated as needed to treat shock signs. Reassessment of cardiorespiratory status is needed during and after each fluid bolus. Glucose concentration should be checked early in this lethargic child.

Scenario-Specific Objectives

- **Recognizes signs of compensated and hypotensive shock;** this case illustrates compensated hypovolemic shock (key indicators include anxiety, tachypnea without abnormal labor, tachycardia, cool and mottled skin, delayed capillary refill, and normotension)
- **Summarizes signs and symptoms of hypovolemic shock;** in this scenario, the child has a 3-day history of diarrhea and fever, signs of shock, and poor skin turgor
- **Demonstrates correct interventions for hypovolemic shock;** the most important interventions in this scenario include oxygen administration, administration of one or more boluses of isotonic crystalloid, and careful reassessment during and after each fluid bolus
- **Summarizes how to evaluate systemic (end-organ) perfusion;** indirect indicators of end-organ perfusion include skin temperature/color, level of consciousness, and urine output

---

Evaluate—*Initial Impression* (Pediatric Assessment Triangle)	**Identify**	**Intervene**
Appearance • Anxious, restless **Breathing** • Fast rate, increased respiratory effort **Circulation** • Pale, dry, and significant mottling, especially in hands and feet	• Immediate intervention needed	• Activate the emergency response system. Emergency medical services requests additional assistance if needed. • Administer 100% oxygen by nonrebreathing face mask. • Apply cardiac monitor. • Apply pulse oximeter.

Evaluate—*Primary Assessment* Focused on Assessment Needed to Support Airway, Oxygenation, Ventilation, and Perfusion	**Identify**	**Intervene**

• **A**irway: Patent; no audible abnormal airway sounds (no stridor, no audible wheezing)
• **B**reathing/Ventilation: Respiratory rate about 36/min; minimal intercostal retractions; SpO₂ 92% on room air, increases to 100% with 100% oxygen; lungs clear on auscultation
• **C**irculation/Perfusion: Central pulses fair, peripheral pulses weak; heart rate 140/min; blood pressure 100/80 mm Hg; capillary refill about 4 seconds; cool, mottled hands and feet
 	
Remainder of Primary Assessment performed if airway, ventilation, and perfusion are adequately supported
 	
• **D**isability: Poor skin turgor
• **E**xposure: Temperature 38.0°C (100.4°F); weight 21 kg
	• Compensated shock
	• Sinus tachycardia
		• Obtain vascular access (child has compensated shock, so initial attempt should focus on IV access).
		• Administer a fluid bolus of 20 mL/kg of isotonic crystalloid rapidly via IV.
		  – Assess perfusion and monitor cardiorespiratory status closely during and immediately after each fluid bolus.
		  – Stop fluid bolus if signs of heart failure develop (eg, increased respiratory distress or development of rales or hepatomegaly).
		• Check point-of-care (POC) glucose concentration and treat hypoglycemia, if needed.
		• Assess response to oxygen administration.

Evaluate—*Secondary Assessment*	**Identify**	**Intervene**

Identify Reversible Causes, but Defer Remainder of Secondary Assessment Until After Initial Shock Therapy

SAMPLE history (only to extent needed to evaluate reversible causes)

- *Signs and symptoms:* Diarrhea for 3 days
- *Allergies:* None known
- *Medications:* Methylphenidate
- *Past medical history:* Attention-deficit/hyperactivity disorder
- *Last meal:* No oral intake for 24 hours
- *Events (onset):* 3-day history of low-grade fever and diarrhea; noted to be increasingly lethargic in last 2 hours

Physical examination

- *Repeat vital signs after oxygen and one bolus of 20 mL/kg fluids:* Heart rate 94/min; respiratory rate 30/min; SpO_2 98% with 100% oxygen by nonrebreathing face mask; blood pressure 90/50 mm Hg
- *Head, eyes, ears, nose, and throat/neck:* Mucous membranes dry; neck supple
- *Heart and lungs:* Normal rate, no extra heart sounds or murmurs; lungs sound clear; capillary refill down to 3-4 seconds
- *Abdomen:* No palpable liver edge; nondistended; nontender; diminished bowel sounds
- *Extremities:* Cool hands and feet; weak peripheral pulses; capillary refill 3-4 seconds
- *Back:* Normal
- *Neurologic:* Lethargic; pupils 4 mm, equal, reactive

Identify

- Compensated hypovolemic shock

Intervene

- Repeat bolus of 20 mL/kg of isotonic crystalloid IV/intraosseous (IO) push; repeat if needed to treat persistent shock symptoms.
- Perform careful and frequent cardiorespiratory assessment during and after each fluid bolus.
  - Stop fluid bolus if signs of heart failure develop (increased respiratory distress or development of rales or hepatomegaly).
- Arrange for transfer to the intensive care unit (ICU) (unless child is already in the ICU).

Evaluate—*Diagnostic Assessments*	**Identify/Intervene**

Perform Throughout the Evaluation of the Patient as Appropriate

Lab data

- *Arterial blood gas:* pH 7.18, PCO_2 24 mm Hg, HCO_3 13 mEq/L, PO_2 74 mm Hg
- *Glucose (POC testing)* 70 mg/dL (3.3 mmol/L)
- *Pending:* Electrolytes, blood urea nitrogen/creatinine, serum urea, bicarbonate level, serum lactate
- *Cultures:* Blood, urine
- *Temperature:* 38.0°C (100.4°F)

Imaging

- *Chest x-ray:* Small heart, clear lung fields

Identify/Intervene

- A blood glucose concentration should be checked as soon as reasonably possible in all critically ill children, particularly neonates and infants. Hypoglycemia should be treated immediately.
- Metabolic acidosis should correct with effective treatment of shock.

Re–evaluate–identify–intervene after each intervention.

Debriefing Tool
Testing Case Scenario 1
Hypovolemic Shock (Child)

General Debriefing Principles

- Use the table below to guide your debriefing; also refer to the **Team Dynamics Debriefing Tool.**
- Debriefings are 10 minutes long.
- Address all learning objectives.
- Summarize take-home messages at the end of the debriefing.
- *Encourage:* Students to self-reflect
  Engagement of all participants
- *Avoid:* Mini-lectures and closed-ended questions
  Dominating the discussion

General Management Objectives

- Uses the PALS Systematic Approach Algorithm to assess and appropriately classify a patient
- Provides oxygen appropriately
- Directs delivery of high-quality CPR (including the use of a feedback device) when indicated
- Demonstrates basic airway maneuvers and use of relevant airway device as appropriate
- Demonstrates application of cardiac and respiratory monitors

- Identifies the cardiac rhythm
- Applies appropriate PBLS or PALS algorithms
- Summarizes general indications, contraindications, and doses of relevant drugs
- Discusses principles of family-centered care in pediatric cardiac arrest
- Applies the 8 elements of effective team dynamics
- Performs frequent reassessment

Action	Gather	Analyze	Summarize
	Student Observations	***Done Well***	***Student-Led Summary***
• Assesses ABCDE, including vital signs • Administers 100% oxygen • Applies cardiac monitor and pulse oximeter • Recognizes signs and symptoms of hypovolemic shock • Categorizes shock as compensated • Directs establishment of IV or IO access	• Can you describe the events from your perspective? • How well do you think your treatments worked? • Can you review the events of the scenario (*directed to the Timer/Recorder*)? • What could you have improved? • What did the team do well?	• How were you able to [*insert action here*]? • Why do you think you were able to [*insert action here*]? • Tell me a little more about how you [*insert action here*].	• What are the main things you learned? • Can someone summarize the key points made? • What are the main take-home messages?
• Directs rapid administration of fluid bolus of isotonic crystalloid; monitors for signs of heart failure during and after fluid bolus • Reassesses patient during and in response to interventions, particularly during and after each fluid bolus • Repeats fluid bolus as needed to treat shock • Checks glucose with point-of-care testing	***Instructor Observations*** • I noticed that [*insert action here*]. • I observed that [*insert action here*]. • I saw that [*insert action here*].	***Needs Improvement*** • Why do you think [*insert action here*] occurred? • How do you think [*insert action here*] could have been improved? • What was your thinking while [*insert action here*]? • What prevented you from [*insert action here*]?	***Instructor-Led Summary*** • Let's summarize what we learned… • Here is what I think we learned… • The main take-home messages are… • What are the therapeutic end points during shock management? (Answer: Normalized heart rate; improved peripheral perfusion, mental status, and urine output; normalized blood pressure; correction of metabolic/lactic acidosis) • Which are the indirect signs of improved end-organ function? (Answer: Improved skin blood flow, increased responsiveness/improved level of consciousness, increased urine output, correction of lactic acidosis)

Lower Airway Obstruction
(Child; Asthma)

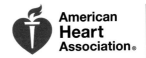

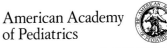

Vital Signs	
Heart rate	150/min
Blood pressure	102/62 mm Hg
Respiratory rate	30/min
SpO₂	88% on room air
Temperature	37°C (98.6°F)
Weight	35 kg
Age	10 years

Scenario Lead-in

Prehospital: You are responding to a 9-1-1 call for a 10-year-old girl with respiratory distress.

ED: A 10-year-old girl is brought in by first responders from her home after her mother called 9-1-1 saying that her daughter had respiratory distress.

General Inpatient Unit: You are called to the room of a 10-year-old girl who is being admitted from the emergency department for respiratory distress.

ICU: You are called to evaluate a 10-year-old girl just admitted to the intensive care unit for respiratory distress.

Scenario Overview and Learning Objectives

Scenario Overview

Emphasis in this scenario is on rapid identification and management of respiratory distress/potential respiratory failure caused by lower airway obstruction/asthma. The provider must quickly recognize signs of distress and provide initial therapy, including administration of 100% oxygen, nebulized albuterol, and oral corticosteroids. Nebulized ipratropium bromide may also be considered. The child improves so acceleration of care is not required. During the debriefing, the student is asked the indications for endotracheal intubation.

Scenario-Specific Objectives

- **Recognizes signs and symptoms of respiratory distress caused by lower airway obstruction;** in this scenario, they include increased respiratory rate and effort, prolonged expiratory time, and wheezing
- **Performs correct initial interventions for lower airway obstruction;** in this scenario, they include administration of oxygen, albuterol nebulizer, corticosteroids, and possibly nebulized ipratropium bromide
- **Discusses importance of obtaining expert consultation if a child with asthma has a history of intensive care unit (ICU) admissions and/or fails to respond to initial interventions**

Evaluate—Initial Impression (Pediatric Assessment Triangle)	Identify	Intervene
Appearance • Anxious; sitting up in bed **Breathing** • Increased rate and effort with retractions **Circulation** • Pink lips and nailbeds; well perfused	• Respiratory distress	• Perform rapid cardiopulmonary assessment. • Administer 100% oxygen by nonrebreathing face mask. • Apply cardiac monitor. • Apply pulse oximeter.

Evaluate—Primary Assessment	Identify	Intervene
• **A**irway: Patent and unobstructed; nasal flaring present; no abnormal upper airway sounds are audible • **B**reathing: Respiratory rate 42/min; substernal retractions; diffuse bilateral expiratory wheezes on auscultation; prolonged expiratory phase; decreased air movement throughout; SpO₂ 88% on room air before provision of 100% oxygen by nonrebreathing face mask • **C**irculation: Heart rate 150/min; pink lips and nailbeds; strong radial pulse; capillary refill 2 seconds; blood pressure 102/62 mm Hg • **D**isability: Anxious, but alert; speaking in 3- to 4-word sentences • **E**xposure: Temperature 37°C (98.6°F); weight 35 kg	• Respiratory distress, possible respiratory failure • Lower airway obstruction	• Allow child to maintain position of comfort. • Assess response to oxygen. • Administer nebulized albuterol and nebulized ipratropium bromide. • Administer oral corticosteroids.

Evaluate—*Secondary Assessment*

SAMPLE history

- **S***igns and symptoms:* Cough; respiratory distress; family members smoke in the house
- **A***llergies:* Molds and grass
- **M***edications:* Inhaler that has not been refilled for several weeks
- **P***ast medical history:* History of asthma; 3 ICU admissions for respiratory failure; asthma poorly controlled due to poor compliance with medical care
- **L***ast meal:* Ate last meal 4 hours ago
- **E***vents (onset):* Cold symptoms for the last 3 days; increased coughing and work of breathing for the past 24 hours

Physical examination

- *Repeat vital signs after oxygen and fluids:* Respiratory rate 24/min; heart rate 132/min; SpO$_2$ 95%; blood pressure 124/76 mm Hg
- *Head, eyes, ears, nose, and throat/neck:* Airway remains patent
- *Heart and lungs:* Expiratory wheezes decreasing in intensity; expiratory phase not as abnormally long; improving air movement; mild substernal retractions
- *Abdomen:* Normal
- *Extremities:* Pulses 2-3+ peripherally; brisk capillary refill
- *Back:* Normal
- *Neurologic:* Remains anxious, but now speaking in complete sentences; no neurologic abnormalities

Identify

- Respiratory distress
- Lower airway obstruction

Intervene

- Assess response to albuterol and ipratropium.
- If wheezing and respiratory distress continue and aeration is not improved, provide continuous nebulized albuterol. Consult a provider with expertise in management of status asthmaticus in children to develop a plan for acceleration of care.
- Check point-of-care (POC) glucose concentration.
- Recognize that further acceleration in care of the asthma does not appear to be needed at this time (child improving), but discuss next steps in care with consulting expert.
- Continue very close observation and consider additional diagnostic testing (eg, chest x-ray).
- Arrange for transfer of child to the ICU (if the child is not already in the ICU).

Evaluate—*Diagnostic Assessments*
Perform Throughout the Evaluation of the Patient as Appropriate

Identify/Intervene

Lab data

- Glucose (POC testing) 128 mg/dL (7.1 mmol/L)

Imaging

- None

- Although laboratory tests are generally not appropriate during immediate management, a blood glucose concentration should be checked as soon as reasonably possible in all critically ill infants and children. Hypoglycemia should be treated immediately.
- Additional testing (eg, chest x-ray) may be performed if child demonstrates any additional respiratory signs or symptoms.

Re–evaluate-identify-intervene after each intervention.

Debriefing Tool
Testing Case Scenario 2
Lower Airway Obstruction (Child; Asthma)

- Use the table below to guide your debriefing; also refer to the **Team Dynamics Debriefing Tool.**
- Debriefings are 10 minutes long.
- Address all learning objectives.
- Summarize take-home messages at the end of the debriefing.
- *Encourage:* Students to self-reflect
  Engagement of all participants
- *Avoid:* Mini-lectures and closed-ended questions
  Dominating the discussion

General Management Objectives

- Uses the PALS Systematic Approach Algorithm to assess and appropriately classify a patient
- Provides oxygen appropriately
- Directs delivery of high-quality CPR (including the use of a feedback device) when indicated
- Demonstrates basic airway maneuvers and use of relevant airway device as appropriate
- Demonstrates application of cardiac and respiratory monitors

- Identifies the cardiac rhythm
- Applies appropriate PBLS or PALS algorithms
- Summarizes general indications, contraindications, and doses of relevant drugs
- Discusses principles of family-centered care in pediatric cardiac arrest
- Applies the 8 elements of effective team dynamics
- Performs frequent reassessment

Action	Gather	Analyze	Summarize
• Directs assessment of ABCDE and vital signs • Directs administration of 100% oxygen • Applies cardiac monitor and pulse oximeter • Recognizes signs and symptoms of lower airway obstruction • Identifies respiratory distress • Initiates therapy for asthma, including continued oxygen administration, nebulized albuterol, and corticosteroids • Directs reassessment of patient in response to each intervention • Summarizes additional therapy to provide if indicated (ie, give nebulized albuterol continuously, administer nebulized ipratropium bromide, consider magnesium sulfate)	***Student Observations*** • Can you describe the events from your perspective? • How well do you think your treatments worked? • Can you review the events of the scenario (*directed to the Timer/Recorder*)? • What could you have improved? • What did the team do well? ***Instructor Observations*** • I noticed that [*insert action here*]. • I observed that [*insert action here*]. • I saw that [*insert action here*].	***Done Well*** • How were you able to [*insert action here*]? • Why do you think you were able to [*insert action here*]? • Tell me a little more about how you [*insert action here*]. ***Needs Improvement*** • Why do you think [*insert action here*] occurred? • How do you think [*insert action here*] could have been improved? • What was your thinking while [*insert action here*]? • What prevented you from [*insert action here*]?	***Student-Led Summary*** • What are the main things you learned? • Can someone summarize the key points made? • What are the main take-home messages? ***Instructor-Led Summary*** • Let's summarize what we learned… • Here is what I think we learned… • The main take-home messages are… • In this scenario, the child improved. If this child continued to deteriorate despite the care provided, and expert consultation was available, what would be the indications for bag-mask ventilation or other airway or ventilation support? (Answer includes decreased level of consciousness; decreased air movement; and decreased wheezing, bradycardia, and pulsus paradoxus.) Note that it is important to seek expert consultation before the patient deteriorates to this point.

Upper Airway Obstruction
(Infant)

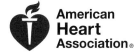

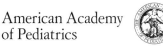

DEDICATED TO THE HEALTH OF ALL CHILDREN™

Scenario Lead-in

Prehospital: You are called to a home in the middle of the night for a 9-month-old infant who is having difficulty breathing. He has had upper respiratory congestion and a low-grade fever for the past 2 days.

ED: A 9-month-old infant presents with sudden onset of noisy breathing during the night. He has had upper respiratory congestion and a low-grade fever for the past 2 days.

General Inpatient Unit: A 9-month-old infant has just been admitted from his pediatrician's office after presenting with difficulty breathing. He has had upper respiratory congestion and a low-grade fever for the past 2 days.

ICU: A 9-month-old infant was extubated 1 hour ago and has developed noisy breathing.

Vital Signs	
Heart rate	140/min
Blood pressure	86/58 mm Hg
Respiratory rate	48/min
SpO$_2$	97% on room air
Temperature	38°C (100.4°F)
Weight	8 kg
Age	9 months

Scenario Overview and Learning Objectives

Scenario Overview

Emphasis in this scenario is on rapid recognition and management of respiratory distress associated with upper airway obstruction. Appropriate therapies include allowing the infant to assume a position of comfort and administering oxygen, nebulized epinephrine, and dexamethasone. The provider must demonstrate frequent reassessment to verify continued improvement in response to therapy and must be able to describe the clinical signs of deterioration that would indicate the need to obtain immediate expert consultation to provide advanced monitoring and care.

Scenario-Specific Objectives

- **Identifies the signs and symptoms of respiratory distress caused by upper airway obstruction;** in this scenario, they include tachypnea, increased respiratory effort, and stridor
- **Recognizes importance of allowing the infant to maintain a position of comfort and for providers to minimize stimulation;** in this scenario, providers should avoid unnecessary venipuncture for laboratory studies and establish an intravenous access only if it is absolutely necessary
- **Performs correct interventions for significant upper airway obstruction;** in this scenario, these include administration of oxygen, nebulized epinephrine, and dexamethasone
- **Reassesses patient frequently to determine response to each intervention**

Evaluate—*Initial Impression* (Pediatric Assessment Triangle)	Identify	Intervene
Appearance • Crying and fussy; being held by parent in attempt to console **Breathing** • Tachypneic with increased work of breathing, occasional stridor **Circulation** • Appears pale and well perfused	• Respiratory distress	• Perform rapid cardiopulmonary assessment. • Apply cardiac monitor. • Apply pulse oximeter.

Evaluate—*Primary Assessment*	Identify	Intervene
• **A**irway: Unobstructed but noisy; high-pitched inspiratory stridor when agitated, stridor minimal but still audible when resting • **B**reathing: Respiratory rate 48/min; suprasternal retractions; transmitted upper airway noises to lung fields, otherwise, lung fields are clear; good aeration bilaterally; no wheezing; SpO$_2$ 97% before oxygen administration and 100% after provision of 30% oxygen by face mask • **C**irculation: Heart rate 140/min; skin pink and well perfused; strong peripheral pulses; capillary refill 2 seconds; blood pressure 86/58 mm Hg • **D**isability: Awake and alert; fussy but consolable • **E**xposure: Temperature 38.0°C (100.4°F); weight 8 kg	• Respiratory distress • Upper airway obstruction	• Administer 30% oxygen by face mask or nasal prongs. Assess response to oxygen. • Allow infant to maintain position of comfort; encourage parent to hold infant. • Give nebulized epinephrine.

Evaluate—*Secondary Assessment*	Identify	Intervene

SAMPLE history

- **S**igns and symptoms: Awoke with barking, seal-like cough; restless; crying; had upper respiratory infection and low-grade fever for the past 2 days
- **A**llergies: None known
- **M**edications: Acetaminophen for fever given by mother 2 hours ago
- **P**ast medical history: Otitis media at 6 and 8 months
- **L**ast meal: Ate well 2 hours ago
- **E**vents (onset): Cold symptoms (nasal discharge; dry, barky cough; low-grade fever) for the last 2 days; symptoms worsen at night but improve during the day

Physical examination

- *Repeat vital signs after oxygen and racemic epinephrine:* Heart rate 158/min; respiratory rate 32/min; SpO₂ 99% on supplementary oxygen; blood pressure 92/66 mm Hg
- *Head, eyes, ears, nose, and throat/neck:* Mild nasal flaring; yellowish nasal discharge; stridor now present with agitation but resolved at rest
- *Heart and lungs:* Lungs clear; transmitted upper airway sounds (less pronounced); suprasternal retractions improved
- *Abdomen:* Normal
- *Extremities:* Normal
- *Back:* Normal
- *Neurologic:* Fussy; cries vigorously; moving all extremities; parent able to console

Identify

- Respiratory distress
- Upper airway obstruction

Intervene

- Reassess cardiorespiratory status after epinephrine administration.
- Attempt to minimize stimulation of the infant.
- Monitor for at least 2 hours for recurrent airway edema/stridor. If signs recur, consider the following:
  - If oxygenation remains adequate, and provider is familiar with its use, consider use of heliox.
  - Be prepared to obtain expert consultation to develop plan of care (expertise is required to perform intubation and provide advanced monitoring and care).
- Administer oral/intravenous/intramuscular corticosteroid (eg, dexamethasone).
- Wean supplementary oxygen as tolerated.

Evaluate—*Diagnostic Assessments* *Perform Throughout the Evaluation of the Patient as Appropriate*	Identify/Intervene

Lab data

- None at his time

Imaging

- Lateral soft tissue neck radiographs are generally not necessary

Identify/Intervene

- Laboratory tests are generally not appropriate during initial stabilization to minimize stimulation and prevent agitation that may be associated with more respiratory distress and respiratory compromise.
- A blood glucose concentration should generally be checked as soon as reasonably possible in all critically ill infants and children. However, this infant has upper airway obstruction, and any agitation can worsen respiratory distress. In addition, the infant is alert and has fed well recently. As a result, in this case, the glucose evaluation should be deferred.

Re-evaluate-identify-intervene after each intervention.

Debriefing Tool
Testing Case Scenario 3
Upper Airway Obstruction (Infant)

- Use the table below to guide your debriefing; also refer to the **Team Dynamics Debriefing Tool.**
- Debriefings are 10 minutes long.
- Address all learning objectives.
- Summarize take-home messages at the end of the debriefing.
- **Encourage:** Students to self-reflect
  Engagement of all participants
- **Avoid:** Mini-lectures and closed-ended questions
  Dominating the discussion

General Management Objectives

- Uses the PALS Systematic Approach Algorithm to assess and appropriately classify a patient
- Provides oxygen appropriately
- Directs delivery of high-quality CPR (including the use of a feedback device) when indicated
- Demonstrates basic airway maneuvers and use of relevant airway device as appropriate
- Demonstrates application of cardiac and respiratory monitors

- Identifies the cardiac rhythm
- Applies appropriate PBLS or PALS algorithms
- Summarizes general indications, contraindications, and doses of relevant drugs
- Discusses principles of family-centered care in pediatric cardiac arrest
- Applies the 8 elements of effective team dynamics
- Performs frequent reassessment

Action	Gather	Analyze	Summarize
	Student Observations	***Done Well***	***Student-Led Summary***
• Directs assessment of ABCDE and vital signs	• Can you describe the events from your perspective?	• How were you able to [*insert action here*]?	• What are the main things you learned?
• Administers humidified oxygen as needed	• How well do you think your treatments worked?	• Why do you think you were able to [*insert action here*]?	• Can someone summarize the key points made?
• Applies cardiac monitor and pulse oximeter	• Can you review the events of the scenario (*directed to the Timer/Recorder*)?	• Tell me a little more about how you [*insert action here*].	• What are the main take-home messages?
• Recognizes signs and symptoms of upper airway obstruction	• What could you have improved?		
• Identifies respiratory distress rather than failure	• What did the team do well?		
• Provides appropriate initial management of upper airway obstruction, including allowing the infant to assume a position of comfort and administering humidified oxygen, nebulized epinephrine, and dexamethasone	***Instructor Observations***	***Needs Improvement***	***Instructor-Led Summary***
	• I noticed that [*insert action here*].	• Why do you think [*insert action here*] occurred?	• Let's summarize what we learned…
	• I observed that [*insert action here*].	• How do you think [*insert action here*] could have been improved?	• Here is what I think we learned…
• Reassesses the infant frequently and evaluates response to interventions	• I saw that [*insert action here*].	• What was your thinking while [*insert action here*]?	• The main take-home messages are…
• Recognizes the need to obtain early expert consultation from practitioners able to provide skilled intubation and advanced monitoring and care		• What prevented you from [*insert action here*]?	• This infant was stable in the scenario. However, if your interventions were not successful, what would be the signs of deterioration and possible indications for bag-mask ventilation or other airway or ventilation support? (Answer: Very rapid or inadequate respiratory rate or irregular breathing pattern; signs of significantly increased work of breathing; decreased breath sounds or aeration; deterioration in level of consciousness, hypoxemia, or cyanosis) Note that advanced expertise is needed for intubation and mechanical ventilation.
			• How would you estimate the correct uncuffed endotracheal tube size? (Answer: Would estimate a tube size about 0.5 mm smaller than typical for length and age)

Asystole
(Child; Arrest)*

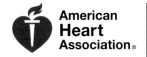

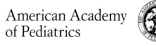

Vital Signs	
Heart rate	CPR in progress
Blood pressure	CPR in progress
Respiratory rate	Bag-mask ventilation (CPR)
SpO₂	Not obtainable
Temperature	Deferred
Weight	23 kg
Age	6 years

Scenario Lead-in

Prehospital: You are dispatched to a house where a 6-year-old boy is pulled from a pool and is pulseless. Parents started CPR and called 9-1-1.

ED: An ambulance is en route to the emergency department with a 6-year-old drowning victim. CPR is ongoing.

General Inpatient Unit: You are called as a member of the rapid response team to see a 6 year old who became limp and unresponsive. Child was admitted for treatment of pneumonia. CPR is in progress.

ICU: You are called to see a 6 year old who became progressively limp and unresponsive. The child was admitted for intravenous antibiotics for pneumonia with an x-ray that showed a possible small pleural effusion 6 hours ago. The remainder of the emergency department workup was unremarkable. CPR is in progress.

Scenario Overview and Learning Objectives

Scenario Overview

This scenario focuses on the identification and management of the child with cardiac arrest and a "nonshockable" rhythm. Emphasis is placed on immediate delivery of high-quality CPR and early administration of epinephrine. The student should identify potential reversible causes of asystole (H's and T's); submersion caused hypoxia and cardiac arrest in this scenario. Although not required for successful completion of the scenario, the instructor may (if time allows) discuss important elements of post–cardiac arrest care, including titration of inspired oxygen concentration to maintain SpO₂ of 94%-99%; targeted temperature management (especially avoidance or aggressive treatment of fever); hemodynamic support; support of airway, ventilation, and perfusion; and support of neurologic and other end-organ function.

Scenario-Specific Objectives

- **Identifies cardiac arrest with a nonshockable rhythm;** in this scenario, the child has asystole
- **Describes correct dose and rationale for epinephrine administration**
- **Summarizes potentially reversible causes of asystole and considers possible reversible causes of cardiac arrest (recalled by conditions beginning with H's and T's);** in this child, submersion and hypoxia are the causes
- **Discusses principles of post–cardiac arrest care;** for this scenario, these include titration of inspired oxygen concentration as tolerated; targeted temperature management (especially prevention of fever); hemodynamic support; support of airway, oxygenation, and ventilation; and support of neurologic and other end-organ function

Evaluate—*Initial Impression* (Pediatric Assessment Triangle)	Identify	Intervene
Appearance • Extremities appear to be limp; no spontaneous movement and no visible reaction to noise **Breathing** • No spontaneous breathing **Circulation** • Cyanotic/pale extremities and lips; severe mottling	• Immediate intervention needed	• Activate the emergency response system. Emergency medical services requests additional assistance if needed. • Check for response (no response) and perform simultaneous check for breathing (none) and carotid or femoral pulse (none). • Immediately begin high-quality CPR.

Evaluate—*Primary Assessment* Deferred to Provide Immediate Basic Life Support	Identify	Intervene
• No response to tap and shout • No breathing • No pulse • Weight 23 kg using color-coded length-based resuscitation tape	• Cardiopulmonary arrest	• Use a CPR feedback device to guide CPR delivery. • When defibrillator arrives, apply pads/leads and turn on monitor. • Identify rhythm (asystole); immediately resume high-quality CPR and check rhythm every 2 minutes. • Obtain vascular access (intravenous [IV]/intraosseous [IO]). • Give epinephrine 0.01 mg/kg (0.1 mL/kg of 0.1 mg/mL concentration) IV/IO during chest compressions. Follow with saline flush. Repeat every 3-5 minutes during cardiac arrest. • Apply pulse oximeter (per local protocol, may be deferred until return of spontaneous circulation [ROSC])

*Could also use as pulseless electrical activity case if needed.

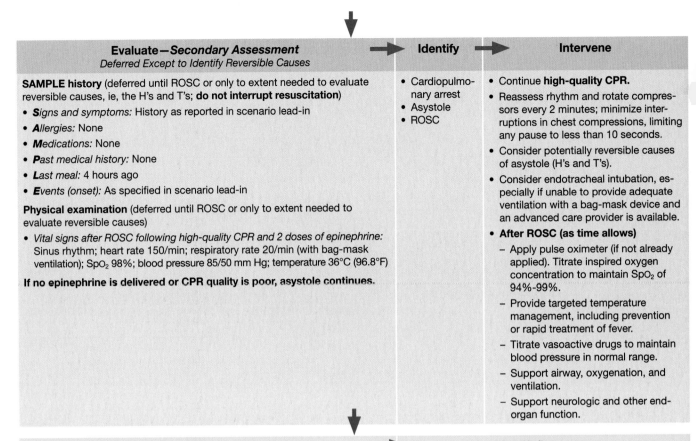

Evaluate—*Secondary Assessment*
Deferred Except to Identify Reversible Causes

SAMPLE history (deferred until ROSC or only to extent needed to evaluate reversible causes, ie, the H's and T's; **do not interrupt resuscitation**)

- **S**igns and symptoms: History as reported in scenario lead-in
- **A**llergies: None
- **M**edications: None
- **P**ast medical history: None
- **L**ast meal: 4 hours ago
- **E**vents (onset): As specified in scenario lead-in

Physical examination (deferred until ROSC or only to extent needed to evaluate reversible causes)

- *Vital signs after ROSC following high-quality CPR and 2 doses of epinephrine:* Sinus rhythm; heart rate 150/min; respiratory rate 20/min (with bag-mask ventilation); SpO_2 98%; blood pressure 85/50 mm Hg; temperature 36°C (96.8°F)

If no epinephrine is delivered or CPR quality is poor, asystole continues.

Identify

- Cardiopulmonary arrest
- Asystole
- ROSC

Intervene

- Continue **high-quality CPR.**
- Reassess rhythm and rotate compressors every 2 minutes; minimize interruptions in chest compressions, limiting any pause to less than 10 seconds.
- Consider potentially reversible causes of asystole (H's and T's).
- Consider endotracheal intubation, especially if unable to provide adequate ventilation with a bag-mask device and an advanced care provider is available.
- **After ROSC (as time allows)**
  - Apply pulse oximeter (if not already applied). Titrate inspired oxygen concentration to maintain SpO_2 of 94%-99%.
  - Provide targeted temperature management, including prevention or rapid treatment of fever.
  - Titrate vasoactive drugs to maintain blood pressure in normal range.
  - Support airway, oxygenation, and ventilation.
  - Support neurologic and other end-organ function.

Evaluate—*Diagnostic Assessments*
Perform Throughout the Evaluation of the Patient as Appropriate

Lab data (as appropriate)
- Blood glucose 108 mg/dL (6 mmol/L) (after ROSC)
- Arterial/venous blood gas, electrolytes, calcium, magnesium

Imaging ROSC
- *Chest x-ray (after ROSC):* Normal heart and lung fields

Identify/Intervene

- Blood work and chest x-ray are not available during the scenario.

Re–evaluate-identify-intervene after each intervention.

Debriefing Tool
Testing Case Scenario 4
Asystole (Child; Arrest)

General Debriefing Principles

- Use the table below to guide your debriefing; also refer to the **Team Dynamics Debriefing Tool.**
- Debriefings are 10 minutes long.
- Address all learning objectives.
- Summarize take-home messages at the end of the debriefing.
- *Encourage:* Students to self-reflect
  Engagement of all participants
- *Avoid:* Mini-lectures and closed-ended questions
  Dominating the discussion

General Management Objectives

- Uses the PALS Systematic Approach Algorithm to assess and appropriately classify a patient
- Provides oxygen appropriately
- Directs delivery of high-quality CPR (including the use of a feedback device) when indicated
- Demonstrates basic airway maneuvers and use of relevant airway device as appropriate
- Demonstrates application of cardiac and respiratory monitors

- Identifies the cardiac rhythm
- Applies appropriate PBLS or PALS algorithms
- Summarizes general indications, contraindications, and doses of relevant drugs
- Discusses principles of family-centered care in pediatric cardiac arrest
- Applies the 8 elements of effective team dynamics
- Performs frequent reassessment

Action	Gather	Analyze	Summarize
	Student Observations	*Done Well*	*Student-Led Summary*
• Identifies cardiac arrest	• Can you describe the events from your perspective?	• How were you able to [*insert action here*]?	• What are the main things you learned?
• Directs immediate initiation of high-quality CPR with the use of a feedback device (if available)	• How well do you think your treatments worked?	• Why do you think you were able to [*insert action here*]?	• Can someone summarize the key points made?
• Directs placement of monitor leads/pads and activation of monitor	• Can you review the events of the scenario (*directed to the Timer/Recorder*)?	• Tell me a little more about how you [*insert action here*].	• What are the main take-home messages?
• Identifies asystole	• What could you have improved?		
• Directs establishment of IV or IO access	• What did the team do well?		
• Directs preparation and administration of 0.01 mg/kg epinephrine (0.1 mL/kg of 0.1 mg/mL concentration) IV/IO bolus at appropriate intervals	*Instructor Observations*	*Needs Improvement*	*Instructor-Led Summary*
• Directs checking rhythm approximately every 2 minutes while minimizing interruptions in chest compressions	• I noticed that [*insert action here*].	• Why do you think [*insert action here*] occurred?	• Let's summarize what we learned…
• Identifies at least 3 potential reversible causes of pulseless electrical activity (recalled by the H's and T's)	• I observed that [*insert action here*].	• How do you think [*insert action here*] could have been improved?	• Here is what I think we learned…
• Performs appropriate re-assessments	• I saw that [*insert action here*].	• What was your thinking while [*insert action here*]?	• The main take-home messages are…
		• What prevented you from [*insert action here*]?	• Of the potential reversible causes of asystole in this patient, which are most likely? (Answer: Hypoxia)
			• Although not covered in this scenario, what are the key elements of post–cardiac arrest care? (Answer should include titration of oxygen; targeted temperature management; hemodynamic support and support of airway, oxygenation, and ventilation; support of neurologic and other end-organ function.)

Pulseless Electrical Activity
(Infant; Arrest)*

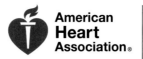

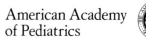

Vital Signs	
Heart rate	CPR in progress
Blood pressure	CPR in progress
Respiratory rate	100% bag-mask ventilation (CPR)
SpO₂	Not obtainable
Temperature	Deferred
Weight	8 kg
Age	9 months

Scenario Lead-in

Prehospital: You are dispatched to a house where a 9-month-old infant with a 2-day history of high fever is now unresponsive.

ED: An ambulance is en route to the emergency department with a 9-month-old infant who was found unresponsive in her crib. There is a 2-day history of high fever. CPR is ongoing.

General Inpatient Unit: You are called as a member of the rapid response team to see a 9 month old who was admitted with sepsis but has now become limp and unresponsive.

ICU: You are called to see a 9 month old who became progressively limp and unresponsive. The infant was admitted with sepsis and was found to be hypotensive at the time of the emergency department visit, though the remainder of the emergency department workup was unremarkable.

Scenario Overview and Learning Objectives

Scenario Overview

This scenario focuses on the identification and management of the infant with cardiac arrest and a "nonshockable" rhythm. Emphasis is placed on immediate delivery of high-quality CPR and early administration of epinephrine. The student should identify potential causes of pulseless electrical activity (PEA) (H's and T's). The infant's history of high fever suggests that sepsis/septic shock and hypovolemia may be the cause of deterioration and arrest. Although not required for successful completion of the scenario, the instructor may (if time allows) discuss important elements of post–cardiac arrest care, including titration of inspired oxygen concentration to maintain SpO₂ of 94%-99%; targeted temperature management (especially avoidance or aggressive treatment of fever); hemodynamic support; support of airway, ventilation, and perfusion; and support of neurologic and other end-organ function.

Scenario-Specific Objectives

- **Identifies cardiac arrest with a nonshockable rhythm;** in this scenario, the infant has PEA
- **Describes correct dose and rationale for epinephrine administration**
- **Summarizes potentially reversible causes of PEA and considers possible reversible causes of cardiac arrest (recalled by conditions beginning with H's and T's);** in this infant, the history of high fever suggests sepsis/septic shock with resultant hypovolemia as a cause
- **Discusses principles of post–cardiac arrest care;** these include titration of inspired oxygen concentration as tolerated; targeted temperature management (especially prevention of fever); hemodynamic support; support of airway, oxygenation, and ventilation; and support of neurologic and other end-organ function

Evaluate—Initial Impression (Pediatric Assessment Triangle)	➡ Identify ➡	Intervene
Appearance • Appears to be limp; no spontaneous movement; no visible reaction to noises **Breathing** • No spontaneous breathing **Circulation** • Cyanotic/pale extremities and lips; severe mottling	• Immediate intervention needed	• Activate the emergency response system. Emergency medical services requests additional assistance if needed. • Check for response (no response) and perform simultaneous check for breathing (none) and brachial pulse (none). • Immediately begin high-quality CPR.

Evaluate—Primary Assessment Deferred to Provide Immediate Basic Life Support	➡ Identify ➡	Intervene
• No response to tap and shout • No breathing • No pulse • Weight 8 kg per color-coded length-based resuscitation tape	• Cardiopulmonary arrest	• Use a CPR feedback device to guide CPR delivery. • When defibrillator arrives, apply pads/leads and turn on monitor. • Identify rhythm (PEA); immediately resume high-quality CPR, and check rhythm every 2 minutes. • Obtain vascular access (intravenous [IV]/intraosseous [IO]). • Give epinephrine 0.01 mg/kg (0.1 mL/kg of 0.1 mg/mL concentration) IV/IO during chest compressions; follow with saline flush. Repeat every 3-5 minutes during cardiac arrest. • Apply pulse oximeter (per local protocol, may be deferred until return of spontaneous circulation [ROSC]).

*Could also use as asystole case if needed.

Evaluate—*Secondary Assessment*	Identify	Intervene
Deferred Except to Identify Reversible Causes		

Evaluate—*Secondary Assessment*
Deferred Except to Identify Reversible Causes

Identify

Intervene

SAMPLE history (deferred until ROSC or only to extent needed to evaluate reversible causes, ie, the H's and T's; **do not interrupt resuscitation**)

- *Signs and symptoms:* History as reported in scenario lead in
- *Allergies:* None
- *Medications:* None
- *Past medical history:* Unremarkable
- *Last meal:* 2 hours ago
- *Events (onset):* As specified in scenario lead-in

Physical examination (deferred until ROSC or only to extent needed to evaluate reversible causes)

- *Vital signs after ROSC following high-quality CPR and 1 dose of epinephrine:* Sinus rhythm; heart rate 170/min; blood pressure 75/50 mm Hg; respiratory rate 20/min with bag-mask ventilation; SpO$_2$ 98%; temperature 36°C (96.8°F)

If no epinephrine is delivered or CPR quality is poor, PEA continues.

- Cardiac arrest
- PEA
- ROSC

- Continue high-quality CPR.
- Reassess rhythm and rotate compressors every 2 minutes while minimizing pauses in compressions, limiting any pause to less than 10 seconds.
- Consider potentially reversible causes of PEA (H's and T's).
- The advanced provider may consider hypovolemia as a cause of PEA in a child with a high likelihood of sepsis and give a fluid bolus of 20 mL/kg isotonic crystalloid.
- Consider endotracheal intubation, especially if unable to provide adequate ventilation with a bag-mask device and an advanced care provider is available.
- **After ROSC (as time allows)**
  - Apply pulse oximeter (if not already applied). Titrate oxygen to maintain SpO$_2$ of 94%-99%.
  - Provide targeted temperature management, including prevention or rapid treatment of fever.
  - Titrate vasoactive drugs to maintain blood pressure in normal range.
  - Support airway, oxygenation, and ventilation.
  - Support neurologic and other end-organ function.
  - Evaluate for possible infection, septic shock.

Evaluate—*Diagnostic Assessments*
Perform Throughout the Evaluation of the Patient as Appropriate

Identify/Intervene

Lab data (as appropriate)

- Blood glucose 108 mg/dL (6 mmol/L) (after ROSC)
- Arterial/venous blood gas, electrolytes, calcium, magnesium, blood culture

Imaging

- *Chest x-ray (after ROSC):* Normal heart and lung fields

- Blood work and chest x-ray are not available during the scenario.

Re–evaluate-identify-intervene after each intervention.

Debriefing Tool
Testing Case Scenario 5
PEA (Infant; Arrest)

General Debriefing Principles

- Use the table below to guide your debriefing; also refer to the **Team Dynamics Debriefing Tool.**
- Debriefings are 10 minutes long.
- Address all learning objectives.
- Summarize take-home messages at the end of the debriefing.
- *Encourage:* Students to self-reflect
  Engagement of all participants
- *Avoid:* Mini-lectures and closed-ended questions
  Dominating the discussion

General Management Objectives

- Uses the PALS Systematic Approach Algorithm to assess and appropriately classify a patient
- Provides oxygen appropriately
- Directs delivery of high-quality CPR (including the use of a feedback device) when indicated
- Demonstrates basic airway maneuvers and use of relevant airway device as appropriate
- Demonstrates application of cardiac and respiratory monitors
- Identifies the cardiac rhythm
- Applies appropriate PBLS or PALS algorithms
- Summarizes general indications, contraindications, and doses of relevant drugs
- Discusses principles of family-centered care in pediatric cardiac arrest
- Applies the 8 elements of effective team dynamics
- Performs frequent reassessment

Action	Gather	Analyze	Summarize
- Identifies cardiac arrest - Directs immediate initiation of high-quality CPR with the use of a feedback device (if available) - Applies cardiac monitor and pulse oximeter - Identifies PEA - Directs establishment of IV or IO access - Directs preparation and administration of 0.01 mg/kg (0.1 mL/kg of 0.1 mg/mL concentration) epinephrine IV/IO bolus at appropriate intervals - Directs checking rhythm approximately every 2 minutes while minimizing interruptions in chest compressions - Identifies at least 3 potential reversible causes of PEA (recalled by the H's and T's) - Performs appropriate reassessments	***Student Observations*** - Can you describe the events from your perspective? - How well do you think your treatments worked? - Can you review the events of the scenario (*directed to the Timer/Recorder*)? - What could you have improved? - What did the team do well? ***Instructor Observations*** - I noticed that [*insert action here*]. - I observed that [*insert action here*]. - I saw that [*insert action here*].	***Done Well*** - How were you able to [*insert action here*]? - Why do you think you were able to [*insert action here*]? - Tell me a little more about how you [*insert action here*]. ***Needs Improvement*** - Why do you think [*insert action here*] occurred? - How do you think [*insert action here*] could have been improved? - What was your thinking while [*insert action here*]? - What prevented you from [*insert action here*]?	***Student-Led Summary*** - What are the main things you learned? - Can someone summarize the key points made? - What are the main take-home messages? ***Instructor-Led Summary*** - Let's summarize what we learned… - Here is what I think we learned… - The main take-home messages are… - Of the potential reversible causes of PEA in this patient, which are most likely? (Answer: Hypovolemia with sepsis) - Although not covered in this scenario, what are the key elements of post–cardiac arrest care? (Answer should include titration of oxygen; targeted temperature management; hemodynamic support and support of airway, oxygenation, and ventilation; support of neurologic and other end-organ function.)

Lung Tissue (Parenchymal) Disease (Child)

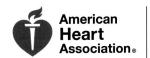

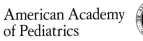

American Academy of Pediatrics

DEDICATED TO THE HEALTH OF ALL CHILDREN™

Vital Signs	
Heart rate	160/min
Blood pressure	110/78 mm Hg
Respiratory rate	38/min
SpO₂	80% on room air
Temperature	38.5°C (101.4°F)
Weight	12 kg
Age	3 years

Scenario Lead-in

Prehospital: You are responding to a 9-1-1 call for a 3-year-old boy in respiratory distress.

ED: A 3-year-old boy is brought in by first responders from his home after his mother called 9-1-1 saying that her child had respiratory distress.

General Inpatient Unit: You are called to the room of a 3-year-old boy who is being admitted from the emergency department for respiratory distress.

ICU: You are evaluating a 3-year-old boy at change of shift with new-onset respiratory distress.

Scenario Overview and Learning Objectives

Scenario Overview

Emphasis in this scenario is on rapid recognition and initial management of respiratory failure associated with lung tissue (parenchymal) disease. Immediate administration of 100% oxygen is required. Signs of respiratory failure indicate the need for assisted ventilation and contacting an advanced provider with appropriate expertise. During debriefing, the method to estimate endotracheal tube size (cuffed and uncuffed) is discussed. Although not required for successful completion of the scenario, the possible use of continuous positive airway pressure (CPAP) or noninvasive ventilation can be addressed with emphasis that such therapy must be provided in appropriate settings where continuous monitoring is provided and intubation equipment and appropriate provider expertise are readily available.

Scenario-Specific Objectives

- **Distinguishes between respiratory distress and respiratory failure;** in this scenario, the child's clinical signs are consistent with respiratory failure
- **Identifies signs of lung tissue disease in a pediatric patient;** in this scenario, the signs of lung tissue disease include tachypnea, increased respiratory effort, grunting, crackles (rales), tachycardia, and hypoxemia despite oxygen administration
- **Implements correct interventions for lung tissue disease;** in this scenario, interventions include administration of a high concentration of oxygen, appropriate monitoring, frequent reassessment, and more advanced support of the child's oxygenation and ventilation (eg, typically with bag-mask ventilation and then with intubation and positive-pressure ventilation)
- **Describes how noninvasive ventilatory support, such as CPAP or noninvasive positive-pressure ventilation, may improve oxygenation in lung tissue disease;** in this scenario, CPAP or noninvasive positive-pressure ventilation may increase alveolar volume and improve matching of ventilation and perfusion (and oxygenation)
- **Recalls the common causes of lung tissue disease;** common causes of lung tissue disease include pneumonia and aspiration

Evaluate—*Initial Impression* *(Pediatric Assessment Triangle)*	Identify	Intervene
Appearance • Lethargic **Breathing** • Rapid respirations; grunting **Circulation** • Pale skin	• Immediate intervention needed	• Administer 100% oxygen by nonrebreathing face mask. • Apply cardiac monitor. • Apply pulse oximeter.

Evaluate—*Primary Assessment* *Focused on Assessment Needed to Support Airway, Oxygenation, Ventilation, and Perfusion*	Identify	Intervene
• **A**irway: Unobstructed but noisy; grunting • **B**reathing: Rapid respirations; moderate intercostal and subcostal retractions; crackles heard over right chest; no stridor or wheezing; expiratory phase is not prolonged; respiratory rate 38/min; SpO₂ 80% on room air and increased to 88% on 100% oxygen via a nonrebreathing face mask • **C**irculation: Heart rate 160/min; pale skin; strong radial pulse; capillary refill 2 seconds; blood pressure 110/78 mm Hg • **D**isability: Arouses to verbal stimuli • **E**xposure: Temperature 38.5°C (101.4°F); weight 12 kg	• Respiratory failure • Lung tissue disease	• Allow child to maintain position of comfort. • Assess response to oxygen.

Evaluate—*Secondary Assessment* *Identify Reversible Causes, but Defer Remainder of Secondary Assessment Until After Stabilization of Airway, Oxygenation, and Ventilation*	Identify	Intervene
SAMPLE history • *Signs and symptoms:* Worsening respiratory distress, cough, and fever for the past 2 days • *Allergies:* None known • *Medications:* None • *Past medical history:* None • *Last meal:* 8 hours ago • *Events (onset):* Child recently diagnosed with influenza **Physical examination** • *Repeat vital signs after oxygen:* Respiratory rate 38/min; heart rate 160/min; SpO$_2$ still 88% with 100% inspired oxygen concentration; blood pressure 110/74 mm Hg • *Head, eyes, ears, nose, and throat/neck:* Normal • *Heart and lungs:* Aeration fair; retractions increasing with occasional grunting; crackles now heard over right chest; central and peripheral pulses remain strong; capillary refill remains 2 seconds • *Abdomen:* Normal • *Extremities:* Normal • *Back:* Normal • *Neurologic:* Lethargic; becoming less responsive; only arouses to painful stimuli	• Respiratory failure • Lung tissue disease	• Begin bag-mask ventilation with 100% oxygen (verify chest rise with ventilation) and contact an advanced provider with appropriate expertise to assist with intubation and initiation of mechanical ventilation. – *Note:* If the child's level of consciousness improves and the child can be continuously monitored, critical care providers may consider a brief trial of noninvasive ventilation support (mask CPAP or noninvasive positive-pressure ventilation) *if* there is equipment and appropriate expertise for rapid intubation immediately available. • Prepare equipment and skilled personnel for endotracheal intubation using a cuffed tracheal tube. • Obtain vascular access. • Obtain arterial/venous blood gas. • Treat fever with antipyretics. • Arrange transfer of the child to an intensive care unit (ICU) (unless the child is already in the ICU). • Consider specific interventions for lung tissue disease (eg, antibiotics for suspected pneumonia).

Evaluate—*Diagnostic Assessments* *Perform Throughout the Evaluation of the Patient as Appropriate*	Identify/Intervene
Lab data • Complete blood count, blood culture, arterial/venous blood gas pending • Glucose (point-of-care testing) 136 mg/dL (7.5 mmol/L) ***Imaging*** • Chest x-ray	• Laboratory tests generally are not appropriate during the first 5-10 minutes when attempting to stabilize a hypoxemic child with severe respiratory distress/respiratory failure. • A blood glucose concentration should be checked as soon as reasonably possible in all critically ill infants and children. Hypoglycemia should be treated immediately. • Chest x-ray shows large right-sided pneumonia with no obvious pleural effusion.

Re–evaluate-identify-intervene after each intervention.

Debriefing Tool
Testing Case Scenario 6
Lung Tissue (Parenchymal) Disease (Child)

- Use the table below to guide your debriefing; also refer to the **Team Dynamics Debriefing Tool.**
- Debriefings are 10 minutes long.
- Address all learning objectives.
- Summarize take-home messages at the end of the debriefing.
- *Encourage:* Students to self-reflect
        Engagement of all participants
- *Avoid:* Mini-lectures and closed-ended questions
        Dominating the discussion

General Management Objectives

- Uses the PALS Systematic Approach Algorithm to assess and appropriately classify a patient
- Provides oxygen appropriately
- Directs delivery of high-quality CPR (including the use of a feedback device) when indicated
- Demonstrates basic airway maneuvers and use of relevant airway device as appropriate
- Demonstrates application of cardiac and respiratory monitors

- Identifies the cardiac rhythm
- Applies appropriate PBLS or PALS algorithms
- Summarizes general indications, contraindications, and doses of relevant drugs
- Discusses principles of family-centered care in pediatric cardiac arrest
- Applies the 8 elements of effective team dynamics
- Performs frequent reassessment

Action	Gather	Analyze	Summarize
• Directs assessment of ABCDE and vital signs • Directs administration of 100% oxygen via nonrebreathing face mask and evaluates response • Applies cardiac monitor and pulse oximeter • Identifies respiratory failure • Identifies signs of lung tissue disease • Evaluates response to 100% oxygen and determines need for additional intervention • Provides or directs provision of bag-mask ventilation • Describes methods to verify that bag-mask ventilation is effective • Directs establishment of intravenous access • Performs frequent reassessment of patient • Identifies need for involvement of advanced provider with expertise in pediatric intubation and mechanical ventilation • Identifies indications for endotracheal intubation	***Student Observations*** • Can you describe the events from your perspective? • How well do you think your treatments worked? • Can you review the events of the scenario (*directed to the Timer/Recorder*)? • What could you have improved? • What did the team do well? ***Instructor Observations*** • I noticed that [*insert action here*]. • I observed that [*insert action here*]. • I saw that [*insert action here*].	***Done Well*** • How were you able to [*insert action here*]? • Why do you think you were able to [*insert action here*]? • Tell me a little more about how you [*insert action here*]. ***Needs Improvement*** • Why do you think [*insert action here*] occurred? • How do you think [*insert action here*] could have been improved? • What was your thinking while [*insert action here*]? • What prevented you from [*insert action here*]?	***Student-Led Summary*** • What are the main things you learned? • Can someone summarize the key points made? • What are the main take-home messages? ***Instructor-Led Summary*** • Let's summarize what we learned… • Here is what I think we learned… • The main take-home messages are… • If this child requires intubation, how would you estimate the appropriate cuffed endotracheal tube size? • Can you explain why CPAP or noninvasive positive-pressure ventilation might improve this child's oxygenation? (Answer: It will increase alveolar ventilation and ventilation-perfusion match.) Discuss why it is important that such care be provided in a setting where continuous monitoring of the child is possible and appropriate expertise is immediately available.

Distributive Shock
(Infant; Septic Shock)

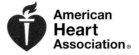

American Heart Association.

life is why™

American Academy of Pediatrics

DEDICATED TO THE HEALTH OF ALL CHILDREN™

Scenario Lead-in

Prehospital: You have been dispatched to transport a 4 month old with a 24-hour history of high fever and lethargy. She has not been feeding well.

ED: You are asked to assess and manage a 4 month old with a 24-hour history of high fever and lethargy. She has not been feeding well.

General Inpatient Unit: You are called to assess a 4 month old who has just been admitted to the ward with a 24-hour history of high fever and lethargy. She has not been feeding well. The intravenous access placed at the time of admission is no longer functioning.

ICU: You are called to the bedside of a 4 month old who has just been admitted to the intensive care unit with a 24-hour history of high fever and lethargy. She has not been feeding well. The intravenous access placed at the time of admission is no longer functioning.

Vital Signs	
Heart rate	192/min
Blood pressure	76/30 mm Hg
Respiratory rate	55/min
SpO$_2$	93% on room air
Temperature	39.0°C (102.2°F)
Weight	5.1 kg
Age	4 months

Scenario Overview and Learning Objectives

Scenario Overview

Emphasis should be on identification of compensated distributive/septic shock. Priorities include immediate establishment of intravenous (IV)/intraosseous (IO) access and administration of fluid bolus(es) of isotonic crystalloid with careful reassessment of cardiorespiratory function during and after each fluid bolus. The provider should recognize the signs of heart failure and stop bolus fluid administration. Within the first hour of identification of signs of septic shock, providers must also administer antibiotics and initiate vasoactive drug therapy if shock persists despite bolus fluid administration. The infant is lethargic, so early point-of-care (POC) glucose check is indicated.

Scenario-Specific Objectives

- **Recognizes compensated vs hypotensive shock;** in this scenario, the infant demonstrates compensated shock (blood pressure is not hypotensive)
- **Recognizes need for early/rapid intervention with bolus administration of isotonic crystalloids and vasoactive drug therapy within the first hour if shock signs/symptoms persist despite bolus fluid administration**
- **Recognizes the need for careful and frequent cardiorespiratory reassessment during and after each fluid bolus;** the provider looks for signs of heart failure (increased respiratory distress or development of rales or hepatomegaly) and stops bolus fluid administration if signs of heart failure develop
- **Recognizes need for early/rapid administration of antibiotics (during the first hour after identification of shock symptoms)**

Evaluate—*Initial Impression* (Pediatric Assessment Triangle)	Identify	Intervene
Appearance • Lethargic, does react to voices in room **Breathing** • Increased rate and effort **Circulation** • Pale, with significant mottling of extremities	• Immediate intervention needed	• Activate the emergency response system. Emergency medical services requests additional assistance if needed. • Administer 100% oxygen by nonrebreathing face mask. • Apply cardiac monitor. • Apply pulse oximeter.

Evaluate—*Primary Assessment* Focused on Assessment Needed to Support Airway, Oxygenation, Ventilation, and Perfusion	Identify	Intervene
• **A**irway: Clear • **B**reathing: Respiratory rate about 55/min; mild subcostal and intercostal retractions; mild nasal flaring; SpO$_2$ 93% on room air, increased to 97% with administration of 100% oxygen; lungs clear to auscultation • **C**irculation: Central pulses fair, peripheral pulses weak; heart rate 192/min; blood pressure 74/30 mm Hg capillary refill 5 seconds; cool and mottled hands and feet • **D**isability: Lethargic • **E**xposure: Rectal temperature 39.0°C (102.2°F); no rash; weight 5.1 kg	• Respiratory distress • Compensated shock (likely septic shock) • Sinus tachycardia	• Obtain vascular access (IV/IO). • Administer a 20 mL/kg bolus of isotonic crystalloid rapidly IV/IO. Reassess during and after fluid bolus. – Stop fluid bolus if signs of heart failure develop (eg, increased respiratory distress or development of rales or hepatomegaly). • Administer antibiotics within the first hour of recognition of shock (if not already done).

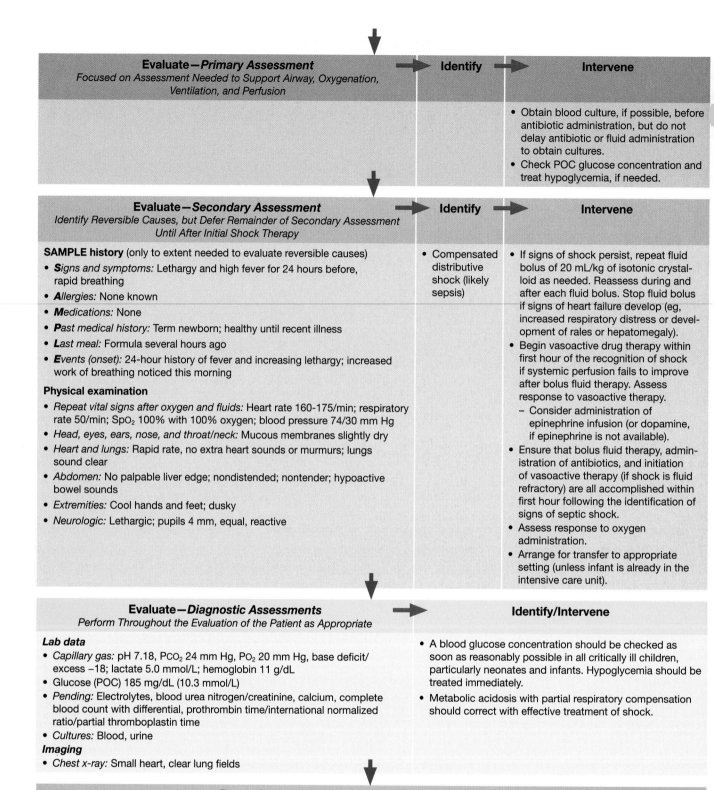

Evaluate—*Primary Assessment*
Focused on Assessment Needed to Support Airway, Oxygenation, Ventilation, and Perfusion

Identify → Intervene

- Obtain blood culture, if possible, before antibiotic administration, but do not delay antibiotic or fluid administration to obtain cultures.
- Check POC glucose concentration and treat hypoglycemia, if needed.

Evaluate—*Secondary Assessment*
Identify Reversible Causes, but Defer Remainder of Secondary Assessment Until After Initial Shock Therapy

SAMPLE history (only to extent needed to evaluate reversible causes)
- **S**igns and symptoms: Lethargy and high fever for 24 hours before, rapid breathing
- **A**llergies: None known
- **M**edications: None
- **P**ast medical history: Term newborn; healthy until recent illness
- **L**ast meal: Formula several hours ago
- **E**vents (onset): 24-hour history of fever and increasing lethargy; increased work of breathing noticed this morning

Physical examination
- *Repeat vital signs after oxygen and fluids:* Heart rate 160-175/min; respiratory rate 50/min; SpO$_2$ 100% with 100% oxygen; blood pressure 74/30 mm Hg
- *Head, eyes, ears, nose, and throat/neck:* Mucous membranes slightly dry
- *Heart and lungs:* Rapid rate, no extra heart sounds or murmurs; lungs sound clear
- *Abdomen:* No palpable liver edge; nondistended; nontender; hypoactive bowel sounds
- *Extremities:* Cool hands and feet; dusky
- *Neurologic:* Lethargic; pupils 4 mm, equal, reactive

Identify → Intervene

- Compensated distributive shock (likely sepsis)

- If signs of shock persist, repeat fluid bolus of 20 mL/kg of isotonic crystalloid as needed. Reassess during and after each fluid bolus. Stop fluid bolus if signs of heart failure develop (eg, increased respiratory distress or development of rales or hepatomegaly).
- Begin vasoactive drug therapy within first hour of the recognition of shock if systemic perfusion fails to improve after bolus fluid therapy. Assess response to vasoactive therapy.
  - Consider administration of epinephrine infusion (or dopamine, if epinephrine is not available).
- Ensure that bolus fluid therapy, administration of antibiotics, and initiation of vasoactive therapy (if shock is fluid refractory) are all accomplished within first hour following the identification of signs of septic shock.
- Assess response to oxygen administration.
- Arrange for transfer to appropriate setting (unless infant is already in the intensive care unit).

Evaluate—*Diagnostic Assessments*
Perform Throughout the Evaluation of the Patient as Appropriate

Identify/Intervene

Lab data
- *Capillary gas:* pH 7.18, PCO$_2$ 24 mm Hg, PO$_2$ 20 mm Hg, base deficit/excess −18; lactate 5.0 mmol/L; hemoglobin 11 g/dL
- Glucose (POC) 185 mg/dL (10.3 mmol/L)
- *Pending:* Electrolytes, blood urea nitrogen/creatinine, calcium, complete blood count with differential, prothrombin time/international normalized ratio/partial thromboplastin time
- *Cultures:* Blood, urine

Imaging
- *Chest x-ray:* Small heart, clear lung fields

- A blood glucose concentration should be checked as soon as reasonably possible in all critically ill children, particularly neonates and infants. Hypoglycemia should be treated immediately.
- Metabolic acidosis with partial respiratory compensation should correct with effective treatment of shock.

Re–evaluate-identify-intervene after each intervention.

Debriefing Tool
Testing Case Scenario 7
Distributive Shock (Infant; Septic Shock)

General Debriefing Principles

- Use the table below to guide your debriefing; also refer to the **Team Dynamics Debriefing Tool.**
- Debriefings are 10 minutes long.
- Address all learning objectives.
- Summarize take-home messages at the end of the debriefing.
- *Encourage:* Students to self-reflect
  Engagement of all participants
- *Avoid:* Mini-lectures and closed-ended questions
  Dominating the discussion

General Management Objectives

- Uses the PALS Systematic Approach Algorithm to assess and appropriately classify a patient
- Provides oxygen appropriately
- Directs delivery of high-quality CPR (including the use of a feedback device) when indicated
- Demonstrates basic airway maneuvers and use of relevant airway device as appropriate
- Demonstrates application of cardiac and respiratory monitors
- Identifies the cardiac rhythm
- Applies appropriate PBLS or PALS algorithms
- Summarizes general indications, contraindications, and doses of relevant drugs
- Discusses principles of family-centered care in pediatric cardiac arrest
- Applies the 8 elements of effective team dynamics
- Performs frequent reassessment

Action	Gather	Analyze	Summarize
• Directs assessment of ABCDE and vital signs • Administers 100% oxygen • Applies cardiac monitor and pulse oximeter • Identifies signs and symptoms of septic shock in an infant • Categorizes shock as compensated • Directs establishment of IV or IO access • Directs rapid administration of 20 mL/kg fluid bolus of isotonic crystalloid • Reassesses patient during and in response to interventions, particularly during and after each fluid bolus; stops fluid bolus if signs of heart failure develop • Repeats fluid bolus as needed to treat shock, with careful reassessment during and after each fluid bolus • Checks glucose with POC testing early in the care of the lethargic infant • Directs early (ie, within first hour after identification of shock) administration of antibiotics • Directs initiation of vasoactive drug therapy within the first hour after the recognition of shock if shock fails to respond to fluid boluses	***Student Observations*** • Can you describe the events from your perspective? • How well do you think your treatments worked? • Can you review the events of the scenario (*directed to the Timer/Recorder*)? • What could you have improved? • What did the team do well? ***Instructor Observations*** • I noticed that [*insert action here*]. • I observed that [*insert action here*]. • I saw that [*insert action here*].	***Done Well*** • How were you able to [*insert action here*]? • Why do you think you were able to [*insert action here*]? • Tell me a little more about how you [*insert action here*]. ***Needs Improvement*** • Why do you think [*insert action here*] occurred? • How do you think [*insert action here*] could have been improved? • What was your thinking while [*insert action here*]? • What prevented you from [*insert action here*]?	***Student-Led Summary*** • What are the main things you learned? • Can someone summarize the key points made? • What are the main take-home messages? ***Instructor-Led Summary*** • Let's summarize what we learned… • Here is what I think we learned… • The main take-home messages are… • What are the therapeutic end points during shock management? (Answer: Normalized heart rate; improved peripheral perfusion, mental status, and urine output; normalized blood pressure; correction of metabolic/lactic acidosis)

Supraventricular Tachycardia
(Adolescent; Stable)

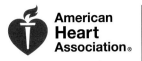

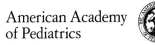

Vital Signs	
Heart rate	235/min
Blood pressure	100/65 mm Hg
Respiratory rate	20/min
SpO₂	94% on room air
Temperature	37.6°C (99.7°F)
Weight	44 kg
Age	12 years

Scenario Lead-in

Prehospital: You are dispatched to a house where a 12-year-old boy has tachypnea and a racing heart.

ED: An ambulance is en route to the emergency department with a 12-year-old boy with tachypnea and a racing heart. An intravenous access has been placed.

General Inpatient Unit: You are called to examine a 12-year-old boy with tachypnea and a racing heart. An intravenous access is in place.

ICU: You are called to the bedside of a 12-year-old boy who says he has a racing heart. He has an intravenous access.

Scenario Overview and Learning Objectives

Scenario Overview

Emphasis should be on recognition and management of supraventricular tachycardia (SVT) in a stable child, including the use of vagal maneuvers and adenosine. Provision of synchronized cardioversion is beyond the scope of this scenario, but discussion regarding indications for synchronized cardioversion, including appropriate dose and safe delivery, should occur during the scenario debriefing. Expert consultation with a pediatric cardiologist is strongly recommended before providing synchronized cardioversion, and synchronized cardioversion preceded by sedation requires expertise to minimize hemodynamic impact of the sedative.

Scenario-Specific Objectives

- **Differentiates between SVT and sinus tachycardia;** the child in this scenario has SVT
- **Describes potential vagal maneuvers used for a child with SVT;** vagal maneuvers used in children include blowing through a narrowed straw or bearing down and grunting
- **Demonstrates the proper rapid bolus technique to administer adenosine**
- **Describes safe administration of synchronized cardioversion (if needed) with the appropriate dose in a patient with SVT**
- **Discusses the reason that expert consultation is advised before performing synchronized cardioversion in a stable child with SVT**

Evaluate—*Initial Impression* (Pediatric Assessment Triangle)	Identify	Intervene
Appearance • Awake; alert; anxious **Breathing** • Increased rate and mildly increased effort **Circulation** • Warm with brisk capillary refill	• No immediate intervention needed	• Proceed to Primary Assessment.

Evaluate—*Primary Assessment*	Identify	Intervene

• **A**irway: Clear
• **B**reathing: Respiratory rate 20/min; SpO₂ 94% before supplementary oxygen administration, 100% when receiving 30% oxygen by face mask; clear lung fields
• **C**irculation: Heart rate 235/min; strong central and peripheral pulses; warm skin; capillary refill about 2 seconds; blood pressure 100/65 mm Hg
• **D**isability: Awake; alert; interactive
• **E**xposure: Temperature 37.6°C (99.7°F); weight 44 kg
	• Narrow-complex tachycardia with a pulse and adequate perfusion (stable)	• Activate the emergency response system. Emergency medical services requests additional assistance if needed.
		• Administer oxygen; titrate to maintain SpO₂ 94%-99%.
		• Apply pads/leads and turn on monitor.
		• Apply pulse oximeter.
		• Establish or verify existing intravenous (IV) access.
		• Guide child to perform vagal maneuvers.
		• Prepare adenosine dose and saline flush.
		  – Record rhythm strip during administration.
		  – Administer first dose of adenosine 0.1 mg/kg (maximum dose: 6 mg) rapid IV push, by rapid saline flush.

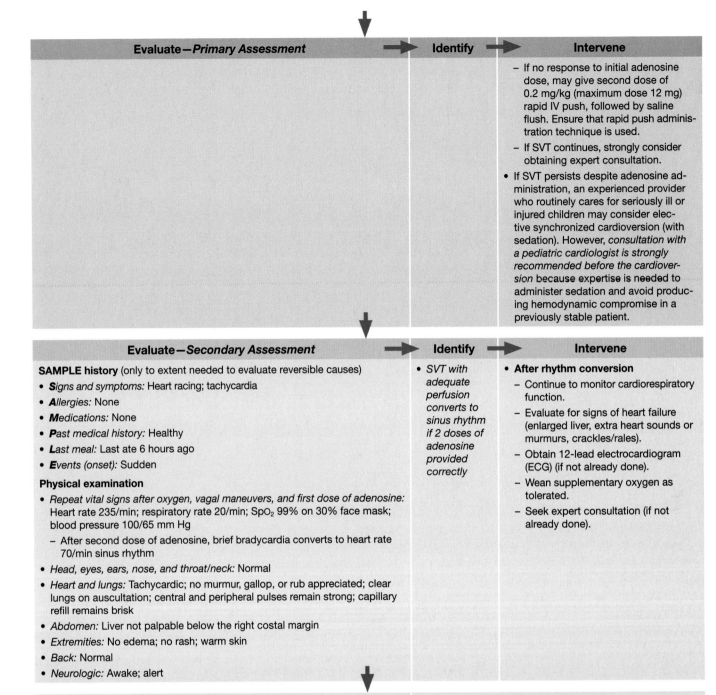

Evaluate—*Primary Assessment* → Identify → Intervene

Intervene

- – If no response to initial adenosine dose, may give second dose of 0.2 mg/kg (maximum dose 12 mg) rapid IV push, followed by saline flush. Ensure that rapid push administration technique is used.
- – If SVT continues, strongly consider obtaining expert consultation.
- If SVT persists despite adenosine administration, an experienced provider who routinely cares for seriously ill or injured children may consider elective synchronized cardioversion (with sedation). However, *consultation with a pediatric cardiologist is strongly recommended before the cardioversion* because expertise is needed to administer sedation and avoid producing hemodynamic compromise in a previously stable patient.

Evaluate—*Secondary Assessment* → Identify → Intervene

SAMPLE history (only to extent needed to evaluate reversible causes)

- **S**igns and symptoms: Heart racing; tachycardia
- **A**llergies: None
- **M**edications: None
- **P**ast medical history: Healthy
- **L**ast meal: Last ate 6 hours ago
- **E**vents (onset): Sudden

Physical examination

- *Repeat vital signs after oxygen, vagal maneuvers, and first dose of adenosine:* Heart rate 235/min; respiratory rate 20/min; SpO₂ 99% on 30% face mask; blood pressure 100/65 mm Hg
  - – After second dose of adenosine, brief bradycardia converts to heart rate 70/min sinus rhythm
- *Head, eyes, ears, nose, and throat/neck:* Normal
- *Heart and lungs:* Tachycardic; no murmur, gallop, or rub appreciated; clear lungs on auscultation; central and peripheral pulses remain strong; capillary refill remains brisk
- *Abdomen:* Liver not palpable below the right costal margin
- *Extremities:* No edema; no rash; warm skin
- *Back:* Normal
- *Neurologic:* Awake; alert

Identify

- SVT with adequate perfusion converts to sinus rhythm if 2 doses of adenosine provided correctly

Intervene

- **After rhythm conversion**
  - – Continue to monitor cardiorespiratory function.
  - – Evaluate for signs of heart failure (enlarged liver, extra heart sounds or murmurs, crackles/rales).
  - – Obtain 12-lead electrocardiogram (ECG) (if not already done).
  - – Wean supplementary oxygen as tolerated.
  - – Seek expert consultation (if not already done).

Evaluate—*Diagnostic Assessments* → Identify/Intervene
Perform Throughout the Evaluation of the Patient as Appropriate

Lab data

- Blood glucose 88 mg/dL
- Electrolytes

Imaging

- Chest x-ray, ECG in SVT and in sinus tachycardia; ideally capture the adenosine dose being given by running a rhythm strip simultaneously

Identify/Intervene

- Although laboratory tests are generally not appropriate during the immediate management, a blood glucose concentration should be checked as soon as reasonably possible in all critically ill children, particularly neonates and infants. Hypoglycemia should be treated immediately.

Re–evaluate-identify-intervene after each intervention.

Debriefing Tool
Testing Case Scenario 8
SVT (Adolescent; Stable)

- Use the table below to guide your debriefing; also refer to the **Team Dynamics Debriefing Tool.**
- Debriefings are 10 minutes long.
- Address all learning objectives.
- Summarize take-home messages at the end of the debriefing.
- *Encourage:* Students to self-reflect
  Engagement of all participants
- *Avoid:* Mini-lectures and closed-ended questions
  Dominating the discussion

General Management Objectives

- Uses the PALS Systematic Approach Algorithm to assess and appropriately classify a patient
- Provides oxygen appropriately
- Directs delivery of high-quality CPR (including the use of a feedback device) when indicated
- Demonstrates basic airway maneuvers and use of relevant airway device as appropriate
- Demonstrates application of cardiac and respiratory monitors

- Identifies the cardiac rhythm
- Applies appropriate PBLS or PALS algorithms
- Summarizes general indications, contraindications, and doses of relevant drugs
- Discusses principles of family-centered care in pediatric cardiac arrest
- Applies the 8 elements of effective team dynamics
- Performs frequent reassessment

Action	Gather	Analyze	Summarize
• Directs assessment of ABCDE and vital signs • Applies cardiac monitor and pulse oximeter • Directs administration of supplementary oxygen • Identifies SVT with stable perfusion and distinguishes it from sinus tachycardia • Knows how to help child perform appropriate vagal maneuvers • Directs establishment of IV/intraosseous access • Directs preparation and administration of correct doses of adenosine using rapid bolus technique • Explains the rationale for expert consultation before synchronized cardioversion if stable child with SVT fails to respond to vagal maneuvers and adenosine • Discusses indications for and safe delivery of correct doses (initial and subsequent) of synchronized cardioversion • Performs frequent reassessment	***Student Observations*** • Can you describe the events from your perspective? • How well do you think your treatments worked? • Can you review the events of the scenario (*directed to the Timer/Recorder*)? • What could you have improved? • What did the team do well? ***Instructor Observations*** • I noticed that [*insert action here*]. • I observed that [*insert action here*]. • I saw that [*insert action here*].	***Done Well*** • How were you able to [*insert action here*]? • Why do you think you were able to [*insert action here*]? • Tell me a little more about how you [*insert action here*]. ***Needs Improvement*** • Why do you think [*insert action here*] occurred? • How do you think [*insert action here*] could have been improved? • What was your thinking while [*insert action here*]? • What prevented you from [*insert action here*]?	***Student-Led Summary*** • What are the main things you learned? • Can someone summarize the key points made? • What are the main take-home messages? ***Instructor-Led Summary*** • Let's summarize what we learned… • Here is what I think we learned… • The main take-home messages are… • The patient in this scenario did not require synchronized cardioversion. Please describe the indications for synchronized cardioversion, the appropriate first and second energy doses, and how to safely deliver synchronized cardioversion.

Testing Case Scenario 9
Supraventricular Tachycardia
(Infant; Unstable)

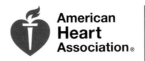

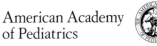

Scenario Lead-in

Prehospital: You are dispatched to a house where a 3-month-old infant has respiratory distress and lethargy.

ED: An ambulance is en route to the emergency department with a 3-month-old infant with respiratory distress and lethargy. An intravenous access has been placed.

General Inpatient Unit: You are called to examine a 3-month-old infant with respiratory distress and lethargy. The infant has an intravenous access in place.

ICU: You are called to the bedside of a 3-month-old infant with respiratory distress and lethargy. The infant has intravenous access.

Vital Signs	
Heart rate	235/min
Blood pressure	50/32 mm Hg
Respiratory rate	60/min
SpO₂	92% on room air
Temperature	37.6°C (99.7°F)
Weight	5 kg
Age	3 months

Scenario Overview and Learning Objectives

Scenario Overview

Emphasis should be on recognition and management of supraventricular tachycardia (SVT) in an unstable patient, including possible rapid bolus administration of adenosine (only if intravenous [IV]/intraosseous [IO] access is readily available) and the safe delivery of synchronized cardioversion using appropriate doses. Vagal maneuvers are performed while preparing adenosine or synchronized cardioversion but should not delay intervention. If time allows, the instructor may briefly discuss the need for expert consultation before administering a precardioversion sedative to an infant with hemodynamic instability.

Scenario-Specific Objectives

- **Differentiates between SVT and sinus tachycardia;** in this scenario, the infant has unstable SVT
- **Describes potential vagal maneuvers used for an infant with SVT;** potential maneuvers used in infants include ice to the face, possible stimulation of gag with soft catheter (if infant hasn't eaten recently)
- **Demonstrates the proper rapid bolus technique to administer adenosine**
- **Discusses indications for synchronized cardioversion;** in this scenario, the infant has poor perfusion, including hypotension, acutely altered mental status, and signs of shock
- **Demonstrates safe delivery of synchronized cardioversion with appropriate dose in a patient with SVT and poor perfusion**

Evaluate—*Initial Impression*
(Pediatric Assessment Triangle)

Appearance
- Lethargic; minimal response to surrounding noises and caregivers

Breathing
- Increased rate and effort, including significant retractions; grunting

Circulation
- Mottled skin

Identify

- Immediate intervention needed

Intervene

- Activate the emergency response system. Emergency medical services requests additional assistance if needed.
- Administer 100% oxygen by nonrebreathing face mask.
- Apply cardiac monitor.
- Apply pulse oximeter.

Evaluate—*Primary Assessment*
Focused on Assessment Needed to Support Airway, Oxygenation, Ventilation, and Perfusion

- **A**irway: Clear
- **B**reathing: Respiratory rate 60/min; moderate intercostal retractions; SpO₂ 92% before supplementary oxygen and 100% after 100% oxygen administered; crackles throughout lung fields
- **C**irculation: Adequate central pulses, weak peripheral pulses; heart rate 235/min; blood pressure 50/32 mm Hg; cool skin; capillary refill about 4 seconds
- **D**isability: Moans and withdraws to pain
- **E**xposure: Weight 5 kg

Temperature 37.6°C (99.7°F)

Identify

- Altered level of consciousness
- Narrow-complex tachycardia/SVT with a pulse and signs of poor perfusion
- Respiratory distress vs respiratory failure
- Hypotensive shock

Intervene

- Establish IV/IO access or verify function of existing access but **do not delay synchronized cardioversion if IV/IO access not readily available.**
- Perform vagal maneuvers if they do not delay adenosine or cardioversion.
- If functional IV is in place or is established immediately, administer adenosine.
  - Begin recording continuous rhythm strip.
  - Give adenosine 0.1 mg/kg (maximum dose: 6 mg) IV/IO by rapid bolus followed by rapid saline flush.
  - If first dose of adenosine is unsuccessful, administer adenosine 0.2 mg/kg rapid bolus (maximum dose: 12 mg) if it can be given more rapidly than providing synchronized cardioversion. Ensure that rapid bolus technique is used to administer the drug.

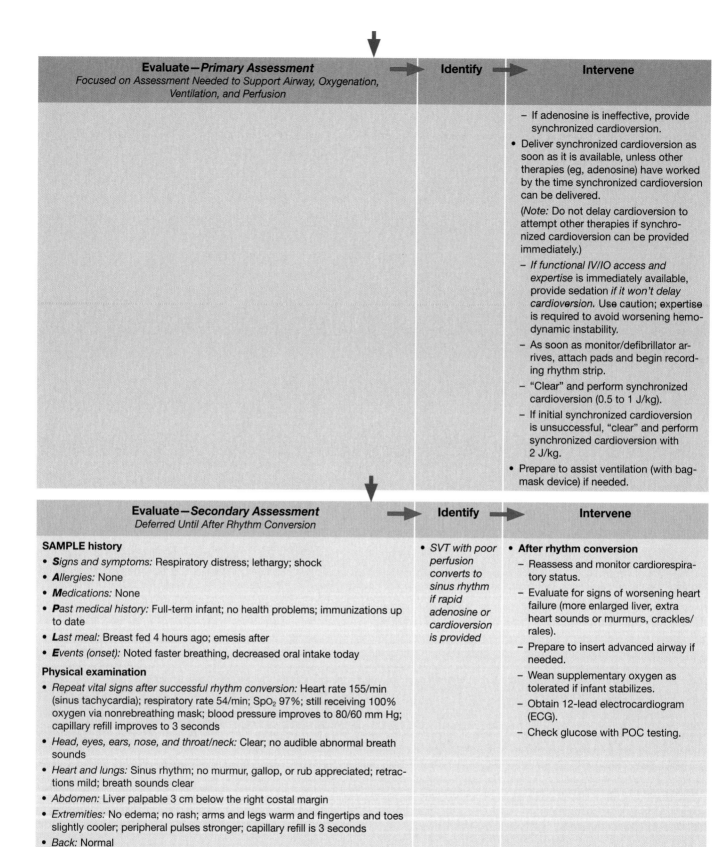

Evaluate—*Primary Assessment* *Focused on Assessment Needed to Support Airway, Oxygenation, Ventilation, and Perfusion*	Identify	Intervene
		– If adenosine is ineffective, provide synchronized cardioversion.
		• Deliver synchronized cardioversion as soon as it is available, unless other therapies (eg, adenosine) have worked by the time synchronized cardioversion can be delivered.
		(*Note:* Do not delay cardioversion to attempt other therapies if synchronized cardioversion can be provided immediately.)
		– *If functional IV/IO access and expertise* is immediately available, provide sedation *if it won't delay cardioversion.* Use caution; expertise is required to avoid worsening hemodynamic instability.
		– As soon as monitor/defibrillator arrives, attach pads and begin recording rhythm strip.
		– "Clear" and perform synchronized cardioversion (0.5 to 1 J/kg).
		– If initial synchronized cardioversion is unsuccessful, "clear" and perform synchronized cardioversion with 2 J/kg.
		• Prepare to assist ventilation (with bag-mask device) if needed.

Evaluate—*Secondary Assessment* *Deferred Until After Rhythm Conversion*	Identify	Intervene
SAMPLE history • **S**igns and symptoms: Respiratory distress; lethargy; shock • **A**llergies: None • **M**edications: None • **P**ast medical history: Full-term infant; no health problems; immunizations up to date • **L**ast meal: Breast fed 4 hours ago; emesis after • **E**vents (onset): Noted faster breathing, decreased oral intake today	• SVT with poor perfusion converts to sinus rhythm if rapid adenosine or cardioversion is provided	• **After rhythm conversion** – Reassess and monitor cardiorespiratory status. – Evaluate for signs of worsening heart failure (more enlarged liver, extra heart sounds or murmurs, crackles/rales). – Prepare to insert advanced airway if needed. – Wean supplementary oxygen as tolerated if infant stabilizes. – Obtain 12-lead electrocardiogram (ECG). – Check glucose with POC testing.

Physical examination

• *Repeat vital signs after successful rhythm conversion:* Heart rate 155/min (sinus tachycardia); respiratory rate 54/min; SpO$_2$ 97%; still receiving 100% oxygen via nonrebreathing mask; blood pressure improves to 80/60 mm Hg; capillary refill improves to 3 seconds

• *Head, eyes, ears, nose, and throat/neck:* Clear; no audible abnormal breath sounds

• *Heart and lungs:* Sinus rhythm; no murmur, gallop, or rub appreciated; retractions mild; breath sounds clear

• *Abdomen:* Liver palpable 3 cm below the right costal margin

• *Extremities:* No edema; no rash; arms and legs warm and fingertips and toes slightly cooler; peripheral pulses stronger; capillary refill is 3 seconds

• *Back:* Normal

• *Neurologic:* Cries with cardioversion; more reactive now in sinus rhythm

• Point-of-care (POC) glucose concentration (see below)

If no adenosine or cardioversion

• *Vital signs:* Heart rate 235/min; respiratory rate 60/min; SpO$_2$ falls to 90%; blood pressure 48/36 mm Hg; weak central and peripheral pulses; cool skin; capillary refill about 5 seconds; mottling more severe

Evaluate—*Diagnostic Assessments* *Perform Throughout the Evaluation of the Patient as Appropriate*		Identify/Intervene

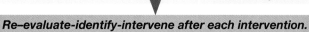

Lab data
- Blood glucose
- Electrolytes

Imaging
- Chest x-ray, ECG in SVT and in sinus tachycardia

- Although laboratory tests are generally not appropriate during the immediate management, a blood glucose concentration should be checked as soon as reasonably possible in critically ill infants and children. Hypoglycemia should be treated immediately.
- Laboratory studies (other than POC glucose testing) are deferred until rhythm is converted and systemic perfusion and hemodynamic function improved.

Re–evaluate-identify-intervene after each intervention.

Debriefing Tool
Testing Case Scenario 9
SVT (Infant; Unstable)

General Debriefing Principles

- Use the table below to guide your debriefing; also refer to the **Team Dynamics Debriefing Tool.**
- Debriefings are 10 minutes long.
- Address all learning objectives.
- Summarize take-home messages at the end of the debriefing.
- *Encourage:* Students to self-reflect
  Engagement of all participants
- *Avoid:* Mini-lectures and closed-ended questions
  Dominating the discussion

General Management Objectives

- Uses the PALS Systematic Approach Algorithm to assess and appropriately classify a patient
- Provides oxygen appropriately
- Directs delivery of high-quality CPR (including the use of a feedback device) when indicated
- Demonstrates basic airway maneuvers and use of relevant airway device as appropriate
- Demonstrates application of cardiac and respiratory monitors

- Identifies the cardiac rhythm
- Applies appropriate PBLS or PALS algorithms
- Summarizes general indications, contraindications, and doses of relevant drugs
- Discusses principles of family-centered care in pediatric cardiac arrest
- Applies the 8 elements of effective team dynamics
- Performs frequent reassessment

Action	Gather	Analyze	Summarize
• Directs assessment of ABCDE and vital signs • Applies cardiac monitor and pulse oximeter • Directs administration of supplementary oxygen • Identifies rhythm as SVT with poor perfusion and distinguishes it from sinus tachycardia • Knows how to perform appropriate vagal maneuvers for an infant	***Student Observations*** • Can you describe the events from your perspective? • How well do you think your treatments worked? • Can you review the events of the scenario (*directed to the Timer/Recorder*)? • What could you have improved? • What did the team do well?	***Done Well*** • How were you able to [*insert action here*]? • Why do you think you were able to [*insert action here*]? • Tell me a little more about how you [*insert action here*].	***Student-Led Summary*** • What are the main things you learned? • Can someone summarize the key points made? • What are the main take-home messages?
• Directs establishment of IV/IO access if it will not delay synchronized cardioversion • Directs preparation and rapid bolus administration of appropriate dose of adenosine • Directs safe delivery of attempted cardioversion at dose of 0.5 J/kg; if ineffective, increases dose to 2 J/kg • Performs frequent reassessments after each intervention	***Instructor Observations*** • I noticed that [*insert action here*]. • I observed that [*insert action here*]. • I saw that [*insert action here*].	***Needs Improvement*** • Why do you think [*insert action here*] occurred? • How do you think [*insert action here*] could have been improved? • What was your thinking while [*insert action here*]? • What prevented you from [*insert action here*]?	***Instructor-Led Summary*** • Let's summarize what we learned… • Here is what I think we learned… • The main take-home messages are… [instructor should ask student to state the indications for synchronized cardioversion] • If time allows, discuss the need for expert consultation before administering a precardioversion sedative to an infant with SVT and hemodynamic instability.

Ventricular Fibrillation
(Child; Arrest)

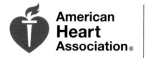

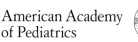

American Heart Association®
life is why™

American Academy of Pediatrics
DEDICATED TO THE HEALTH OF ALL CHILDREN™

Scenario Lead-in

Prehospital: You are en route to a school where a 7 year old suddenly collapsed in the gym. The teacher started CPR and called 9-1-1.

ED: You are called to evaluate a 7-year-old child who suddenly collapsed after saying he was dizzy while playing vigorously. CPR is in progress.

General Inpatient Unit: You are called as a member of the rapid response team to see a 7 year old who suddenly became limp and gray. The child was admitted for observation after syncope at playground. CPR is in progress.

ICU: You are called to see a 7 year old who suddenly became limp and gray. The child was admitted for observation after collapsing at basketball practice. CPR is in progress.

Vital Signs	
Heart rate	CPR in progress
Blood pressure	CPR in progress
Respiratory rate	No spontaneous breathing
SpO$_2$	100% bag-mask ventilation (CPR)
Temperature	Deferred
Weight	25 kg
Age	7 years

Scenario Overview and Learning Objectives

Scenario Overview

This scenario focuses on the identification and management of the child with cardiac arrest and a "shockable" rhythm. Emphasis is placed on immediate delivery of high-quality CPR and integration of shock delivery while minimizing interruptions in CPR. One shock, followed by CPR, and then (when VF persists) a second shock, followed by CPR + epinephrine, and then (when VF persists) a third shock, followed by CPR + antiarrhythmic (amiodarone or lidocaine) are administered before return of spontaneous circulation (ROSC). Identification of potential causes (H's and T's) should be discussed during debriefing.

Insertion of advanced airway and post-ROSC care are beyond the scope of this scenario. Post-ROSC care is addressed with the asystole scenario.

Scenario-Specific Objectives

- **Identifies cardiac arrest with a shockable rhythm;** in this scenario, the child has ventricular fibrillation (VF)
- **Demonstrates safe shock delivery with appropriate dose and minimal interruption of chest compressions;** the correct initial dose is 2 J/kg, second shock is 4 J/kg, and subsequent doses are at least 4 J/kg (maximum 10 J/kg)
- **Describes correct dose and rationale for epinephrine administration**
- **Uses appropriate antiarrhythmic in VF/pulseless ventricular tachycardia (VT);** the 2015 AHA Guidelines Update for CPR and ECC noted that either amiodarone or lidocaine was equally acceptable
- **Identifies reversible causes of persistent VF;** during the debriefing, the student should be asked to recall possible reversible causes of cardiac arrest (recalled by conditions beginning with H's and T's)

Evaluate—*Initial Impression* (Pediatric Assessment Triangle)	Identify	Intervene
Appearance • Extremities appear to be limp; no spontaneous movement; no visible reaction to noise **Breathing** • No spontaneous breathing **Circulation** • Cyanotic/pale extremities and lips; overall gray color	• Immediate intervention needed	• Activate the emergency response system. Emergency medical services requests additional assistance if needed. • Check for response (no response) and perform simultaneous check for breathing (none) and carotid or femoral pulse (none). • Immediately begin high-quality CPR.

Evaluate—*Primary Assessment* Deferred to Initiate Provide Immediate Basic Life Support, and Then Focused on Assessment Needed to Support Airway, Oxygenation, Ventilation, and Perfusion	Identify	Intervene
• Should verify appearance, breathing, and circulation support • Monitor reveals VF • Weight 25 kg per color-coded length-based resuscitation tape	• Cardiopulmonary arrest • VF cardiac arrest	• Use a CPR feedback device, if available, to guide CPR delivery. • When defibrillator arrives, apply pads/leads and turn on monitor. • Identify rhythm (VF, shockable). • Attempt defibrillation with 2 J/kg as soon as possible. • Resume high-quality CPR immediately after shock delivery. • Obtain vascular access (intravenous [IV]/intraosseous [IO]). • Apply pulse oximeter (per local protocol, may be deferred until ROSC).

Evaluate—*Secondary Assessment*	**Identify**	**Intervene**
Deferred Except to Identify Reversible Causes		

	Identify	**Intervene**

SAMPLE history (deferred until ROSC or only to extent needed to evaluate reversible causes, ie, the H's and T's; **do not interrupt resuscitation**)
 	
• **S**igns and symptoms: Child suddenly became limp; no precursors
• **A**llergies: Penicillin
• **M**edications: Adderall
• **P**ast medical history: Attention-deficit disorder/attention-deficit/hyperactivity disorder
• **L**ast meal: 2 hours ago
• **E**vents (onset): As specified in scenario lead-in
 	
Physical examination (deferred until ROSC or only to extent needed to evaluate reversible causes)
 	
• **ROSC occurs after** high-quality CPR, 3 shocks delivered, 1 dose of epinephrine and 1 antiarrhythmic (amiodarone or lidocaine). Scenario can be shortened with ROSC after 2 shocks and 1 dose of epinephrine, with debriefing discussion of antiarrhythmic.
• Sinus rhythm; heart rate 130/min; respiratory rate 20/min with bag-mask ventilation; SpO$_2$ 100% during bag-mask ventilation with 100% oxygen; blood pressure 92/60 mm Hg; temperature 36.1°C (97.0°F)
	• Cardiopulmonary arrest
	• VF
	• ROSC
		• Continue high-quality CPR; reassess rhythm and every 2 minutes.
		• If a shockable rhythm persists at next rhythm check, give second shock of 4 J/kg, followed by immediate CPR.
		• Prepare epinephrine 0.01 mg/kg (0.1 mL/kg of 0.1 mg/mL concentration) IV/IO and administer during chest compressions.
		  – Repeat every 3-5 minutes during cardiac arrest.
		• If shockable rhythm persists at next rhythm check, deliver shock, resume CPR, and prepare and administer antiarrhythmic drug for persistent VF/pulseless VT during chest compressions.
		  – Amiodarone 5 mg/kg IV/IO bolus (maximum single dose 300 mg) *or* lidocaine 1 mg/kg IV/IO.
		  – Any subsequent shocks should be at dose of 4 J/kg or higher (maximum: 10 J/kg or standard adult dose for that defibrillator).
		• Consider endotracheal intubation, especially if unable to provide adequate ventilation with a bag-mask device and an advanced care provider is available.

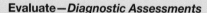

Evaluate—*Diagnostic Assessments*	**Identify/Intervene**
Perform Throughout the Evaluation of the Patient as Appropriate	
Lab data *(as appropriate)* • Rapid bedside blood glucose 96 mg/dL (5.3 mmol/L) (after ROSC) • Arterial/venous blood gas, electrolytes, calcium, magnesium, consider toxicology studies ***Imaging*** • *Chest x-ray (after ROSC):* Normal heart and lung fields	• Blood work and chest x-ray are not available during the scenario.

Re–evaluate-identify-intervene after each intervention.

Debriefing Tool
Testing Case Scenario 10
VF (Child; Arrest)

General Debriefing Principles

- Use the table below to guide your debriefing; also refer to the **Team Dynamics Debriefing Tool.**
- Debriefings are 10 minutes long.
- Address all learning objectives.
- Summarize take-home messages at the end of the debriefing.
- *Encourage:* Students to self-reflect
    Engagement of all participants
- *Avoid:* Mini-lectures and closed-ended questions
    Dominating the discussion

General Management Objectives

- Uses the PALS Systematic Approach Algorithm to assess and appropriately classify a patient
- Provides oxygen appropriately
- Directs delivery of high-quality CPR (including the use of a feedback device) when indicated
- Demonstrates basic airway maneuvers and use of relevant airway device as appropriate
- Demonstrates application of cardiac and respiratory monitors

- Identifies the cardiac rhythm
- Applies appropriate PBLS or PALS algorithms
- Summarizes general indications, contraindications, and doses of relevant drugs
- Discusses principles of family-centered care in pediatric cardiac arrest
- Applies the 8 elements of effective team dynamics
- Performs frequent reassessment

Action	Gather	Analyze	Summarize
- Identifies cardiac arrest - Directs immediate initiation of high-quality CPR with the use of a feedback device (if available) and monitors quality throughout resuscitation - Directs placement of monitor leads/pads and activation of monitor - Identifies VF cardiopulmonary arrest - Directs safe performance of first shock of 2 J/kg - After each shock, directs immediate resumption of high-quality CPR, beginning with chest compressions - Directs establishment of IV or IO access - If VF persists at second rhythm check, directs safe delivery of a second shock, using a dose of 4 J/kg; any subsequent shocks should use a dose of 4 J/kg or higher (maximum 10 J/kg or standard adult dose) - Directs preparation and administration of appropriate IV/IO dose (0.01 mg/kg [0.1 mL/kg of the 0.1 mg/mL concentration]) of epinephrine at appropriate intervals - After each shock, directs immediate resumption of CPR, beginning with compressions - If VF persists at third rhythm check, directs that antiarrhythmic with appropriate dose (amiodarone 5 mg/kg or lidocaine 1 mg/kg) be administered when compressions resume - Performs appropriate reassessments	***Student Observations*** - Can you describe the events from your perspective? - How well do you think your treatments worked? - Can you review the events of the scenario (*directed to the Timer/Recorder*)? - What could you have improved? - What did the team do well? ***Instructor Observations*** - I noticed that [*insert action here*]. - I observed that [*insert action here*]. - I saw that [*insert action here*].	***Done Well*** - How were you able to [*insert action here*]? - Why do you think you were able to [*insert action here*]? - Tell me a little more about how you [*insert action here*]. ***Needs Improvement*** - Why do you think [*insert action here*] occurred? - How do you think [*insert action here*] could have been improved? - What was your thinking while [*insert action here*]? - What prevented you from [*insert action here*]?	***Student-Led Summary*** - What are the main things you learned? - Can someone summarize the key points made? - What are the main take-home messages? ***Instructor-Led Summary*** - Let's summarize what we learned… - Here is what I think we learned… - The main take-home messages are… - If the child's VF failed to respond to the therapies given, what else should you consider? (Answer: H's and T's—ie, reversible causes) - If a third shock is needed, what dose is used? (Answer: 4 J/kg or higher; maximum 10 J/kg or adult dose for that defibrillator)

Obstructive Shock
(Child; Hypotensive; Tension Pneumothorax)

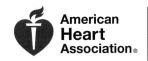

American Heart Association® life is why™

American Academy of Pediatrics
DEDICATED TO THE HEALTH OF ALL CHILDREN™

Scenario Lead-in

Prehospital: You are on scene with an 8-year-old boy. He was intubated with an oral-tracheal tube because of depressed mental status, and then he suddenly deteriorated and is being manually ventilated by another care provider. An intravenous catheter is in place.

ED: An 8-year-old boy is being transported by emergency medical services. He has been intubated with an oral-tracheal tube for decreased level of consciousness (a Glasgow Coma Scale Score of 4). He suddenly deteriorated and is being manually ventilated through the endotracheal tube. An intravenous catheter is in place.

General Inpatient Unit: You are called to the room of an 8-year-old boy who was just intubated by the rapid response team for pneumonia and hypoxemia. An oral-tracheal tube was placed. As the team was preparing to transport him to the intensive care unit, the child suddenly deteriorated and is being manually ventilated through the endotracheal tube. An intravenous catheter is in place.

ICU: You are called to the room of an 8-year-old boy who is intubated and mechanically ventilated. He has suddenly deteriorated and is being manually ventilated through the endotracheal tube. An intravenous catheter is in place.

Vital Signs	
Heart rate	140/min
Blood pressure	80/54 mm Hg
Respiratory rate	Manual ventilation
SpO$_2$	68% on 100% oxygen
Temperature	37.2°C (99.0°F)
Weight	20 kg
Age	8 years

Scenario Overview and Learning Objectives

Scenario Overview

Emphasis is placed on immediate recognition of respiratory failure and signs of obstructive shock. The provider should use the DOPE (Displacement of the tube, Obstruction of the tube, Pneumothorax, Equipment failure) mnemonic to quickly identify a tension pneumothorax as the cause and then must perform immediate needle decompression followed by chest tube insertion. Emphasize the importance of performing the needle decompression before obtaining a chest x-ray.

Scenario-Specific Objectives

- **Recognizes compensated vs hypotensive shock;** this case illustrates hypotensive shock (key indicators in this case include hypotension, tachycardia, and decreased level of consciousness)
- **Summarizes signs and symptoms of obstructive shock;** key indicators in this case include signs of shock combined with evidence of tension pneumothorax
- **Summarizes the elements of the DOPE mnemonic for an intubated patient with sudden deterioration;** in this scenario, displacement of tube, obstruction of tube, and equipment failure should be ruled out before needle decompression
- **Demonstrates correct interventions for tension pneumothorax;** in this scenario, interventions include needle decompression, a chest x-ray, and chest tube insertion
- **Discusses conditions under which fluid bolus administration would be appropriate for treatment of obstructive shock;** although fluid resuscitation is not needed in this scenario, bolus fluid administration may be helpful for cardiac tamponade, until pericardiocentesis can be performed and in massive pulmonary embolus

Evaluate—*Initial Impression* *(Pediatric Assessment Triangle)*	Identify	Intervene
Appearance • No spontaneous movement; flaccid extremities; no visible reaction to noise **Breathing** • Orally intubated; poor chest wall movement with manual ventilation using a resuscitation bag **Circulation** • Pale skin; dusky mucous membranes	• Immediate intervention needed	• Activate the emergency response system. Emergency medical services requests additional assistance if needed. • Continue manual ventilation with 100% oxygen. • Apply cardiac monitor. • Apply pulse oximeter.

Evaluate—*Primary Assessment* *Focused on Assessment Needed to Restore Patent Airway, Oxygenation, Ventilation, and Perfusion*	Identify	Intervene
• **Airway:** Orally intubated with a 6.0 cuffed endotracheal tube (ETT); secured at 18 cm at the lip • **Breathing:** Manually ventilated; asymmetric chest rise, absent breath sounds on the right; increasing inspiratory pressure needed to produce chest expansion; SpO$_2$ 68% despite receiving 100% inspired oxygen. As student evaluates using DOPE mnemonic, provide the following responses to student queries and actions:	• Respiratory failure and hypotensive shock	• Analyze rhythm (sinus tachycardia). • Assess response to oxygen and manual ventilation (no change). • Check waveform capnography (if applicable).

Evaluate—*Primary Assessment* *Focused on Assessment Needed to Support Airway, Oxygenation, Ventilation, and Perfusion*	Identify	Intervene
– Displacement: Depth of insertion unchanged; breath sounds present on left; exhaled CO_2 still detectable – Obstruction: Normal breath sounds on left; *if ETT is withdrawn slightly to detect and treat possible left main stem intubation, there is no change in the breath sounds, chest rise, or resistance to manual ventilation* – Pneumothorax (consistent with current clinical picture) – Equipment failure: Ruled out by switching to manual ventilation with bag • *Circulation:* Heart rate 140/min; weak pulses; capillary refill 5 seconds; blood pressure 80/54 mm Hg • *Disability:* Unconscious; pupils equal and reactive to light • *Exposure:* Temperature 37.2°C (99.0°F); weight 20 kg	• Probable tension pneumothorax and obstructive shock	• Rule out endotracheal tube displacement and obstruction and equipment failure. • Perform needle decompression on right side (inserting an 18- to 20-gauge over-the-needle catheter over the top of the child's third rib, second intercostal space in the midclavicular line). • Obtain chest x-ray and insert chest tube.

Evaluate—*Secondary Assessment* *Identify Reversible Causes, but Defer Remainder of Secondary Assessment Until Effective Ventilation Established (After Needle Thoracostomy)*	Identify	Intervene

SAMPLE history (only to extent needed to evaluate reversible causes)
• *Signs and symptoms:* Orally intubated for respiratory failure; sudden deterioration
• *Allergies:* None known
• *Medications:* None
• *Past medical history:* None
• *Last meal:* Nothing by mouth
• *Events (onset):* Sudden deterioration in intubated patient
 	
Physical examination
• *Repeat vital signs after oxygen:* Heart rate 175/min; manual ventilation at 24 breaths/min
  – If needle decompression performed: SpO_2 85% and rising; blood pressure increases to 110/65 mm Hg; capillary refill 3 seconds
  – If needle decompression *not* performed: SpO_2 58% and falling; blood pressure becomes undetectable and cardiac arrest develops; capillary refill extremely prolonged
• *Head, eyes, ears, nose, and throat/neck*
  – If needle decompression performed: Normal
  – If needle decompression *not* performed: Jugular vein distention
• *Heart and lungs*
  – If needle decompression performed: Breath sounds equal bilaterally and there is decreased resistance to manual ventilation
  – If needle decompression *not* performed: Breath sounds absent on right
• *Abdomen:* Normal
• *Extremities*
  – If needle decompression performed: 2+ central and peripheral pulses, capillary refill 3 seconds
  – If needle decompression *not* performed: No palpable pulses, capillary refill extremely prolonged
• *Back:* Normal
• *Neurologic:* Unconscious
	• Respiratory failure
	• Hypotensive obstructive shock (corrects when needle decompression performed; if needle decompression is *not* performed, pulseless arrest develops)
	• Tension pneumothorax
		• Reassess cardiorespiratory function (particularly ventilation and perfusion); immediate improvement should be noted following needle decompression.
		• Verify that intravenous catheter remains patent.
		• Check glucose with point-of-care (POC) testing.
		• Arrange for transfer to intensive care unit (ICU) (if child is not already in ICU) for closer monitoring and treatment of underlying conditions.

Evaluate—*Diagnostic Assessments* *Perform Throughout the Evaluation of the Patient as Appropriate*	Identify/Intervene
Lab data • *Pending:* Arterial blood gas or venous blood gas *Imaging* • Chest radiograph (should not delay intervention until chest x-ray performed)	• Laboratory diagnostic testing is deferred until treatment of the tension pneumothorax. • A blood glucose concentration should be checked as soon as reasonably possible in all critically ill children, particularly neonates and infants. Hypoglycemia should be treated immediately. • *Note:* Needle decompression is performed before obtaining chest x-ray (ie, the chest x-ray should follow needle decompression but can precede chest tube insertion).

Re–evaluate-identify-intervene after each intervention.

Debriefing Tool

Testing Case Scenario 11
Obstructive Shock (Child; Hypotensive; Tension Pneumothorax)

General Debriefing Principles

- Use the table below to guide your debriefing; also refer to the **Team Dynamics Debriefing Tool.**
- Debriefings are 10 minutes long.
- Address all learning objectives.
- Summarize take-home messages at the end of the debriefing.
- *Encourage:* Students to self-reflect
     Engagement of all participants
- *Avoid:* Mini-lectures and closed-ended questions
     Dominating the discussion

General Management Objectives

- Uses the PALS Systematic Approach Algorithm to assess and appropriately classify a patient
- Provides oxygen appropriately
- Directs delivery of high-quality CPR (including the use of a feedback device) when indicated
- Demonstrates basic airway maneuvers and use of relevant airway device as appropriate
- Demonstrates application of cardiac and respiratory monitors
- Identifies the cardiac rhythm
- Applies appropriate PBLS or PALS algorithms
- Summarizes general indications, contraindications, and doses of relevant drugs
- Discusses principles of family-centered care in pediatric cardiac arrest
- Applies the 8 elements of effective team dynamics
- Performs frequent reassessment

Action	Gather	Analyze	Summarize
• Assesses ABCDE, including vital signs • Applies cardiac monitor and pulse oximeter • Identifies signs and symptoms of obstructive shock • Categorizes as hypotensive shock • Verbalizes DOPE mnemonic for intubated patient who deteriorates • Identifies tension pneumothorax • Describes performance of needle decompression for tension pneumothorax • Reassesses patient's response to needle decompression	***Student Observations*** • Can you describe the events from your perspective? • How well do you think your treatments worked? • Can you review the events of the scenario (*directed to the Timer/Recorder*)? • What could you have improved? • What did the team do well?	***Done Well*** • How were you able to [*insert action here*]? • Why do you think you were able to [*insert action here*]? • Tell me a little more about how you [*insert action here*].	***Student-Led Summary*** • What are the main things you learned? • Can someone summarize the key points made? • What are the main take-home messages?
	Instructor Observations • I noticed that [*insert action here*]. • I observed that [*insert action here*]. • I saw that [*insert action here*].	***Needs Improvement*** • Why do you think [*insert action here*] occurred? • How do you think [*insert action here*] could have been improved? • What was your thinking while [*insert action here*]? • What prevented you from [*insert action here*]?	***Instructor-Led Summary*** • Let's summarize what we learned… • Here is what I think we learned… • The main take-home messages are… • Name 2 additional causes of obstructive shock. (Answer: Cardiac tamponade, massive pulmonary embolism, and closure of the ductus arteriosus in infants with ductal-dependent congenital heart lesions) • Please highlight key aspects of the management of cardiac tamponade (fluid bolus and pericardiocentesis), massive pulmonary embolus (oxygen, ventilatory support, fluid bolus, and expert consultation) and ductal closure in neonates with ductal-dependent congenital heart disease (prostaglandin infusion and expert consultation).

(continued)

(continued)

Action	Gather	Analyze	Summarize
			• What are the therapeutic end points during shock management? (Answer: Normalized heart rate; improved peripheral perfusion, mental status, and urine output; normalized blood pressure; correction of metabolic/lactic acidosis)

Cardiogenic Shock
(Adolescent; Myocarditis)

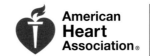
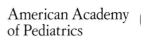

American Heart Association®
life is why™

American Academy of Pediatrics
DEDICATED TO THE HEALTH OF ALL CHILDREN™

Scenario Lead-in

Prehospital: You are dispatched to transport a 16 year old who had a sudden onset of chest pain and shortness of breath at school. He has visible signs of increased work of breathing and cold extremities, and he is very pale. He experienced flu-like symptoms a few days before.

ED: Emergency medical services arrives with a 16 year old who today at school complained of severe chest pain and shortness of breath. He has a history of flu-like symptoms a few days before. He is in obvious respiratory distress, has cold extremities, and is very pale. The emergency medical services providers were unable to obtain an intravenous access.

General Inpatient Unit: As a member of the rapid response team, you respond to a 16 year old who was admitted after being evaluated for chest pain and shortness of breath. He is in obvious respiratory distress, has cold extremities, and is very pale. The intravenous access that was placed on admission has infiltrated.

ICU: You are called to the bedside of a 16 year old who was directly admitted to the intensive care unit with a sudden onset of chest pain. He is pale and hypotensive, demonstrates increased work of breathing, and appears confused and agitated. He has no intravenous access in place.

Vital Signs	
Heart rate	140/min
Blood pressure	86/40 mm Hg
Respiratory rate	35/min
SpO$_2$	89% on room air
Temperature	Not obtained
Weight	82 kg
Age	16 years

Scenario Overview and Learning Objectives

Scenario Overview

Emphasis is on identification and rapid treatment of hypotensive cardiogenic shock. Priorities include immediate establishment of vascular (intravenous [IV]) access and careful administration of a small bolus of isotonic crystalloid over 10-20 minutes, with careful reassessment of cardiorespiratory function during and after the fluid bolus. The provider should identify signs of worsening heart failure during the administration of the fluid bolus and should stop bolus fluid administration. The patient requires inotropic therapy to improve cardiac function and vasoactive drug therapy to improve blood pressure and systemic perfusion. Expert consultation from a pediatric cardiologist and further diagnostic studies (including echocardiography) are needed.

Scenario-Specific Objectives

- **Differentiates compensated vs hypotensive shock;** in this scenario, the child is hypotensive, so has hypotensive shock
- **Differentiates the signs and symptoms of cardiogenic shock from other types of shock;** in this scenario, the combination of signs of hypotensive shock with signs of heart failure point to likely cardiogenic shock
- **Provides correct interventions for cardiogenic shock;** in this scenario, these interventions include establishment of cardiac monitoring and pulse oximetry, careful bolus administration of isotonic crystalloids, careful reassessment during and after each fluid bolus and initiation, and titration of inotropic/vasoactive drugs
- **Describes correct volume and duration of fluid bolus administration for cardiogenic shock and describes possible negative effects of excessive and/or rapid fluid bolus administration;** in this scenario, the fluid bolus of 5-10 mL/kg of isotonic crystalloid should be administered over 10 to 20 minutes (excessive fluid administration can worsen heart failure/cardiogenic shock)

Evaluate—*Initial Impression* (Pediatric Assessment Triangle)	Identify	Intervene
Appearance • Seems confused, keeps repeating that he feels very tired **Breathing** • Labored breathing with moderate to severe intercostal and subcostal retractions, coughing, and grunting **Circulation** • Pale, very mottled extremities	• Immediate intervention needed	• Activate emergency response system, if appropriate. • Administer 100% oxygen by nonrebreathing face mask. • Apply cardiac monitor. • Apply pulse oximeter.

Evaluate—Primary Assessment *Focused on Assessment Needed to Support Airway, Oxygenation, Ventilation, and Perfusion*	**Identify**	**Intervene**
• *Airway:* Patent and maintainable • *Breathing:* Respiratory rate 35/min; substantial and intercostal retractions, nasal flaring, and grunting; SpO₂ 89% on room air, increases to 94% with administration of 100% oxygen via nonrebreathing mask • *Circulation:* Central pulses present, peripheral pulses weak and thready; heart rate 140/min; blood pressure 86/40 mm Hg capillary refill 4 seconds; cold extremities; bilateral lower extremity peripheral edema noted • *Disability:* Disoriented to place and time; states he is very tired and light-headed • *Exposure:* Jugular vein distention and peripheral edema noted; weight 82 kg	• Respiratory distress • Hypotensive cardiogenic shock • Sinus tachycardia	• Obtain vascular (IV/intraosseous [IO]) access (attempt IV access first). • Administer a fluid bolus of 5-10 mL/kg of isotonic crystalloid over 10-20 minutes. • Perform careful and frequent re-assessment of adolescent during and after fluid bolus. Stop fluid bolus if signs of heart failure develop (eg, worsening respiratory status, development of rales or hepatomegaly). • Check glucose using point-of-care testing.

Evaluate—Secondary Assessment *Identify Reversible Causes, but Defer Remainder of Secondary Assessment Until After Initial Shock Therapy*	**Identify**	**Intervene**
SAMPLE history (only to extent needed to evaluate reversible causes) • *Signs and symptoms:* Increased work of breathing, chest pain, and lethargy • *Allergies:* No known allergies • *Medications:* None • *Past medical history:* No past history of illness • *Last meal:* Poor intake for last 12 hours • *Events (onset):* Flu-like symptoms 2 days before **Physical examination** • *Repeat vital signs after oxygen and first fluid bolus:* Heart rate 155/min; respiratory rate 45/min; SpO₂ 90% with 100% oxygen; blood pressure 80/40 mm Hg • *Head, eyes, ears, nose, and throat/neck:* Mucous membranes dry; distended jugular vein; peripheral edema • *Heart and lungs:* Rapid rate; heart sounds; crackles and retractions worsening • *Abdomen:* Liver edge palpable at 5 cm below right costal margin; nondistended abdomen; hypoactive bowel sounds • *Extremities:* Cold arms and feet; mottled; weak peripheral pulses; capillary refill 5 seconds • *Back:* Normal • *Neurologic:* Lethargic; pupils 4 mm, equal, reactive	• Hypotensive cardiogenic shock • Worsening respiratory distress after fluid bolus • Possible respiratory failure	• Stop fluid bolus administration (signs of heart failure worsening). • Begin appropriate inotropic/vasoactive infusions and assess response. • Assess response to oxygen administration. • Administer continuous positive airway pressure or other positive-pressure ventilation support if hypoxemia and respiratory distress continue. • Obtain 12-lead electrocardiogram. • Obtain cardiology consultation and echocardiogram if available. • Arrange for transfer to intensive care unit for closer monitoring if adolescent is not already in intensive care unit.

Evaluate—Diagnostic Assessments *Perform Throughout the Evaluation of the Patient as Appropriate*	**Identify/Intervene**
Lab data • Arterial blood gas pH 7.18; PCO₂ 22 mm Hg; HCO₃ 10 mEq/L; PO₂ 70 mm Hg; lactate 5.5 mmol/L • Glucose (point-of-care testing) 80 mg/dL (4.4 mmol/L) • *Pending:* Electrolytes, blood urea nitrogen/creatinine, calcium, complete blood count with differential, prothrombin time/international normalized ratio/partial thromboplastin time • *Cultures:* Blood, urine *Imaging* • *Chest x-ray:* Cardiomegaly; increased pulmonary vascular markings	• A blood glucose concentration should be checked as soon as reasonably possible in all critically ill children, particularly neonates and infants. Hypoglycemia should be treated immediately. • Arterial blood gas confirms metabolic acidosis due to low cardiac output. • Chest x-ray shows cardiomegaly and pulmonary edema consistent with heart failure/cardiogenic shock. • Obtain echocardiogram when available.

Re–evaluate-identify-intervene after each intervention.

Debriefing Tool
Testing Case Scenario 12
Cardiogenic Shock (Adolescent; Myocarditis)

General Management Objectives

- Uses the PALS Systematic Approach Algorithm to assess and appropriately classify a patient
- Provides oxygen appropriately
- Directs delivery of high-quality CPR (including the use of a feedback device) when indicated
- Demonstrates basic airway maneuvers and use of relevant airway device as appropriate
- Demonstrates application of cardiac and respiratory monitors
- Identifies the cardiac rhythm
- Applies appropriate PBLS or PALS algorithms
- Summarizes general indications, contraindications, and doses of relevant drugs
- Discusses principles of family-centered care in pediatric cardiac arrest
- Applies the 8 elements of effective team dynamics
- Performs frequent reassessment

Action	Gather	Analyze	Summarize
• Directs assessment of ABCDE and vital signs • Applies cardiac monitor and pulse oximeter • Administers 100% oxygen • Recognizes signs and symptoms of cardiogenic shock • Categorizes shock as hypotensive • Directs establishment of IV or IO access • Directs administration of a 5-10 mL/kg bolus of isotonic crystalloid IV/IO over 10-20 minutes • Reassesses patient during and in response to interventions, particularly during and after each fluid bolus • Identifies signs of worsening heart failure and stops bolus fluid administration • Identifies need for initiation of inotropic/vasoactive support: titrates to improve cardiac function and systemic perfusion • Obtains expert consultation from a pediatric cardiologist and obtains an echocardiogram or other diagnostic studies as recommended by cardiologist	***Student Observations*** • Can you describe the events from your perspective? • How well do you think your treatments worked? • Can you review the events of the scenario (*directed to the Timer/Recorder*)? • What did the team do extremely well? • What did the team find challenging? ***Instructor Observations*** • I noticed that [*insert action here*]. • I observed that [*insert action here*]. • I saw that [*insert action here*].	***Done Well*** • How were you able to [*insert action here*]? • Why do you think you were able to [*insert action here*]? • Tell me a little more about how you [*insert action here*]. ***Needs Improvement*** • Why do you think [*insert action here*] occurred? • How do you think [*insert action here*] could have been improved? • What was your thinking while [*insert action here*]? • What prevented you from [*insert action here*]?	***Student-Led Summary*** • What are the main things you learned? • Can someone summarize the key points made? • What are the main take-home messages? ***Instructor-Led Summary*** • Let's summarize what we learned… • Here is what I think we learned… • The main take-home messages are… • What are the therapeutic end points during shock management? (Answer: Normalized heart rate; improved peripheral perfusion, mental status, and urine output; normalized blood pressure; correction of metabolic/lactic acidosis)

Disordered Control of Breathing Disease (Child)

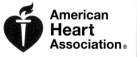

American Heart Association
life is why™

American Academy of Pediatrics
DEDICATED TO THE HEALTH OF ALL CHILDREN™

Scenario Lead-in

Prehospital: You respond to a 9-1-1 call for a 4 year old having a seizure with respiratory distress.

ED: Emergency medical services arrives with a 4-year-old boy brought from his home after mother called 9-1-1 because her child had a seizure with respiratory distress.

General Inpatient Unit: You are called to the room of a 4-year-old boy who is being admitted after having a seizure with respiratory distress.

Vital Signs	
Heart rate	130/min
Blood pressure	98/62 mm Hg
Respiratory rate	8/min
SpO₂	80% on room air
Temperature	39.7°C (103.5°F)
Weight	17 kg
Age	4 years

Scenario Overview and Learning Objectives

Scenario Overview

Emphasis of this scenario is on recognition and immediate management of a child with respiratory failure and disordered control of breathing (inadequate respiratory rate and effort), upper airway obstruction by the tongue, and decreased level of consciousness after a seizure. This child requires immediate bag-mask ventilation with 100% oxygen. During debriefing, discuss with the student the indications for intubation in this patient and methods to estimate appropriate cuffed and uncuffed endotracheal tube sizes.

Scenario-Specific Objectives

- **Identifies respiratory distress vs respiratory failure;** in this scenario, respiratory failure is present
- **Summarizes signs of disordered control of breathing;** in this scenario, the child demonstrated inadequate spontaneous respiratory effort with very slow, irregular, and shallow breaths
- **Recalls causes of disordered control of breathing;** common causes include drugs, increased intracranial pressure, and seizures
- **Discusses correct interventions for disordered control of breathing;** in this scenario, interventions include opening the airway and provision of bag-mask ventilation with 100% oxygen

---

Evaluate—*Initial Impression* (Pediatric Assessment Triangle)	Identify	Intervene
Appearance • Lethargic; eyes closed; no visible reaction to his mother's voice or noises in environment **Breathing** • Very slow respiratory rate with minimal chest rise; snoring **Circulation** • Pink skin	• Immediate intervention needed	• Activate the emergency response system. Emergency medical services requests additional assistance if needed. • Position the child to open the airway. • Begin bag-mask ventilation with 100% oxygen. • Apply cardiac monitor. • Apply pulse oximeter.

Evaluate—*Primary Assessment* Focused on Assessment Needed to Support Airway, Oxygenation, Ventilation, and Perfusion	Identify	Intervene
• **Airway:** Snoring respirations when child lying on his back, relieved when airway opened • **Breathing:** Spontaneous respiratory rate 8/min; shallow and irregular; SpO₂ 80% on room air, increases to 99% with bag-mask ventilation with 100% oxygen at a rate of 20/min • **Circulation:** Heart rate 130/min; dusky (before bag-mask ventilation with 100% oxygen); strong radial pulse; capillary refill 2 seconds; blood pressure 98/62 mm Hg • **Disability:** Lethargic; responsive to painful stimuli • **Exposure:** Temperature 39.7°C (103.5°F); weight 17 kg	• Respiratory failure (inadequate respiratory rate and effort)	• Verify chest rise with bag-mask ventilation and monitor response to bag-mask ventilation with oxygen. • Continue bag-mask ventilation with 100% oxygen and monitor for increase in child's spontaneous respiratory effort—match ventilation with child's effort if possible. • Consider insertion of nasopharyngeal airway. • Establish vascular access (intravenous). • Treat fever with antipyretic.

Evaluate—*Secondary Assessment*	**Identify**	**Intervene**

Identify Reversible Causes, but Defer Remainder of Secondary Assessment Until After Stabilization of Airway, Oxygenation, and Ventilation

SAMPLE history

- *Signs and symptoms:* Fever, upper respiratory infection symptoms for the last 3 days
- *Allergies:* None known
- *Medications:* Acetaminophen given by mother 2 hours ago
- *Past medical history:* None—no history of previous seizure disorder
- *Last meal:* Ate 3 hours ago
- *Events (onset):* Abrupt onset of tonic-clonic seizure lasting approximately 5 minutes

Physical examination

- *Repeat vital signs with assisted ventilation with 100% oxygen:* Respiratory rate 26/min with bag-mask ventilation now assisting the child's spontaneous respiratory effort; heart rate 136/min; SpO$_2$ 99% with inspired oxygen concentration of 100%; blood pressure 94/58 mm Hg
- *Head, eyes, ears, nose, and throat/neck:* Airway clear
- *Heart and lungs:* Clear breath sounds; good chest rise and fall with assisted ventilation; rate and depth of spontaneous breaths increasing
- *Abdomen:* Normal
- *Extremities:* No edema; no rash
- *Back:* Normal
- *Neurologic:* Becoming more responsive and more difficult to arouse

Identify:

- Respiratory failure (inadequate respiratory rate and effort)
- Disordered control of breathing

Intervene:

- Closely monitor patient's level of consciousness, spontaneous respiratory effort, and airway protective mechanisms (ability to cough to protect airway).
- As child's spontaneous respiratory effort improves, provide bag-mask ventilation that assists the child's spontaneous respiratory effort.
- Once the child's spontaneous respiratory rate and depth are adequate, cease bag-mask ventilation and provide non-rebreathing mask with 100% oxygen.
- Perform frequent reassessment to ensure that child continues to demonstrate adequate respiratory rate and effort and airway protective mechanisms.
- Wean supplementary oxygen concentration as tolerated.
- If slow, irregular, inadequate breathing recurs, resume bag-mask ventilation with 100% oxygen and obtain expert consultation to plan for advanced airway insertion and support of ventilation.
- Check glucose using point-of-care testing.
- Arrange for transfer of the child to a higher level of care for evaluation, observation, and care.

Evaluate—*Diagnostic Assessments*	**Identify/Intervene**

Perform Throughout the Evaluation of the Patient as Appropriate

Lab data

- Glucose (bedside) 166 mg/dL (9.2 mmol/L)
- Electrolytes; blood urea nitrogen/creatinine; complete blood count with differential; blood culture

Imaging

- Chest x-ray ordered

Identify/Intervene:

- A blood glucose concentration should be checked as soon as reasonably possible in all critically ill infants and children. This child has had a seizure and decreased level of consciousness, so it is especially important to check the glucose. Hypoglycemia should be treated immediately.
- It is not always possible to obtain an arterial blood gas.

Re–evaluate-identify-intervene after each intervention.

Debriefing Tool
Testing Case Scenario 13
Disordered Control of Breathing Disease (Child)

General Management Objectives

- Uses the PALS Systematic Approach Algorithm to assess and appropriately classify a patient
- Provides oxygen appropriately
- Directs delivery of high-quality CPR (including the use of a feedback device) when indicated
- Demonstrates basic airway maneuvers and use of relevant airway device as appropriate
- Demonstrates application of cardiac and respiratory monitors
- Identifies the cardiac rhythm
- Applies appropriate PBLS or PALS algorithms
- Summarizes general indications, contraindications, and doses of relevant drugs
- Discusses principles of family-centered care in pediatric cardiac arrest
- Applies the 8 elements of effective team dynamics
- Performs frequent reassessment

Action	Gather	Analyze	Summarize
	Student Observations	***Done Well***	***Student-Led Summary***
• Directs assessment of ABCDE and vital signs	• Can you describe the events from your perspective?	• How were you able to [*insert action here*]?	• What are the main things you learned?
• Provides or directs bag-mask ventilation with 100% oxygen	• How well do you think your treatments worked?	• Why do you think you were able to [*insert action here*]?	• Can someone summarize the key points made?
• Applies cardiac monitor and pulse oximeter	• Can you review the events of the scenario (*directed to the Timer/Recorder*)?	• Tell me a little more about how you [*insert action here*].	• What are the main take-home messages?
• Identifies respiratory failure	• What could you have improved?		
• Identifies signs of disordered control of breathing	• What did the team do well?		
• Directs establishment of intravenous access			
• Performs frequent reassessment of patient	***Instructor Observations***	***Needs Improvement***	***Instructor-Led Summary***
• Describes methods to verify that bag-mask ventilation is effective	• I noticed that [*insert action here*].	• Why do you think [*insert action here*] occurred?	• Let's summarize what we learned…
• Identifies need for involvement of advanced provider with expertise in pediatric intubation and mechanical ventilation	• I observed that [*insert action here*].	• How do you think [*insert action here*] could have been improved?	• Here is what I think we learned…
• Summarizes specific interventions for disordered control of breathing	• I saw that [*insert action here*].	• What was your thinking while [*insert action here*]?	• The main take-home messages are…
		• What prevented you from [*insert action here*]?	• What would be the indications for endotracheal intubation in a child with disordered control of breathing? (Answer: Inadequate spontaneous respiratory effort and/or failure to maintain a patent airway)
			• If the child requires intubation, how would you estimate the size of cuffed and uncuffed endotracheal tube to use?

Bradycardia
(Infant; Hypoxia, Cardiopulmonary Failure)

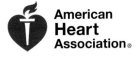

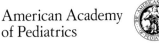

Scenario Lead-in

Prehospital: You are dispatched to the home of a 3-month-old infant with difficulty breathing.

ED: You are working in the emergency department and are asked to see a 3-month-old infant with difficulty breathing brought in by his parents.

General Inpatient Unit: You are a member of the emergency response team called to evaluate a 3-month-old infant admitted earlier in the day with difficulty breathing.

ICU: You are asked to see a 3-month-old infant admitted earlier in the day with difficulty breathing.

Vital Signs	
Heart rate	45/min
Blood pressure	Not obtainable
Respiratory rate	4/min
SpO₂	Not obtainable
Temperature	39.6°C (103.2°F)
Weight	5.7 kg
Age	3 months

Scenario Overview and Learning Objectives

Scenario Overview

Emphasis should be on identification of cardiopulmonary failure and management of hypoxic bradycardia associated with shock and likely lung tissue disease. Priorities include immediate bag-mask ventilation with 100% oxygen. Chest compressions are also required and epinephrine is administered. The heart rate rises and perfusion improves. The provider should also be able to discuss the preparation for insertion of an endotracheal tube and the method to estimate appropriate cuffed and uncuffed tube size. The experienced PALS provider may discuss possible delivery of a fluid bolus to treat persistent shock (the infant is febrile with little oral intake. However, this discussion is beyond the scope of the scenario and is not required for successful scenario completion.

Scenario-Specific Objectives

- **Demonstrates the support of oxygenation and ventilation in a patient with hypoxic bradycardia**
- **Recognizes indications for CPR in a bradycardic patient;** in this scenario, compressions are needed in addition to bag-mask ventilation because, despite oxygenation and ventilation, the infant has a heart rate less than 60/min with signs of poor perfusion
- **States 3 causes of bradycardia;** these include hypoxia (most common), vagal stimulation, heart block, and drug overdose
- **Describes appropriate indications for and dose of epinephrine for bradycardia**

Evaluate—*Initial Impression* (Pediatric Assessment Triangle)	Identify	Intervene
Appearance • No visible reaction to noises, caregivers **Breathing** • Very slow respiratory rate; grunting **Circulation** • Pale; cyanotic	• Immediate intervention needed	• Activate the emergency response system. Emergency medical services requests additional assistance if needed. • Check for response (no response) and perform simultaneous check for breathing (still very slow) and brachial pulse (very slow). • Begin bag-mask ventilation with 100% oxygen. • Apply cardiac monitor. • Apply pulse oximeter.

Evaluate—*Primary Assessment* Focused on Assessment Needed to Support Airway, Oxygenation, Ventilation, and Perfusion	Identify	Intervene
• **A**irway: Clear • **B**reathing: Respiratory rate 4/min; SpO₂ not obtainable; severe intercostal and subcostal retractions; nasal flaring; grunting; very poor air entry bilaterally; scattered wheezes • **C**irculation: Heart rate 45/min (sinus bradycardia) after short period of bag-mask ventilation; peripheral pulses absent, weak central pulses; extremities cool with sluggish capillary refill; unable to obtain blood pressure using noninvasive blood pressure measurement • **D**isability: Unresponsive • **E**xposure: Temperature 39.6°C (103.2°F); weight 5.7 kg; no rashes	• Cardiopulmonary failure • Sinus bradycardia	• Continue bag-mask ventilation with 100% oxygen. • Begin chest compressions when heart rate does not increase to 60/min or greater and signs of poor perfusion persist despite bag-mask ventilation with 100% oxygen. • Obtain vascular access (intravenous [IV]/intraosseous [IO]). • Administer epinephrine 0.01 mg/kg (0.1 mL/kg of the 0.1 mg/mL concentration) IV/IO followed by a rapid saline flush.

Evaluate—*Secondary Assessment* *Identify Reversible Causes, but Defer Remainder of Secondary Assessment Until Heart Rate 60/min or Greater With Adequate Perfusion*	**Identify**	**Intervene**
SAMPLE history (only to extent needed to evaluate reversible causes) • *Signs and symptoms:* Cough; nasal secretions; respiratory distress • *Allergies:* None • *Medications:* None • *Past medical history:* Previously well • *Last meal:* Took 1 oz from a bottle 8 hours ago • *Events (onset):* Upper respiratory infection symptoms for 2 days; worsening respiratory distress and lethargy today **Physical examination** • *Repeat vital signs after CPR and epinephrine bolus:* Heart rate increases to 130/min; SpO$_2$ 92% with bag-mask ventilation at a rate of 16-20/min with 100% oxygen; blood pressure 63/42 mm Hg • *Head, eyes, ears, nose, and throat/neck:* Apnea • *Heart and lungs:* No murmur; reduced air entry with positive-pressure ventilation; diffuse crackles/wheezes; weak peripheral pulses, stronger central pulses; capillary refill 4-5 seconds • *Abdomen:* Soft; no organomegaly • *Extremities:* Unremarkable • *Back:* Unremarkable • *Neurologic:* Lethargic; difficult to rouse • Point-of-care (POC) glucose concentration (see below)	• Cardiopulmonary failure	• Discontinue chest compressions when heart rate 60/min or greater (and rising) and perfusion improves. • Continue bag-mask ventilation with 100% oxygen at a rate of 16-20/min. • Prepare for advanced airway placement. • The experienced PALS provider may consider administration of a fluid bolus of 20 mL/kg of isotonic crystalloid. Reassess during and after fluid bolus. Stop fluid bolus if signs of heart failure (worsening respiratory distress, or development of hepatomegaly or rales) develop. Repeat fluid bolus as needed to treat signs of hypovolemic shock.

Evaluate—*Diagnostic Assessments* *Perform Throughout the Evaluation of the Patient as Appropriate*	**Identify/Intervene**
Lab data • Blood glucose 75 mg/dL • A blood gas (arterial, venous, or capillary) is not indicated in the immediate management of this infant. **Imaging** • A chest x-ray may be considered after intubation and stabilization to assess lung fields as well as confirming appropriate endotracheal tube positioning.	• A blood glucose concentration should be checked as soon as reasonably possible in critically ill infants and children. Hypoglycemia should be treated immediately. • Laboratory studies (other than POC glucose testing) deferred until effective bag-mask ventilation and heart rate are established and shock resuscitation has begun.

Re–evaluate-identify-intervene after each intervention.

Debriefing Tool
Testing Case Scenario 14
Bradycardia (Infant; Hypoxia, Cardiopulmonary Failure)

General Debriefing Principles

- Use the table below to guide your debriefing; also refer to the **Team Dynamics Debriefing Tool.**
- Debriefings are 10 minutes long.
- Address all learning objectives.
- Summarize take-home messages at the end of the debriefing.
- *Encourage:* Students to self-reflect
    Engagement of all participants
- *Avoid:* Mini-lectures and closed-ended questions
    Dominating the discussion

General Management Objectives

- Uses the PALS Systematic Approach Algorithm to assess and appropriately classify a patient
- Provides oxygen appropriately
- Directs delivery of high-quality CPR (including the use of a feedback device) when indicated
- Demonstrates basic airway maneuvers and use of relevant airway device as appropriate
- Demonstrates application of cardiac and respiratory monitors
- Identifies the cardiac rhythm
- Applies appropriate PBLS or PALS algorithms
- Summarizes general indications, contraindications, and doses of relevant drugs
- Discusses principles of family-centered care in pediatric cardiac arrest
- Applies the 8 elements of effective team dynamics
- Performs frequent reassessment

Action	Gather	Analyze	Summarize
• Directs assessment of ABCDE and vital signs • Identifies bradycardia associated with cardiorespiratory compromise/failure • Directs initiation of bag-mask ventilation with 100% oxygen • Applies cardiac monitor and pulse oximeter • Reassesses heart rate and perfusion after initiation of bag-mask ventilation with oxygen • Recognizes indications to provide high-quality CPR (chest compressions plus ventilation) for the bradycardic patient • Directs establishment of IV or IO access • Directs or discusses administration of 0.01 mg/kg (0.1 mL/kg of the 0.1 mg/mL concentration) epinephrine IV/IO bolus • Discusses preparation for advanced airway placement • Performs frequent reassessment	***Student Observations*** • Can you describe the events from your perspective? • How well do you think your treatments worked? • Can you review the events of the scenario (*directed to the Timer/Recorder*)? • What could you have improved? • What did the team do well? ***Instructor Observations*** • I noticed that [*insert action here*]. • I observed that [*insert action here*]. • I saw that [*insert action here*].	***Done Well*** • How were you able to [*insert action here*]? • Why do you think you were able to [*insert action here*]? • Tell me a little more about how you [*insert action here*]. ***Needs Improvement*** • Why do you think [*insert action here*] occurred? • How do you think [*insert action here*] could have been improved? • What was your thinking while [*insert action here*]? • What prevented you from [*insert action here*]?	***Student-Led Summary*** • What are the main things you learned? • Can someone summarize the key points made? • What are the main take-home messages? ***Instructor-Led Summary*** • Let's summarize what we learned… • Here is what I think we learned… • The main take-home messages are… • In addition to hypoxia, what are 3 other causes of bradycardia in infants and children? • This scenario did not include advanced airway insertion. In preparing for intubation, how would you estimate the correct cuffed and uncuffed endotracheal tube size for this infant?

Team Dynamics Debriefing Tool

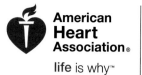

- Use the table below to guide your debriefing.
- Observe and record elements of team dynamics.
- Identify 2 or 3 elements of team dynamics to discuss per debriefing session.

Action	Gather	Analyze	Summarize
Closed-Loop Communication	**Student Observations**	**Done Well**	**Student-Led Summary**
• Orders acknowledged and confirmed when given • Orders announced when executed	• Can you describe the events from your perspective? • How well do you think your treatments worked? • Can you review the events of the scenario? (*directed to the Timer/Recorder*) • What could you have improved? • What did the team do well?	• How were you able to [*insert action here*]? • Why do you think you were able to [*insert action here*]? • Tell me a little more about how you [*insert action here*].	• What are the main things you learned? • Can someone summarize the key points made? • What are the main take-home messages?
Clear Messages			
• Team members speak clearly • Orders are questioned when doubt exists			
Clear Roles	**Instructor Observations**	**Needs Improvement**	**Instructor-Led Summary**
• All team members have appropriate roles • Roles are reallocated when appropriate	• I noticed that [*insert action here*]. • I observed that [*insert action here*]. • I saw that [*insert action here*].	• Why do you think [*insert action here*] occurred? • How do you think [*insert action here*] could have been improved? • What was your thinking while [*insert action here*]? • What prevented you from [*insert action here*]?	• Let's summarize what we learned… • Here is what I think we learned… • The main take-home messages are…
Knowing One's Limitations			
• Calls for assistance • Seeks advice when appropriate			
Knowledge Sharing			
• Sharing information between team members • Asks for ideas and suggestions			
Constructive Intervention			
• Identifies priorities • Questions colleagues who make mistakes			
Reevaluation and Summarizing			
• Reevaluates patient • Summarizes patient condition and treatment plan			
Mutual Respect			
• Speaks in a professional, friendly tone of voice • Provides positive feedback			

Appendix C

ECG Rhythms

ECG Rhythms A–C

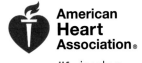

A

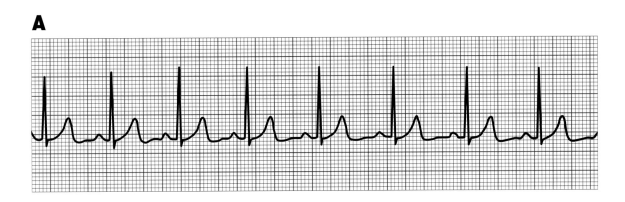

B

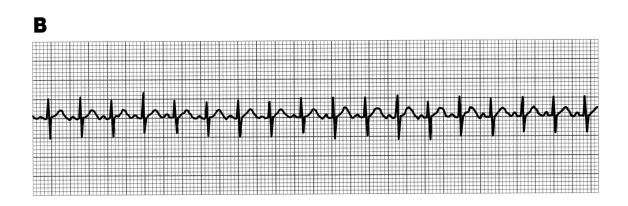

C

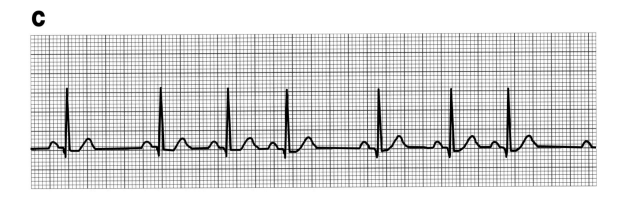

ECG Rhythms
Identification of A–C

A. Sinus rhythm

B. Sinus tachycardia

C. Sinus arrhythmia

ECG Rhythms D–F

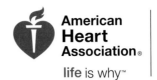 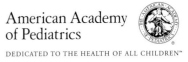

D

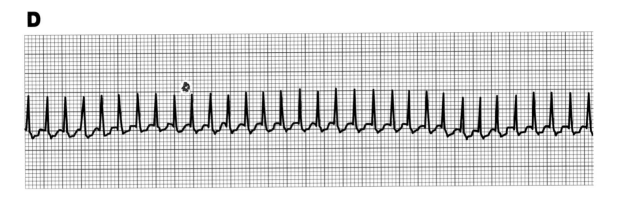

E

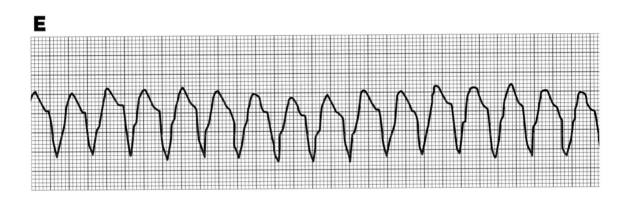

F

Drug administered

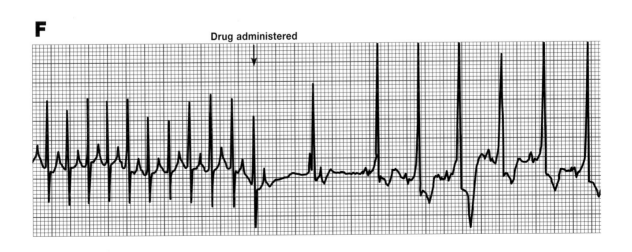

ECG Rhythms
Identification of D–F

D. Narrow-complex tachycardia

E. Wide-complex tachycardia

F. SVT converting to sinus rhythm with adenosine administration

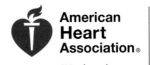
Pediatric Advanced Life Support

G

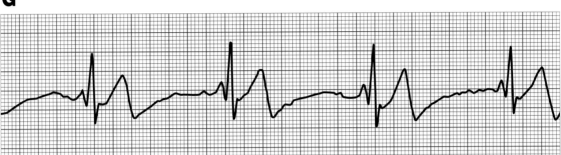

H

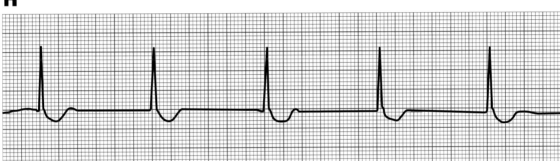

I

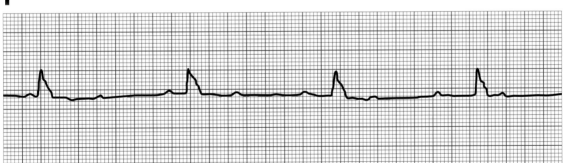

J

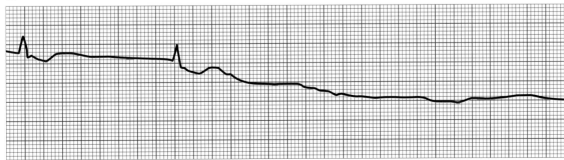

ECG Rhythms
Identification of G–J

G. Sinus bradycardia

H. Junctional bradycardia

I. Complete heart block with ventricular escape rhythm

J. Agonal rhythm progressing to asystole

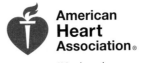

K

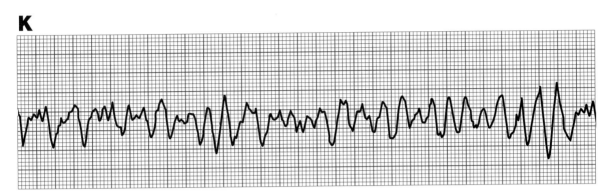

L

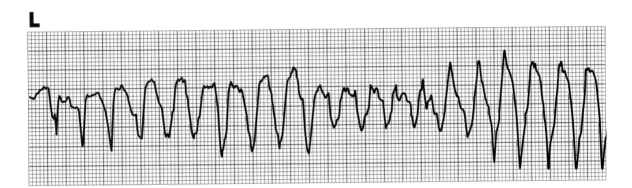

M

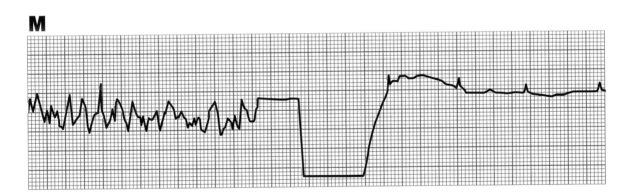

N

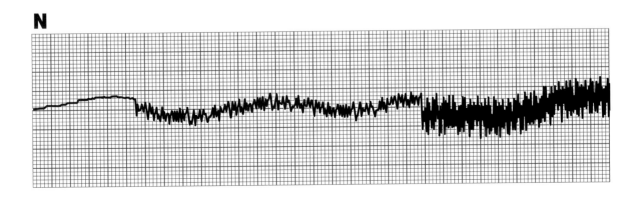

ECG Rhythms
Identification of K–N

K. Ventricular fibrillation

L. Torsades de pointes

M. VF converted to organized rhythm after defibrillation (successful shock)

N. Asystole with superimposed muscle artifact followed by 60-cycle (60-Hz) artifact

Part 6

PALS Lesson Plans

Lessons are numbered for labeling and convenience only.

PALS
Lesson Plans

Precourse Preparation

Instructor Tips

- Prepare well with strong messaging and anticipating questions/challenges before they arise. The time you invest in this part of your preparation is priceless
- Have a plan for possible challenges
  - Instructor manual does not arrive
  - Equipment failure/malfunctions
  - Extra batteries

30 to 60 Days Before Course

- Determine course specifics
  - Target audience
  - Number of students
  - Special needs or equipment
- Review and reserve equipment
- Schedule room as soon as dates are determined
- Schedule additional instructors, if needed

Activity	Recommended Size or Ratio
Large-group interactions	The size of the group is limited by the size of the room and the number of video monitors or projection screens
Learning stations	6:1 up to a maximum of 8:1 • The student-to-instructor ratio should be 6:1 up to a maximum of 8:1 (with additional time as needed)

Optional

Instructors or Training Centers may consider offering a PALS preparation course days or weeks before the PALS Course to ensure that students understand the concepts outlined in the course manual. In addition, the Student Website contains the Precourse Self-Assessment and supplementary information for precourse preparation. Students must be knowledgeable in the following areas:

- ECG rhythm identification
- Pharmacology
- Practical application

At Least 3 Weeks Before Course

- Confirm room reservations and setups
- Send students precourse letters with student materials
- Ensure that students understand that precourse preparation is necessary for successful participation in the PALS Course
- For the PALS Course, ensure that students are aware of the requirements to complete the online Precourse Self-Assessment with a score of 70% or higher, print their score sheet, and bring it to the course

- Confirm additional instructors
- **Research local treatment protocols and prepare for discussion**

Day Before Course

- Set up the room
- Coordinate the plan with additional instructors, if needed for class size
- Ensure that all equipment is available and tested for operation
  - Have extra batteries on hand for equipment
- Check with the Training Center Coordinator to determine any Training Center–specific paperwork needed
- Ensure that all course paperwork is in order, such as
  - PALS course roster
  - Testing checklists
  - Learning station competency checklists
- Ensure that all instructors understand which stations to teach and the course rotation schedule

Day of Course

- Make sure all equipment is working
- Greet students as they arrive to make them feel at ease
- Have students fill out the course roster. Rosters may vary between Training Centers; refer to the Instructor Network (**www.ahainstructornetwork.org**)
- Required: Collect the students' Precourse Self-Assessment certificate (with score of 70% or higher)
  - Refer to the *PALS Instructor Manual* if a student does not come with a printed copy of his or her Precourse Self-Assessment certificate

PALS Equipment List

Equipment and Supplies	Quantity Needed	Learning/Testing Station Equipment Needed
Paperwork		
Precourse letter	1/student	Precourse
Course roster	1/course	Beginning of course
Name tags	1/student and instructor	All
Course agenda	1/student and instructor	End of course
Course completion card	1/student	All
PALS Provider Manual	1/student and instructor	All
PALS Instructor Manual with Lesson Plans	1/instructor	All
Instructor case scenarios	1/instructor	All

(continued)

(continued)

Equipment and Supplies	Quantity Needed	Learning/Testing Station Equipment Needed
Team role labels	1 set/station to identify team role for each student	All small group stations
Skills station competency checklists	1/student and instructor	BLS and skills stations
PALS Course Progress Checklist	1/instructor	All
Cardiac, shock, and respiratory practice scenario checklists	1/student	Airway Management Learning Station, Vascular Access Learning Station, and Rhythm Disturbances/Electrical Therapy Learning Station
Child and infant BLS skills testing checklists	1 of each/student	Child and Infant High-Quality BLS
ECC Handbook (optional)	1/student and instructor	Optional; all
PALS algorithms/flowcharts	1 set/station	All
PALS Exam	1/student	Exam
Blank exam answer sheet	1/student	Exam
Exam answer key/annotated answer key	1/course	Exam
Algorithm posters	1/course	Cardiac case scenario discussions, Rhythm Disturbances/Electrical Therapy Learning Station
Institution-based documentation form	1/course	Cardiac case scenario discussions
Learning station competency checklists	1/student	Child and Infant High-Quality BLS, Airway Management Learning Station, Rhythm Disturbances/Electrical Therapy Learning Station, Vascular Access Learning Station
Audiovisual Equipment		
TV with DVD player or computer with video player and projection screen	1/station	Course Overview, Overview of PALS Science, Child and Infant High-Quality BLS Practice and Testing, Airway Management Learning Station, Rhythm Disturbances/Electrical Therapy Learning Station, Vascular Access Learning Station, Systematic Approach, Team Dynamics

(continued)

(continued)

Equipment and Supplies	Quantity Needed	Learning/Testing Station Equipment Needed
Course video	1	Course Overview, Overview of PALS Science, Child and Infant High-Quality BLS Practice and Testing, Airway Management Learning Station, Rhythm Disturbances/Electrical Therapy Learning Station, Vascular Access Learning Station, Systematic Approach, Team Dynamics
CPR and AED Equipment		
BLS feedback device recommended	1/station	Child and Infant High-Quality BLS Practice and Testing, Rhythm Disturbances/Electrical Therapy Learning Station, cardiac case scenario discussions
Child CPR manikin with shirt*	1/every 3 students	Child and Infant High-Quality BLS Practice and Testing, Rhythm Disturbances/Electrical Therapy Learning Station, cardiac case scenario discussions, shock case scenario discussions
Infant CPR manikin*	1/every 3 students	Child and Infant High-Quality BLS Practice and Testing, Management of Cardiac Emergencies Learning Station, cardiac case scenario discussions, shock case scenario discussions
Child airway manikin or intubation head	1/every 3 students	Airway Management Learning Station, respiratory case scenario discussions
Infant airway manikin or intubation head	1/every 3 students	Airway Management Learning Station, respiratory case scenario discussions
Stopwatch/timing device	1/instructor	High-Quality BLS Practice and Testing
Countdown timer	1/instructor	High-Quality BLS Practice and Testing
AED trainer with adult and child AED training pads	1/every 3 students	High-Quality BLS Practice and Testing, Rhythm Disturbances/Electrical Therapy Learning Station, cardiac case scenario discussions
CPR backboard	1/every 3 students	High-Quality BLS Practice and Testing, cardiac case scenario discussions
Stools to stand on for CPR	1/every 3 students	High-Quality BLS Practice and Testing, cardiac case scenario discussions
Airway and Ventilation		
Infant airway manikin or intubation head	1/every 3 students	Airway Management Learning Station, respiratory case scenario discussions

(continued)

Equipment and Supplies	Quantity Needed	Learning/Testing Station Equipment Needed
Child pocket mask and infant pocket mask	1/every 3 students or 1/student	High-Quality BLS Practice and Testing, respiratory case scenario discussions
1-way valve	1/student	High-Quality BLS Practice and Testing, respiratory case scenario discussions
Bag-mask devices • 450 to 500 mL for infants and young children • 1000 mL or larger for older children and adolescents	1/every 3 students	High-Quality BLS Practice and Testing, Rhythm Disturbances/Electrical Therapy Learning Station, respiratory case scenario discussions, shock case scenario discussions
Nonrebreathing mask with reservoir	1/station	Airway Management Learning Station, respiratory case scenario discussions, shock case scenario discussions
Nasal cannula	1/station	Airway Management Learning Station, respiratory case scenario discussions
High-flow nasal cannula (optional)	1/station	Airway Management Learning Station, respiratory case scenario discussions
Simple oxygen mask	1/station	Airway Management Learning Station, respiratory case scenario discussions
Suction catheters	1 set of multiple sizes/station	Airway Management Learning Station, respiratory case scenario discussions
Nebulizer setup	1 set/station	Airway Management Learning Station, respiratory case scenario discussions
Waveform capnography equipment*	Pictures can be used to represent this technology	Airway Management Learning Station, Rhythm Disturbances/Electrical Therapy Learning Station, respiratory case scenario discussions, cardiac case scenario discussions, shock case scenario discussions
Stethoscope	1/every manikin	Airway Management Learning Station, respiratory case scenario discussions, shock case scenario discussions
Color-coded length-based resuscitation tape	1/station	Airway Management Learning Station, Rhythm Disturbances/Electrical Therapy Learning Station, respiratory case scenario discussions, cardiac case scenario discussions, shock case scenario discussions, Vascular Access Learning Station

(continued)

9

(continued)

Equipment and Supplies	Quantity Needed	Learning/Testing Station Equipment Needed
Towel	1/every 3 students	Airway Management Learning Station, respiratory case scenario discussions
Exhaled CO_2 detector: adult, child, and infant	1/station	Airway Management Learning Station, respiratory case scenario discussions, shock case scenario discussions
Tube holder or tape, pediatric	1/every manikin	Airway Management Learning Station, respiratory case scenario discussions
Rhythm Recognition and Electrical Therapy		
Cardiac monitor with ECG leads, electrodes, and pads (infant, child/adult)	1 set/station	Rhythm Disturbances/Electrical Therapy Learning Station, cardiac case scenario discussions
Rhythm generator	1/course	Rhythm Disturbances/Electrical Therapy Learning Station, cardiac case scenario discussions
AED trainer	1/station	Rhythm Disturbances/Electrical Therapy Learning Station, cardiac case scenario discussions
Color-coded length-based resuscitation tape		Rhythm Disturbances/Electrical Therapy Learning Station
BLS feedback devices recommended		Rhythm Disturbances/Electrical Therapy Learning Station
Waveform capnography recommended		Rhythm Disturbances/Electrical Therapy Learning Station
Equipment and Medications		
IO manikin	1 (with replacement bones)	Vascular Access Learning Station, shock case scenario discussions
IO drill and needles recommended	1 drill, various needle sizes	Vascular Access Learning Station, shock case scenario discussions
IO manual needles	3/station	Vascular Access Learning Station, shock case scenario discussions
Respiratory medications: resuscitation drugs or drug cards • Albuterol • Ipratropium • Epinephrine 1 mg/mL racemic (2.25%) • IM epinephrine 1 mg/mL	1/student	Respiratory case scenario discussions

(continued)

(continued)

Equipment and Supplies	Quantity Needed	Learning/Testing Station Equipment Needed
Cardiac medications: resuscitation drugs or drug cards • Adenosine • Amiodarone • Atropine sulfate • Epinephrine 0.1 mg/mL • Glucose • Lidocaine • Magnesium sulfate		Cardiac case scenario discussions
Shock medications: resuscitation drugs or drug cards • Atropine sulfate • Epinephrine 0.1 mg/mL • Fluids • Glucose • Inotropes • Vasopressors		Shock case scenario discussions
Fluid bag	1	Vascular Access Learning Station, shock case scenario discussions
3-way stopcock	1	Vascular Access Learning Station, shock case scenario discussions
60-cc locking syringe	1	Vascular Access Learning Station, shock case scenario discussions
Syringes	2-3/station	Vascular Access Learning Station, shock case scenario discussions
Advanced Airways (must choose endotracheal tube and at least 1 supraglottic device)		
Oropharyngeal airways	Various infant/child sizes/1 each	High-Quality BLS Practice and Testing, respiratory case scenario discussions, Airway Management Emergencies Learning Station
Supraglottic airways	Various samples sizes	Airway Management Learning Station, respiratory case scenario discussions
MDI, spacers, and mouth piece/mask	1 set/station	Airway Management Learning Station, respiratory case scenario discussions
Water-soluble lubricant	1/station	Airway Management Learning Station, respiratory case scenario discussions
Laryngoscope handle	1 adult and 1 child size/ every 3 students	Airway Management Learning Station, respiratory case scenario discussions

(continued)

(continued)

Equipment and Supplies	Quantity Needed	Learning/Testing Station Equipment Needed
Laryngoscope blades	Multiple straight and curved blades	Airway Management Learning Station, respiratory case scenario discussions
Endotracheal tubes, cuffed and uncuffed with stylet	Various sizes that fit airway manikin	Airway Management Learning Station, respiratory case scenario discussions
Safety		
Sharps container (if using real needles)	1/station	Vascular Access Learning Station, shock case scenario discussions
Cleaning Supplies for Use Between Student Practice and After Course		
Manikin cleaning supplies	As needed between students	High-Quality BLS Practice and Testing, Airway Management Learning Station, Rhythm Disturbances/Electrical Therapy Learning Station, Vascular Access Learning Station, respiratory case scenario discussions, cardiac case scenario discussions, shock case scenario discussions

*Directive feedback devices.

Instructor Notes

_____

_____

_____

_____

Next
Course Introduction

Lesson
Course Introduction

Instructor Tips

- Knowing what you want to communicate, why it's important, and what you want to have happen as a result is critical to the success of your presentation
- Be willing to adjust your Lesson Plans to the students' learning needs
- Introductions: Use the class roster or other visual aids (flip chart, whiteboard) to help keep track of the students in the course (eg, name, scope of practice, workplace)

Discussion

In a large group, with all students, discuss the following:

- Introduce yourself and additional instructors, if needed
- Invite students to introduce themselves and ask them to provide the following information:
  - Name
  - Occupation
  - Specialty
  - Place of practice
- As students are introducing themselves, document occupation, specialty, etc; this will assist instructors when tailoring future case scenarios and lessons
- Explain that the course is interactive, and discuss use of the following checklists:
  - BLS skills testing checklists (2)
    - Child
    - Infant
  - Learning station competency checklists (3)
    - Respiratory
    - Cardiac
    - Shock
  - Case scenario testing checklists (3)
    - Respiratory
    - Cardiac
    - Shock
- Explain that parts of the course are somewhat physically strenuous
  - For example, Lesson 4 involves CPR, which will require you to perform a number of compressions that could be physically strenuous
- Ask that anyone with a medical concern, such as knee or back problems, speak with one of the instructors

- Explain the layout of the building, including bathrooms and fire exits
- Advise students where AEDs can be found in the building
- Tell students to silence cell phones
  - If a call needs to be answered, tell students to answer in the hallway
- Tell the students, "We are scheduled to end at _____"

Instructor Notes

_____

_____

_____

_____

Next

Life Is Why Activity
(Optional)

Lesson 1
Life Is Why™ Activity (Optional)

5 minutes

Instructor Tips

- Before facilitating this lesson, complete the Life Is Why activity in the Instructor Manual. Have your "_____ Is Why" prepared to share with students

- You can make additional copies of the Life Is Why activity from the Instructor Manual for students who do not bring their Provider Manual to class

Play Life Is Why Video

- Play video (found in the video menu)

Discussion

- To engage the class, after viewing the Life Is Why video, take 2 to 3 minutes to share your Why with the class, based on your completed Life Is Why activity in the Instructor Manual

- Then, encourage students to participate in the following activity:

  – Have students find the "_____ Is Why" page in their Provider Manual and follow the directions. Tell students:

    - Complete this activity by filling in the blank with the word that describes your Why

    - Tell your family and friends about your "_____ Is Why," and ask them to discover their Why

AHA Life Is Why Icon

- Tell students that throughout their Provider Manual, they will find information that correlates what they are learning in this course to Life Is Why and the importance of cardiovascular care. This information is identified by the Life Is Why heart-and-torch icon

- Remind students that what they are learning today has an impact on the mission of the American Heart Association

Instructor Notes

_____

_____

_____

_____

Next
Course Overview

Lesson 2
Course Overview

5 minutes

Instructor Tips

- Be sensitive to the agenda timeline and, as much as possible, use suggested times for each lesson
- Keep in mind that some students learn differently and you may need to use a variety of teaching techniques (eg, some learners are visual learners, some learners are auditory learners, and some learners are kinesthetic learners)
- Allow yourself a few minutes before and after lunch and/or at the end of day to give students the opportunity to ask questions that they may not have felt comfortable asking in a large group setting
- **Items in boldface on all Lesson Plans have greater importance**

Play Course Overview Video

In a large group, with all students

- Play the video

Discussion

In a large group, with all students, discuss the following:

- **At no time was medical care delayed for the purpose of obtaining videos. All children received timely and appropriate medical care, and parents provided consent before recording**
- Be certain students understand major course concepts
    - Importance of high-quality CPR to patient survival
    - Integration of high-quality BLS with pediatric interventions and effective team dynamics

- Tell students that they will be taking their *PALS Provider Manual* with them to every station throughout the course
- Remind students about course completion requirements
    - **PALS course completion requirements**
        - Actively participate in, practice, and complete the skills stations and learning stations
        - Pass skills tests in child CPR and AED and infant CPR
        - Pass an exam with a minimum score of 84%
        - Perform satisfactorily as a Team Leader in both of the following:
            - A cardiac case scenario
            - Either a respiratory or a shock case scenario

Next
Science of Pediatric Resuscitation

Lesson 3
Science of Pediatric Resuscitation

10 minutes

Instructor Tips

- After playing the video, be sure to emphasize how this new information will fit in with the providers' clinical practice

- Assure students that this information will be reinforced throughout the course

- To optimize the content learned from the video, try to tie in science updates to what was learned in the video and how it can be used in the students' scope of practice

Play Science of Pediatric Resuscitation Video

- In a large group, with all students, play the video

Discussion

- Briefly answer students' questions (refer to the Summary of High-Quality CPR Components table on the next page)

- If there are no student questions, consider asking questions to highlight key concepts

(continued)

Summary of High-Quality CPR Components for BLS Providers— Comparison of Key Elements of Child and Infant BLS

Component	Adults and Adolescents	Children (Age 1 Year to Puberty)	Infants (Age Less Than 1 Year, Excluding Newborns)
Scene safety	Make sure the environment is safe for rescuers and the victim		
Recognition of cardiac arrest	Check for responsiveness No breathing or only gasping (ie, no normal breathing) No definite pulse felt within 10 seconds (Breathing and pulse check can be performed simultaneously in less than 10 seconds)		
Activation of emergency response system	If you are alone with no mobile phone, leave the victim to activate the emergency response system and get the AED before beginning CPR Otherwise, send someone and begin CPR immediately; use the AED as soon as it is available	***Witnessed collapse*** Follow steps for adults and adolescents on the left ***Unwitnessed collapse, single rescuer*** Give 2 minutes of CPR Leave the victim to activate the emergency response system and get the AED Return to the child or infant and resume CPR; use the AED as soon as it is available	
Compression-ventilation ratio *without advanced airway*	*1 or 2 rescuers* 30:2	*1 rescuer* 30:2 *2 or more rescuers* 15:2	
Compression-ventilation ratio *with advanced airway*	Continuous compressions at a rate of 100-120/min Give 1 breath every 6 seconds (10 breaths/min)		
Compression rate	100-120/min		
Compression depth	At least 2 inches (5 cm)*	At least one third AP diameter of chest About 2 inches (5 cm)	At least one third AP diameter of chest About 1½ inches (4 cm)
Hand placement	2 hands on the lower half of the breastbone (sternum)	2 hands or 1 hand (rescuer can use either method on small child) on the lower half of the breastbone (sternum)	*1 rescuer* 2 fingers in the center of the chest, just below the nipple line *2 or more rescuers* 2 thumb–encircling hands in the center of the chest, just below the nipple line
Chest recoil	Allow full recoil of chest after each compression; do not lean on the chest after each compression		
Minimizing interruptions	Limit interruptions in chest compressions to less than 10 seconds		

*Compression depth should be no more than 2.4 inches (6 cm).

Abbreviations: AED, automated external defibrillator; AP, anteroposterior; CPR, cardiopulmonary resuscitation.

(continued)

(continued)

Instructor Notes

_____

_____

_____

_____

Next

Learning/Testing Station:
Child High-Quality BLS
Practice

Lesson 4A
Learning/Testing Station:
Child High-Quality BLS Practice

25 minutes

Learning Objective

- Recognize cardiopulmonary arrest early and begin CPR within 10 seconds

Instructor Tips

- Play the video without interruption; if you have additional comments, wait until the end of the video
- Consider using a stopwatch or timing device during testing to ensure accurate and objective assessments
- Familiarize yourself with the skills testing checklist (refer to "Part 3: Testing and Remediation" in the *PALS Instructor Manual* for information on how to use skills testing checklists)

Play Basic Life Support Video

- Play the video
- Video will instruct students to position themselves for practice and then pause automatically

Practice While Watching: Child 1-Rescuer CPR

- **Resume video**
- Ensure that students pay attention to the video as they practice CPR
- Use of directive feedback devices is recommended
- Give positive and corrective feedback
- Use a stopwatch or timer to familiarize students with being timed during compressions
- Tell students that they will practice with the Child High-Quality BLS testing video and will rotate roles
- Have students position themselves in front of manikins
    - 2 to 3 students per manikin
    - Each student must have a 1-way valve
- Emphasize the following concepts:
    - Students' shoulders should be positioned directly over the manikin's sternum with straight arms
    - Push hard, push fast (proper rate and depth)
        - Depress chest at least one third the diameter of the chest (5 cm in most children)
        - Rate of 100 to 120 compressions/min
    - Let the chest return to the normal position between compressions (recoil); no pressure should be applied to the chest during recoil (ie, do not lean on the patient)
    - Minimize the number and duration of compression interruptions
- Video will pause automatically; replay for practice or **resume video**

Practice While Watching: Bag-Mask Device for a Child

- **Resume video**
  - Students practice
  - Give correction and feedback
- Demonstrate appropriate ventilation rate and volume
  - Deliver 1 breath every 6 seconds
  - Deliver breath until chest rise is visible
- Video will pause automatically; replay for practice or **resume video**

Students Practice: AED

- Video will explain the use of an AED and then pause automatically for practice
- Instructor demonstrates correct AED use
- Answer any questions students have about AEDs
- Place students in groups to practice the use of an AED
- Confirm that each student can operate the AED effectively
- Video will pause automatically

Students Practice: Putting It All Together

- Students should practice compressions, bag-mask ventilation, and AED skills
- After practice, test students

Instructor Notes

_____

_____

_____

_____

_____

Next

Learning/Testing Station:
Child High-Quality BLS
Testing—Testing Details

Lesson 4B
Learning/Testing Station:
Child High-Quality BLS Testing—
Testing Details

15 minutes

Instructor Tips

- Use a stopwatch or feedback device—which is highly recommended—during testing to ensure accurate and objective assessments

- Familiarize yourself with the Child CPR and AED Skills Testing Checklist (refer to "Part 3: Testing and Remediation" in the *PALS Instructor Manual* for information on how to use skills testing checklists)

- Complete the Child CPR and AED Skills Testing Checklist for each student during this portion of the lesson

Skills Testing

- **Test students one at a time**
- Ask students who are not testing to practice on another manikin
- Consider matching one of the scenarios on the skills testing checklist to each student's scope of practice
- Each student must demonstrate the entire sequence of 2-rescuer CPR and AED **without instructor prompting**
- Carefully observe the student being tested for appropriate
    - Compression rate (use a stopwatch)
    - Compression depth
        - For example, check the depth of compressions with a feedback device, which is highly recommended
- If a student is unsuccessful (based on checklist requirements), refer him or her for immediate remediation
    - Each student may retest 1 additional time during this station
    - If a student remains unsuccessful after a second attempt, ensure that the student receives formal remediation at the end of the course (refer to "Part 3: Testing and Remediation" in the *PALS Instructor Manual*)
- Complete the Child CPR and AED Skills Testing Checklist for each student
- Summarize the importance of high-quality CPR to patient survival

Instructor Notes

Next

Learning/Testing Station: Infant High-Quality BLS Practice

Lesson 5A
Learning/Testing Station:
Infant High-Quality BLS Practice

20 minutes

Learning Objective

- Recognize cardiopulmonary arrest early and begin CPR within 10 seconds

Instructor Tips

- Use a stopwatch or feedback device—which is highly recommended—during testing to ensure accurate and objective assessments

- Familiarize yourself with the Infant CPR Skills Testing Checklist (refer to "Part 3: Testing and Remediation" in the *PALS Instructor Manual* for information on how to use skills testing checklists)

- Complete the skills testing checklist for each student during this portion of the lesson

Play Basic Life Support Video

- **Play the video**

- Video will instruct students to position themselves for practice and then pause automatically

Practice While Watching: Infant Compressions

- Have students position themselves in front of manikins

  - 2 to 3 students per manikin

- Play the video

  - Ensure that students pay attention to the video as they practice CPR

  - Use of directive feedback devices is recommended

  - Give positive and corrective feedback

  - Use a stopwatch or timer to familiarize students with being timed during compressions

  - Tell students that they will practice with the High-Quality BLS testing video and will rotate roles

- Video will pause automatically; replay for practice or **resume video**

Practice While Watching: Infant 2-Rescuer CPR

- Play the video
  - Ensure that students pay attention to the video as they practice CPR
  - Use of directive feedback devices is recommended
  - Give positive and corrective feedback
  - Use a stopwatch or timer to familiarize students with being timed during compressions
  - Tell students that they will practice with the High-Quality BLS testing video and will rotate roles
- Have students position themselves in front of manikins
  - 2 to 3 students per manikin
- Video will pause automatically; replay for practice or **resume video**

Students Practice: Putting It All Together

- When video pauses, students will practice compressions along with bag-mask ventilation skills
- After practice, test students

Instructor Notes

Next

Learning/Testing Station: Infant High-Quality BLS Testing — Testing Details

Lesson 5B
Learning/Testing Station:
Infant High-Quality BLS Testing—
Testing Details

15 minutes

Instructor Tips

- Use a stopwatch or feedback device—which is highly recommended—during testing to ensure accurate and objective assessments
- Review the Infant CPR Skills Testing Checklist before testing students (refer to "Part 3: Testing and Remediation" in the *PALS Instructor Manual* for information on how to use skills testing checklists)
- Complete the skills testing checklist for each student while he or she is completing the test

---

Skills Testing

- **Test students one at a time**
- Ask students who are not testing to practice on another manikin
- Consider matching one of the scenarios on the skills testing checklist to your student's scope of practice
- Each student must demonstrate the entire sequence of 2-rescuer CPR **without instructor prompting**
- Carefully observe the student being tested for appropriate:
  - Compression rate (use a stopwatch)
  - Compression depth
    - For example, check the speed of chest compressions with a stopwatch or feedback device, which is highly recommended
- If a student is unsuccessful (based on checklist requirements), refer him or her for immediate remediation
  - Each student may retest 1 additional time during this station
  - If a student remains unsuccessful after a second attempt, ensure that the student receives formal remediation at the end of the course (refer to "Part 3: Testing and Remediation" in the *PALS Instructor Manual*)
- Complete the Infant CPR Skills Testing Checklist for each student
- Summarize the importance of high-quality CPR to patient survival

---

Instructor Notes

Next

Learning/Testing Station:
Child and Infant Choking
(Optional)

Lesson 6
Learning/Testing Station:
Child and Infant Choking (Optional)

20 minutes

Learning Objective

• Perform high-quality CPR per AHA BLS recommendations

Instructor Tips

• Play the video without interruption; if you have additional comments, wait until the end of the video

Play Relief of Choking Video

• **Play the video**
• Video will demonstrate choking interventions for children and infants

Practice While Watching: Relief of Choking in an Infant

• **Play the video**
• Ensure that students pay attention to the video as they practice choking intervention techniques
• Use of directive feedback devices is recommended
• Give positive and corrective feedback
• Tell students that they will practice infant choking interventions

Discussion: Debrief

• Were there any specific elements you found difficult?
• If you were asked to perform the same skills again, is there anything you would do differently?
  – What?
  – Why?

Instructor Notes

_____

_____

_____

_____

Next

Overview of Systematic Approach Model

Lesson 7A
Overview of Systematic Approach Model

45 minutes

Learning Objective

- Differentiate between patients who do and do not require immediate intervention

Instructor Tips

- Ask students to use the *PALS Provider Manual* in this lesson to help further engage them and help with retention of information
- Draw or reference the PAT before presenting patient cases
- Make sure not to interrupt the video. If you have any comments to add, write them down and discuss them at the end of the video. Students do not learn well when they are trying to listen to 2 things at once
- **Consider watching the videos before teaching this lesson to become familiar with the content**

Instructor Note

When facilitating this lesson, keep in mind that each element of the systematic approach is designed to lay the foundation for the next. Be intentional to not progress beyond the individual elements of the systematic approach; ie, don't progress into primary assessment information in the PAT case discussion videos because the primary assessment content will be covered in the next lesson

Ask Students to Open the *PALS Provider Manual* to Part 3

Play Systematic Approach Video

- **Play the video**
- The video automatically pauses on a patient for the instructor to identify the components of PAT related to this patient
  - Video will discuss evaluate-identify-intervene, initial impression—PAT, and primary assessment
- Initial impression and primary assessment are the evaluation tools used to evaluate the patient, identify medical emergencies, and provide appropriate interventions
- The PAT and primary assessment are performed in a systematic order to address medical emergencies from the most critical to the least critical
- When you are performing the PAT and primary assessment, interventions must be provided as medical emergencies are identified **before** you proceed with the assessment (see instructor note about **life-threatening conditions**)
- Advise students to refer to the PAT in Part 3 of the *PALS Provider Manual* for the next 3 videos

Instructor Note: Life-Threatening Conditions

- If during any part of this sequence you find that a patient has a **life-threatening condition**, correction of those conditions takes precedence over establishing baseline vital sign measures, such as blood pressure or pulse oximetry. When the primary assessment is completed, and after life-threatening problems have been addressed, the healthcare provider proceeds to the secondary assessment

- Always remember that a **life-threatening condition** is present if the child is unresponsive or apneic; has inadequate or labored breathing; or is mottled, gray, pale, or cyanotic. If these are present, immediately call for help and begin lifesaving treatment. If there is no **life-threatening condition**, you proceed with the primary assessment

Evaluate-Identify-Intervene Algorithm

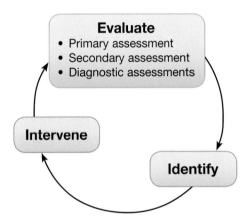

Initial Impression—Pediatric Assessment Triangle

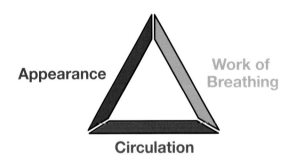

Initial Impression—Pediatric Assessment Triangle*
Appearance
From the doorway, your initial observation of the patient
Caregiver observes
• Abnormal tone
• Decreased interaction
• Inconsolable
• Abnormal look/gaze
• Abnormal speech/cry

(continued)

Work of Breathing

- Abnormal audible sounds
- Abnormal positioning
- Retractions or use of accessory muscles
- Nasal flaring
- Apnea/gasping
- Absent, inadequate, or increased respiratory effort

Circulation to the Skin

- Pallor
- Mottling
- Dusky
- Cyanosis
- Bruising or petechiae

*If the patient is unresponsive, not breathing, or only gasping, initiate the BLS algorithm. Students can refer to Part 2 of the *PALS Provider Manual*.

Video will automatically pause on the patient.

Systematic Approach video 1: Blonde, 18-month-old child with pacifier

	Instructor discussion
	Systematic Approach video 1: Blonde, 18-month-old child with pacifier
1	Draw or tell students to reference and focus on the initial impression—PAT; then play video 1 clip
2	**When video pauses,** ask students the following questions (these questions are focused on the initial impression): *Answers are provided to help guide discussion if students have difficulty answering any questions* **1.** What is the patient's appearance? • Awake but decreased interaction **2.** What is the patient's work of breathing? • Increased work of breathing • Tachypnea • Retractions (suprasternal, intercostal, and subcostal) • Nasal flaring • Abdominal breathing **3.** What is this patient's color? • Pale **4.** Does this patient need immediate intervention? • Yes; this infant looks ill and, despite oxygen administration, has tachypnea and increased work of breathing ***Instructor note:*** This child appears to be very ill. It is important to perform a focused primary assessment and be prepared to interrupt the assessment to provide immediate intervention if signs of respiratory failure or shock are detected

Resume Video

Video will automatically pause on the patient.

Systematic Approach video 2: 3-year-old child in yellow shirt

	Instructor discussion
	Systematic Approach video 2: 3-year-old child in yellow shirt
1	Draw or tell students to reference and focus on the initial impression—PAT; then play video 2 clip

2	**When video pauses,** ask students the following questions (these questions are focused on the initial impression):
	Answers are provided to help guide discussion if students have difficulty answering any questions
	1. What is the patient's appearance?
	  • Increased interaction
	2. What is the patient's work of breathing?
	  • No abnormal/audible breath sounds
	  • Normal position
	  • No nasal flaring
	3. What is this patient's color?
	  • Pink mucous membranes
	4. Does this patient need immediate intervention?
	  • No

Resume Video

Video will automatically pause on the patient.

Systematic Approach video 3: Infant in car seat

	Instructor discussion
	Systematic Approach video 3: Infant in car seat
1	Draw or tell students to reference and focus on the initial impression—PAT; then play video 3 clip

2	**When video pauses,** ask students the following questions (these questions are focused on the initial impression):
	Answers are provided to help guide discussion if students have difficulty answering any questions
	1. What is the patient's appearance?
	  • Decreased interaction
	  • Altered level of consciousness
	2. What is the patient's work of breathing?
	  • Increased work of breathing
	  • Abdominal breathing
	  • Abnormal audible inspiratory sounds (stridor)
	3. What is this patient's color?
	  • Pale to gray
	4. Does this patient need immediate intervention?
	  • Yes; the stridor indicates upper airway obstruction, and the pale, gray color likely indicates hypoxemia. The infant should be positioned to open the airway, and oxygen should be administered while additional assessment is performed

Play Primary Assessment Video

- Play the video
- Video will automatically pause on the patient for the instructor to identify the components of the PAT and primary assessment as they relate to the patient
- Advise students to refer to the PAT and the Primary Assessment section in the *PALS Provider Manual* for the next 3 lessons

Primary Assessment

A	**Airway** *Assessment* • Is the airway maintainable? • Is the airway clear? • If no to any of these, below are the interventions* *Interventions* • Maintain airway patency by positioning, using OPA • Suction as indicated • Advanced airway (eg, supraglottic airway or endotracheal tube) • If inserting an advanced airway, verify correct placement with waveform capnography
B	**Breathing** *Assessment* • Adequate depth and rate of respirations • Equal, adequate bilateral chest rise • Absence of noisy breathing (eg, grunting, stridor, wheezing) • No use of accessory muscles, no nasal flaring • Normal/appropriate oxygen saturation by pulse oximetry* *Interventions* • Provide high-flow O_2 • Use bag-mask device with or without OPA • Consider need for advanced airway • Avoid excessive ventilation
C	**Circulation** *Assessment* • Peripheral and/or central pulse • Heart rate • Blood pressure* • Capillary refill—peripheral and/or central • Skin color and temperature • Level of consciousness *Interventions* • Obtain IV/IO access • Consider need for fluid resuscitation
D	**Disability** *Assessment* • Quickly assess for responsiveness, level of consciousness, and pupil response to light • AVPU: Alert, Voice, Painful, and Unresponsive • Check point-of-care glucose

(continued)

	Interventions • Consider need for spinal motion restrictions • Correct hypoglycemia • Consider naloxone for acute opioid toxicity
E	**Exposure** **Assessment** • Remove clothing to perform a physical examination (anterior and posterior), looking for obvious signs of trauma, bleeding, burns, unusual markings, rashes, or medical alert bracelets • Temperature **Interventions** • Maintain normothermia • Control bleeding • Decontamination

*If at any part of this sequence you find that a patient has a **life-threatening condition**, correction of that condition takes precedence over completing the elements of the primary assessment. After life-threatening problems have been addressed and the primary assessment is completed, proceed to the secondary assessment.

Video will automatically pause on the patient.

Primary Assessment video 1: Patient with dragon nebulizer

	Instructor discussion
	Primary Assessment video 1: Patient with dragon nebulizer
1	Draw or tell students to reference and focus on the initial impression—PAT and the Primary Assessment section in the *PALS Provider Manual*; then play video 1 clip

2	**When video pauses,** ask students the following questions (these questions are focused on the initial impression—PAT):
	Answers are provided to help guide discussion if students have difficulty answering any questions
	1. What is the patient's appearance?
	  • Decreased interaction
	2. What is the patient's work of breathing?
	  • Increased work of breathing
	  • Tachypnea
	  • Retractions
	  • Audible wheezes
	  • Prolonged expiratory phase
	3. What is this patient's color?
	  • Lips pale; slightly dusky
	  • No mottling or pallor
	4. Does this patient need immediate intervention?
	  • Yes; this child has significant respiratory distress and wheezing. He needs immediate intervention with albuterol and then reassessment to evaluate response to the albuterol to determine if further intervention is urgently needed

(continued)

(continued)

3	**Discuss Airway and Breathing of primary assessment** *Instructor note:* **Only Airway and Breathing are assessed in this video. Circulation, Disability, and Exposure will appear later in the video and on subsequent parts of the Lesson Plan**
4	Tell students to focus on Airway (A) and Breathing (B) of the primary assessment; then **resume video 1 clip**

5	**When video pauses,** ask students to focus on Airway and Breathing
	Ask students:
	1. **A:** Is the airway maintainable?
	   • Yes, the airway is maintainable
	2. **B:** Is the breathing adequate?
	   • No, increased work of breathing, which includes
	     – Tachypnea (respiration: 68/min)
	     – Retractions
	     – Prolonged expiratory phase
	     – Audible inspiratory and expiratory wheezes; wheezes and diminished breath sounds heard with auscultation
	     – SpO$_2$: 90% to 92%
	
	Instructor note: Slight variations in the sequence of the primary assessment may be reasonable based on the patient condition and the clinical setting. Immediate life threats should be rapidly identified and treated before continuing with the primary assessment. Baseline vital signs, including blood pressure and oxygen saturation by pulse oximetry, are important to identify and treat **life-threatening conditions**. However, providers should not delay simple and quick lifesaving treatments, such as a jaw thrust or applying pressure to a site of hemorrhage, to perform technical assessments such as measuring blood pressure or applying a monitor

Resume Video

Video will automatically pause on the patient.

Primary Assessment video 2: Infant in blanket with ECG leads

	Instructor discussion
	Primary Assessment video 2: Infant in blanket with ECG leads
1	Draw or tell students to reference and focus on the initial impression—PAT and the Primary Assessment section in the *PALS Provider Manual*; then play video 2 clip
2	**When video pauses,** ask students the following questions (these questions are focused on the initial impression—PAT): *Answers are provided to help guide discussion if students have difficulty answering any questions*

(continued)

1. What is the patient's appearance?
   - Occasionally fussy/irritable
   - Sleeping
2. What is the patient's work of breathing?
   - Irregular respirations; shallow breaths with occasional deep breaths (gasps)
   - Intercostal, subcostal, and suprasternal retractions
3. What is this patient's color?
   - Cyanotic
4. Does this patient need immediate intervention?
   - Yes

Instructor note: If students do not recognize the need for immediate intervention, be sure to reinforce the information below. This infant has a **life-threatening condition** and should be taken from the mother's arms. The infant requires immediate bag-mask ventilation with 100% oxygen. Then follow Systematic Approach and BLS algorithms as indicated

3 | Tell students to focus on the primary assessment; then **resume video 2 clip**

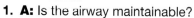

4 | **When video pauses,** ask students to focus on the parts of the primary assessment (Airway [A], Breathing [B], Circulation [C], Disability [D], and Exposure [E]) that will help identify and treat problems with airway, ventilation, and perfusion

Ask students:

1. **A:** Is the airway maintainable?
   - No, an intervention is needed
   - Infant is unable to support his head
2. **B:** Is the breathing adequate?
   - No, infant requires bag-mask ventilation with oxygen
   - Breath sounds clear
   - SpO_2: 69% to 71%
3. **C:** Is the infant perfusing adequately?
   - No
   - Poor skin turgor with tenting
   - Central pulses weak; peripheral pulses absent
   - Heart rate: 70/min, falling to 64/min, and then falling
   - Blood pressure: 80/48 mm Hg
   - Capillary refill: 4 seconds

This infant has a **life-threatening condition** that requires immediate intervention. What is the condition? [Hypoxemia with compensated shock] What are the potential causes? [Dehydration, possible infection]

We need to focus the remainder of the primary assessment on factors that will help us identify and treat the cause of the hypoxemia with compensated shock.

4. **D:** What's the infant's level of consciousness?
   - Sleepy; occasionally irritable
5. **E:** What is the infant's temperature?
6. **E:** Is the infant hypothermic or hyperthermic?
   - Afebrile (98.9°F/37.2°C)
7. **E:** Are there any obvious signs of trauma?
   - No obvious signs of trauma

5 | Ask students:
1. What is your assessment?
   - Cardiopulmonary failure (inadequate ventilation and oxygenation with bradycardia; infant is also dehydrated)

(continued)

(continued)

2. What immediate interventions are needed?
   - Maintain an airway
   - Begin immediate bag-mask ventilation with oxygen
   - Establish IV/IO access and administer an isotonic crystalloid bolus of 20 mL/kg over 5 to 20 minutes. Reassess perfusion during and after fluid bolus, and stop fluid bolus if signs of heart failure develop (including worsening respiratory distress or development of rales or hepatomegaly)

Resume Video

Video will automatically pause on the patient.

Primary Assessment video 3: Infant with 12-lead stickers

	Instructor discussion
	Primary Assessment video 3: Infant with 12-lead stickers
1	Draw or tell students to reference and focus on the initial impression—PAT and the Primary Assessment section in the *PALS Provider Manual*; then play video 3 clip
2	**When video pauses,** ask students the following questions (these questions are focused on the initial impression—PAT): *Answers are provided to help guide discussion if students have difficulty answering any questions* 1. What is the patient's appearance? • Awake with spontaneous movements; sucking pacifier 2. What is the patient's work of breathing? • Tachypnea • Mild retractions 3. What is this patient's color? • Pink, with no mottling 4. Does this patient need immediate intervention? • No
3	Tell students to focus on the primary assessment; then **resume video 3 clip**
4	**When video pauses,** ask students to focus on the primary assessment (Airway [A], Breathing [B], Circulation [C], Disability [D], and Exposure [E]) Ask students: 1. **A:** Is the airway maintainable? • Yes, no need for intervention 2. **B:** Is the breathing adequate? • Increased work of breathing • Tachypnea (respiration: 70/min) • Breath sounds clear 3. **C:** Is the infant perfusing adequately? • Yes • Central and peripheral pulses strong • Heart rate: 219 to 229/min • Blood pressure: 90/54 mm Hg • Capillary refill: 2 seconds 4. **D:** What's the infant's level of consciousness? • Awake and moving hands spontaneously

(continued)

(continued)

5. **E:** What is the infant's temperature?
   - Normal: 98.6°F/37°C
6. **E:** Are there any obvious signs of trauma?
   - No trauma

5	Ask students:
	1. What is your assessment?
	   • Respiratory distress, tachycardia with adequate perfusion (stable)
	2. What interventions do you anticipate?
	   • Administer oxygen, vagal maneuvers, adenosine, or cardioversion, depending on the patient's clinical status. If patient remains stable, expert consultation is strongly recommended before synchronized cardioversion is performed

Instructor Notes

_____

_____

_____

_____

Next

Secondary Assessment

Lesson 7B
Secondary Assessment

15 minutes

Learning Objective
- Differentiate between patients who do and do not require immediate intervention

Instructor Tips
- Make sure not to interrupt the video. If you have any comments to add, write them down and discuss them at the end of the video
- For SAMPLE activity below, reference scenarios provided on Instructor CD to give to students, or use optional sample lead-in provided below to facilitate activity

Ask Students to Open the *PALS Provider Manual* to Part 3

Play PALS Secondary Assessment Video
- Play the video

Discussion
- Review the table below
- Consider reviewing each section of SAMPLE with examples to gauge student comprehension

Secondary Assessment

Signs and symptoms	Signs and symptoms at onset of illness, such as • Breathing difficulty (eg, cough, rapid breathing, increased respiratory effort, breathlessness, abnormal breathing pattern, chest pain on deep inhalation) • Wheezing • Tachypnea • Tachycardia • Diaphoresis • Decreased level of consciousness • Agitation, anxiety • Fever • Headache • Decreased oral intake • Diarrhea, vomiting • Abdominal pain • Bleeding • Fatigue • Time course of symptoms

(continued)

(continued)

Allergies	• Medications, foods, latex, etc • Associated reactions
Medications	• Patient medications, including over-the-counter medications, vitamins, inhalers, and herbal supplements • Last dose and time of recent medications • Medications that can be found in the child's environment
Past medical history	• Health history (eg, premature birth, previous illnesses, hospitalizations) • Significant underlying medical problems (eg, asthma, chronic lung disease, congenital heart disease, arrhythmia, congenital airway abnormality, seizures, head injury, brain tumor, diabetes, hydrocephalus, neuromuscular disease) • Past surgeries • Immunization status
Last meal	• Time and nature of last intake of liquid or food (including breast or bottle feeding in infants) • Elapsed time between last meal and presentation of current illness can affect treatment and management of the condition (eg, possible anesthesia, possible intubation)
Events	• Events leading to current illness or injury (eg, onset sudden or gradual, type of injury) • Hazards at scene • Treatment during interval from onset of disease or injury until evaluation • Estimated time of onset (if out-of-hospital onset)

Students Practice (Optional Activity if Time Permits)

Practice a systematic method to determine relevant patient information as related to presenting symptoms

• Group students into pairs

• Explain that this is a 5- to 10-minute exercise to practice the SAMPLE mnemonic

• Instruct students to use the SAMPLE tool in the *PALS Provider Manual* (see table above)

• Using the patient introductions provided, assign one student as the patient/caregiver and the other as the provider

• After the introduction by the provider, have the patient/caregiver provide the required elements of each part of SAMPLE when asked by the provider

• Instruct the patient/caregiver to create a believable presenting patient story

Optional sample lead-in: Parent brings in an 18-month-old child who has difficulty breathing. Patient is tachypneic with audible wheezes and copious amounts of nasal drainage. For additional scenarios, please refer to the Instructor CD and/or the Instructor Network

Discussion

After this activity, bring closure to the group activity by asking open-ended questions, such as

- Were you able to get a complete picture of your patient?
- Did you ask all the appropriate questions?
  - If not, what did you miss?
- Were you able to ask follow-up questions?

Instructor Notes

Next
Team Dynamics

Lesson 8
Team Dynamics

15 minutes

Instructor Tips

• Clearly communicate the objective of this Lesson Plan to help students gain a better understanding of the lesson

• This Team Dynamics lesson is a great way to further engage your students

  – Change the inflection in your voice and also change your pace to help change the energy level in the room

Ask Students to Open the *PALS Provider Manual* to Part 5

Play Team Dynamics Video

• Play the video

• Video will automatically pause after "Poor Team Dynamics"

Discussion

• **When video pauses**, ask students the following questions:

  – What poor team dynamics were observed?

  – What behaviors were observed?

Resume Video

• Refer to table below to help identify effective team behaviors

• Elements of effective team dynamics

  – Roles

    ▪ Clear roles and responsibilities

    ▪ Knowing your limitations

    ▪ Constructive intervention

  – What to communicate

    ▪ Knowledge sharing

    ▪ Summarizing and reevaluation

- How to communicate
  - Closed-loop communication
  - Clear messages
  - Mutual respect
- Remind students that they will be functioning as Team Leaders and other roles in the learning and testing stations, and they will need to apply these concepts

Element	Effective Team Dynamics: Team Leader	Effective Team Dynamics: Team Members
1. Clear roles and responsibilities	• Clearly define all roles of team members in the clinical setting • Assign roles and responsibilities according to competence and the scope of practice of each team member • Distribute assignments evenly so that resources (skills) of team members are used as efficiently and effectively as possible	• Seek out and perform tasks that are clearly defined and appropriate to level of competence • Inform the Team Leader if the role or requested task is too difficult based on experience or competence • Be prepared to assist with tasks as needed
2. Knowing your limitations	• Call for assistance early rather than waiting until the patient deteriorates and it is too late to get the help needed • Ask other team members to help if one team member is having difficulty completing tasks • Seek advice from more experienced personnel when the patient's condition worsens despite initial treatment	
3. Constructive intervention	• Intervene if a team member is preparing to perform an incorrect action • Take corrective action to ensure that team members are performing the correct tasks in the appropriate sequence • Reassign a team member if that team member is not able to perform assigned tasks	• Ask the Team Leader or a team member to verify an action if you think a team member is about to make a mistake • Suggest an alternative drug, drug dose, or therapy if you observe an error in the drug, drug dose, or therapy ordered or prepared for administration
4. Knowledge sharing	• Encourage an environment of information sharing, and ask for suggestions if uncertain of the next best interventions • Ask for opinions and suggestions from team members about reversible causes of arrest and factors that may be limiting the effectiveness of the resuscitation attempt • Ask if anything has been overlooked (eg, IV access should have been obtained or drugs should have been administered) • Consider all clinical signs that are relevant to treatment	• Share information with other team members • Try to identify factors that may be limiting the effectiveness of the resuscitation attempt

(continued)

(continued)

5. **Summarizing and reevaluation**	• Ask for suggestions from team members about differential diagnoses and factors that may be contributing to unsuccessful resuscitative efforts • Frequently review the drugs and treatments administered and the patient's response with the team • Change the treatment strategy when new information or patient response (or failure to respond) suggests the need for such a change • Inform arriving personnel of the patient's current status and plans for further action	• Clearly draw attention to significant changes in the patient's clinical condition and increase monitoring frequency (eg, blood pressure measurements) when the patient's condition deteriorates
6. **Closed-loop communication**	• Listen for verbal confirmation that requests are heard and understood • Await confirmation that the previous task has been completed (eg, "Vascular access in place") before assigning another task • Confirm receipt of a completed assignment (eg, "Good, now that the IV is in, give 1 mg of epinephrine")	• Confirm that the request is heard and understood (eg, "I'll start the IV") • Inform the Team Leader when a task begins or ends (eg, "The IV is in") • Verify orders for drugs or other treatments before administration (eg, "Did you want the 5 mg/kg of IV amiodarone given now?")
7. **Clear messages**	• Provide clear messages and orders to specific team members • Encourage team members to speak clearly and distinctly • Request clarification of any ambiguous messages • Speak in a calm and normal tone of voice • Outline next steps so the team can understand/anticipate what you will need next	• Repeat the medication order • Clarify an order if it is ambiguous or not understood
8. **Mutual respect**	• Speak in a respectful, controlled tone of voice • Provide feedback to team members • Intervene if team members begin to raise their voices or speak disrespectfully • Remember, all team members are trying to perform well despite the stress present during the attempted resuscitation	• Speak in friendly, controlled tone of voice • Remember, the Team Leader and all team members are trying to perform well despite the stress present during the attempted resuscitation

Roles and Responsibilities of Team Dynamics

Positions for 6-Person High-Performance Teams*

Resuscitation Triangle Roles

 Compressor

- Assesses the patient
- Does 5 cycles of chest compressions
- Alternates with AED/Monitor/ Defibrillator every 5 cycles or 2 minutes (or earlier if signs of fatigue set in)

AED/Monitor/ Defibrillator

- Brings and operates the AED/monitor/defibrillator
- Alternates with Compressor every 5 cycles or 2 minutes (or earlier if signs of fatigue set in), ideally during rhythm analysis
- If a monitor is present, places it in a position where it can be seen by the Team Leader (and most of the team)

Airway

- Opens the airway
- Provides bag-mask ventilation
- Inserts airway adjuncts as appropriate

The team owns the code. No team member leaves the triangle except to protect his or her safety.

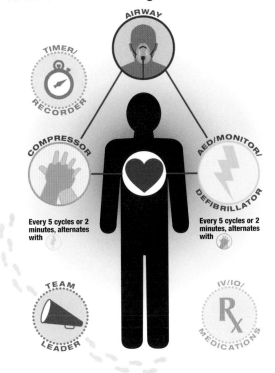

Every 5 cycles or 2 minutes, alternates with

Every 5 cycles or 2 minutes, alternates with

*This is a suggested team formation. Roles may be adapted to local protocol.

Leadership Roles

Team Leader

- **Every resuscitation team must have a defined leader**
- Assigns roles to team members
- Makes treatment decisions
- Provides feedback to the rest of the team as needed
- Assumes responsibility for roles not assigned

IV/IO/Medications

- An ACLS provider role
- Initiates IV/IO access
- Administers medications

Timer/Recorder

- Records the time of interventions and medications (and announces when these are next due)
- Records the frequency and duration of interruptions in compressions
- Communicates these to the Team Leader (and the rest of the team)

Discussion

- When video ends, ask students the following questions:
  - What good team dynamics were observed?
  - What behaviors were observed?

Instructor Notes

Next

Management of Respiratory Emergencies

Lesson 9A
Management of Respiratory Emergencies

15 minutes

- Differentiate between respiratory distress and failure

Instructor Tips

- These video-based lessons are designed to allow you to challenge students, whether they are novice or experienced providers. Adjust the difficulty of your questions based on the knowledge level of the students in the course

- Before playing this video, have your questions ready for upper airway obstruction, lower airway obstruction, lung tissue disease, and disordered control of breathing

Ask Students to Open the *PALS Provider Manual* to Part 7

Play Management of Respiratory Emergencies Video

- Play the video
- Review the signs, symptoms, and treatments of the 4 types of respiratory emergencies: upper airway obstruction, lower airway obstruction, lung tissue disease, and disordered control of breathing

Instructor Notes

_____

_____

_____

_____

Next
Respiratory Video Case Discussions

Lesson 9B
Respiratory Video Case Discussions

25 minutes

Learning Objective

• Perform early interventions for respiratory distress and failure

Instructor Tips

• During all video discussions, use the video titles to help you understand each case

  – Make sure to facilitate full discussion, which includes the PAT and primary assessment, before disclosing the final diagnosis of the case

• Encourage students to work together to answer questions and allow for self-discovery

• When discussing the video, be sure to allow students to lead this discussion by asking what they observed during the video segment

• Students are often hesitant to answer questions at first. Before this lesson, write down questions to help prompt discussion. These video-based lessons are designed to allow you to challenge students, whether they are novice or experienced providers. Adjust the difficulty of your questions based on the knowledge level of the students in the course

Play PALS Respiratory Video Case Discussion

Video will automatically pause on the patient.

Respiratory video case discussion 1: 3-year-old child with nasal cannula, in diaper, lying on mother's chest (child with special healthcare needs)—*lung tissue disease*

	Instructor discussion
	Respiratory video case discussion 1: 3-year-old child with nasal cannula, in diaper, lying on mother's chest (child with special healthcare needs)—*lung tissue disease*
1	Draw or tell students to reference and focus on the initial impression—PAT and the Primary Assessment section in the *PALS Provider Manual*; then play video 1 clip
2	**When video pauses,** ask students the following questions (these questions are focused on the initial impression—PAT): *Answers are provided to help guide discussion if students have difficulty answering any questions* 1. What is the patient's appearance? • Lethargic • Sleeping; no reaction to noises 2. What is the patient's work of breathing? • Increased work of breathing • Tachypnea • Retractions • Nasal flaring 3. What is this patient's color? • Pink mucous membranes • No mottling; skin color consistent

(continued)

(continued)

	4. Does this patient need immediate intervention? • No
3	Tell students to focus on the primary assessment; then **resume video 1 clip**
4	**When video pauses,** ask students to focus on the primary assessment (Airway [A], Breathing [B], Circulation [C], Disability [D], and Exposure [E]) Ask students: **1. A:** Is the airway maintainable? • Yes **2. B:** What is the patient's work of breathing? • Increased work of breathing • Decreased breath sounds • Tachypnea (respiratory rate: 38/min) • Retractions • Head bobbing • Nasal flaring • Breath sounds: expiratory wheezes; fine crackles in lung bases • SpO$_2$: 94% to 95% (note that oxygen administration is occurring) **3. C:** Is the child perfusing adequately? • Yes • Pink mucous membranes • Strong central and peripheral pulses • Heart rate: 136 to 138/min • Blood pressure: 92/62 mm Hg • Brisk capillary refill: under 2 seconds **4. D:** What's the child's level of consciousness? • Lethargic • Decreased tone • Check pupils for symmetry and reactivity **5. D:** *Instructor note:* If you had a patient who looked like this, what would you check? • Glucose: 105 mg/dL **6. E:** What is the child's temperature? • Temperature: 102.6°F/39°C **7. E:** Are there any obvious signs of trauma? • No obvious signs of trauma
5	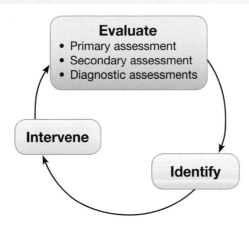

(continued)

(continued)

6	Ask students:
	1. What is your assessment?
	• Respiratory distress caused by lung tissue disease (Identify section of Systematic Approach Algorithm)
	• **Instructor note:** Have students refer to the Pediatric Management of Respiratory Emergencies Flowchart
	2. What interventions do you anticipate?
	• Administer oxygen and IV antibiotics; observe for worsening respiratory distress or hypoxemia (Intervene section of Systematic Approach Algorithm)
	Instructor Note: Optional Scenario for Advanced-Level Providers
	This scenario can be changed by reducing the patient's O_2 saturation to 79%. Patient is now in respiratory failure and requires airway support, including bag-mask ventilation and consideration of an airway adjunct (*Note:* an OPA is used only if child has no cough or gag reflex). Discuss indications for advanced airway insertion (ie, if respiratory failure develops), but emphasize the need to consult a provider experienced in pediatric intubation and mechanical ventilation *before* the child requires intubation

Resume Video

Video will automatically pause on the patient.

Respiratory video case discussion 2: 2-year-old shirtless boy in green shoes—*lower airway obstruction*

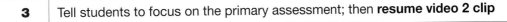

	Instructor discussion
	Respiratory video case discussion 2: 2-year-old shirtless boy in green shoes—*lower airway obstruction*
1	Draw or tell students to reference and focus on the initial impression—PAT and the Primary Assessment section in the *PALS Provider Manual*; then play video 2 clip
2	**When video pauses,** ask students the following questions (these questions are focused on the initial impression—PAT):
	Answers are provided to help guide discussion if students have difficulty answering any questions
	1. What is the patient's appearance?
	• Alert
	• Interactive
	2. What is the patient's work of breathing?
	• Tachypnea
	• **Audible wheezes**
	• Retractions
	• **Prolonged expiratory phase**
	3. What is this patient's color?
	• Pink lips
	• No mottling or other visible evidence of poor perfusion
	4. Does this patient need immediate intervention?
	• No
3	Tell students to focus on the primary assessment; then **resume video 2 clip**

(continued)

(continued)

4 | **When video pauses,** ask students to focus on the primary assessment (Airway [A], Breathing [B], Circulation [C], Disability [D], and Exposure [E])
Ask students:
1. **A:** Is the airway maintainable?
   - Yes
2. **B:** Is breathing adequate?
   - Tachypnea (respiratory rate: 50/min)
   - Audible wheezes; wheezes and diminished breath sounds heard on auscultation
   - Retractions
   - Prolonged expiratory phase
   - SpO_2: 96% to 97%
3. **C:** Is the child perfusing adequately?
   - Yes
   - Strong central and peripheral pulses
   - Heart rate: 136 to 138/min (sinus tachycardia)
   - Blood pressure: 91/76 mm Hg
   - Capillary refill: 2 seconds
4. **D:** What's the child's level of consciousness?
   - Alert
   - Glucose deferred to minimize agitation
5. **E:** What is the child's temperature?
   - Normothermic (temperature: 98.7°F/37.1°C)
6. **E:** Are there any obvious signs of trauma or infection?
   - No obvious signs of trauma or infection (ie, no skin rash)

5 |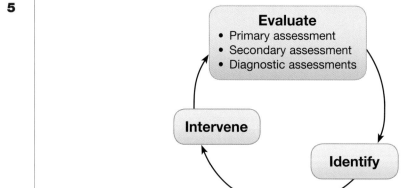

6 | Ask students:
1. What is your assessment?
   - Respiratory distress caused by lower airway obstruction (Identify section of Systematic Approach Algorithm)
   - ***Instructor note:*** Have students refer to the Pediatric Management of Respiratory Emergencies Flowchart
2. What interventions do you anticipate?
   - Administer albuterol nebulizer treatment; administer continuously if needed (Intervene section of Systematic Approach Algorithm)
   - Administer ipratropium bromide
   - Administer corticosteroids

Resume Video

Video will automatically pause on the patient.

Respiratory video case discussion 3: 3-year-old, dark-haired boy with gray shorts with mother—*upper airway obstruction*

	Instructor discussion
	Respiratory video case discussion 3: 3-year-old, dark-haired boy with gray shorts with mother—*upper airway obstruction*
1	Draw or tell students to reference and focus on the initial impression—PAT and the Primary Assessment section in the *PALS Provider Manual*; then play video 3 clip
2	**When video pauses,** ask students the following questions (these questions are focused on the initial impression—PAT): *Answers are provided to help guide discussion if students have difficulty answering any questions* **1.** What is the patient's appearance? • Alert; irritable but consolable **2.** What is the patient's work of breathing? • Audible inspiratory stridor • Severe subcostal retractions • Nasal flaring **3.** What is this patient's color? • Pink mucous membranes; no mottling **4.** Does this patient need immediate intervention? • No
3	Tell students to focus on the primary assessment; then **resume video 3 clip**
4	**When video pauses,** ask students to focus on the primary assessment (Airway [A], Breathing [B], Circulation [C], Disability [D], and Exposure [E]) Ask students: **1. A:** Is the airway maintainable? • Yes, but must be watched closely. Positioning may relieve or reduce obstruction **2. B:** Is breathing adequate? • Yes, with risk of deterioration • Respiratory rate: 23/min • Audible inspiratory stridor • Retractions • Nasal flaring • SpO_2: 95% to 96%

(continued)

(continued)

3. **C:** Is the child perfusing adequately?
   - Yes
   - Strong central and peripheral pulses
   - Heart rate: 107 to 109/min (sinus tachycardia)
   - Blood pressure: 94/50 mm Hg
   - Capillary refill: less than 2 seconds
4. **D:** What's the child's level of consciousness?
   - Alert
   - Irritable but consolable
   - Glucose deferred to minimize agitation
5. **E:** What is the child's temperature?
   - Normothermic (temperature: 98.9°F/37.2°C)
6. **E:** Are there any obvious signs of trauma?
   - No obvious signs of trauma

5

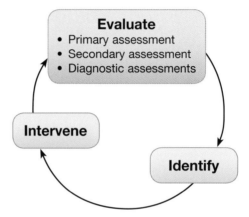

6 Ask students:
1. What is your assessment?
   - Respiratory distress caused by upper airway obstruction (Identify section of Systematic Approach Algorithm)
   - *Instructor note:* Have students refer to the Pediatric Management of Respiratory Emergencies Flowchart and a color-coded length-based tape for appropriate drug doses
2. What interventions do you anticipate?
   - Administer racemic epinephrine nebulizer treatment (Intervene section of Systematic Approach Algorithm)
   - Administer corticosteroid (dexamethasone)
   - Avoid painful interventions or any cause of agitation

Next

Learning Station: Airway Management

Lesson 9C
Learning Station: Airway Management

20 minutes

Instructor Tips

- Encourage students to use their Pocket Reference Cards or ECC Handbook early on during the cases, but to become less reliant on those resources as the cases progress.
- When debriefing students
  - Ask your audience open-ended questions that focus on their perspective to engage their minds and increase energy focus

Students Practice

- Have students position themselves in front of manikins
- Students will complete respiratory skills check and demonstrate the following skills as listed on the skills station competency checklist (use Airway Management Skills Station Competency Checklist):
  - Verbalizes difference between high-flow and low-flow O_2 delivery systems
  - Verbalizes maximum nasal cannula flow rate (4 L/min)
  - Opens airway by using head tilt–chin lift and jaw-thrust maneuvers
  - After ROSC from cardiac arrest, titrates FiO_2 to maintain oxygen saturation at 94% to 99%
  - Verbalizes different indications for an OPA
  - Selects correct size OPA
  - Inserts OPA correctly
  - Evaluates breathing after insertion of an OPA
  - Suctions with an OPA in place; states suctioning not to exceed 10 seconds
  - Selects correct mask size for ventilations
  - Attaches bag-mask device, creates seal by using the E-C clamp technique, opens airway, and ventilates effectively
  - Gives 2 breaths (approximately 1 second for each) causing chest rise with bag-mask device
- Provide feedback as needed
- Evaluate each student's performance of skills and indicate evaluation results on the PALS Course Progress Checklist

Next
Management of Shock Emergencies

Lesson 10A
Management of Shock Emergencies

15 minutes

Learning Objective

• Differentiate between compensated and decompensated (hypotensive) shock

Instructor Tips

• Make sure not to interrupt the video. If you have any comments to add, write them down and discuss them at the end of the video. Students do not learn well when they are trying to listen to 2 things at once

• **Before playing this video, have your questions ready for hypovolemic, distributive, obstructive, and cardiogenic shock**

Advise Students to Open the *PALS Provider Manual* to Part 9

Play Management of Shock Emergencies Video

• Play the video

• **Review the signs, symptoms, and treatments of the 4 types of shock emergencies: hypovolemic, distributive, obstructive, and cardiogenic shock**

Instructor Notes

_____

_____

_____

_____

Next
Shock Video Case Discussions

Lesson 10B
Shock Video Case Discussions

25 minutes

Instructor Tips

- During all video discussions, use the video titles to help you understand each case. Make sure to facilitate a full discussion that includes the PAT and primary assessment before disclosing the final diagnosis of the case
- This lesson provides a great way to further engage the students
  - Change the inflection in your voice and also change your pace to help change the energy level in the room
- Encourage students to work together and be prepared to answer questions
- Make sure that each student has successfully mastered all of the skills before moving forward

Play PALS Shock Video Case Discussion

Video will automatically pause on the patient.

Shock video case discussion 1: 12-month-old child with G-tube—*hypovolemic shock*

	Instructor discussion
	Shock video case discussion 1: 12-month-old child with G-tube—*hypovolemic shock*
1	Draw or tell students to reference and focus on the initial impression—PAT and the Primary Assessment section in the *PALS Provider Manual*; then play video 1 clip

2	**When video pauses,** ask students the following questions (these questions are focused on the initial impression—PAT):
	Answers are provided to help guide discussion if students have difficulty answering any questions
	1. What is the patient's appearance?
	  • Sleeping and lethargic
	2. What is the patient's work of breathing?
	  • Mild increased work of breathing
	  • Mild suprasternal and subcostal retractions
	  • Mildly tachypneic
	3. What is this patient's color?
	  • Pale, particularly lips
	  • No mottling or cyanosis
	4. Does this patient need immediate intervention?
	  • Yes; child has decreased level of consciousness and tachypnea with increased work of breathing and pallor. Immediate evaluation focusing on airway, ventilation, and perfusion is required

(continued)

(continued)

Instructor note: If students do not recognize the need for immediate intervention, be sure to reinforce the information below. This child has a **life-threatening condition** and requires immediate bag-mask ventilation with 100% oxygen. Then follow Systematic Approach and BLS algorithms as indicated

3	Tell students to focus on the primary assessment; then **resume video 1 clip**

4

When video pauses, ask students to focus on the parts of the primary assessment (Airway [A], Breathing [B], Circulation [C], Disability [D], and Exposure [E]) that will help identify and treat problems with airway, ventilation, and perfusion

Ask students:

1. **A:** Is the airway maintainable?
   - Yes, no audible airway sounds or sounds of airway secretions
2. **B:** Is breathing adequate?
   - Yes
   - Mild retractions and distress but good chest rise without much increased work of breathing
   - Respiratory rate: 30 to 32/min
   - SpO_2: 95%
3. **C:** Is the child perfusing adequately?
   - No
   - Pale
   - Strong central pulses; weak peripheral pulses
   - Heart rate: 170 to 172/min (sinus tachycardia)
   - Blood pressure: 82/55 mm Hg
   - Capillary refill (check to medial side of left foot): 9 seconds or more

This child has a **life-threatening condition** that requires immediate intervention. What is the condition? [Compensated shock] What are the potential causes? [Dehydration, sepsis, trauma]

We need to focus the remainder of the primary assessment on factors that will help us identify and treat the cause of the compensated shock.

4. **D:** What's the child's level of consciousness?
   - Lethargic (briefly opens eyes to voice and touch but quickly falls back asleep)
   - Pupils 3 mm equal and briskly reactive to light bilaterally
   - Withdraws all extremities appropriately
5. **E:** What is the child's temperature?
   - Normothermic (temperature: 102.4°F/39.1°C)
6. **E:** Are there any rashes or obvious signs of trauma?
   - No rashes
   - No obvious signs of trauma
   - Mucous membranes very dry

5

Ask students:

1. What is your assessment?
   - Compensated hypovolemic shock with respiratory distress (mild)
   - ***Instructor note:*** Have students refer to "Part 9: Management of Shock" in the *PALS Provider Manual*, a color-coded length-based tape, and appropriate drug doses
2. What interventions do you anticipate?
   - Establish IV/IO access; administer fluid bolus of 20 mL/kg of isotonic crystalloid (typically normal saline). Perform careful reassessment during and after the fluid bolus. Stop bolus fluid administration if signs of heart failure develop (worsening respiratory distress or development of rales or hepatomegaly). Repeat the fluid bolus as needed to treat signs of shock
   - Check point-of-care glucose concentration as soon as possible

Resume Video

Video will automatically pause on the patient.

Shock video case discussion 2: 17-year-old female adolescent in red shirt—*distributive shock*

		Instructor discussion
		Shock video case discussion 2: 17-year-old female adolescent in red shirt— *distributive shock*
	1	Draw or tell students to reference and focus on the initial impression—PAT and the Primary Assessment section in the *PALS Provider Manual*; then play video 2 clip
	2	**When video pauses,** ask students the following questions (these questions are focused on the initial impression—PAT): *Answers are provided to help guide discussion if students have difficulty answering any questions* 1. What is the patient's appearance? • Lethargic; opens eyes occasionally but falls immediately back to sleep 2. What is the patient's work of breathing? • Mild tachypnea 3. What is this patient's color? • Very pale 4. Does this patient need immediate intervention? • Yes (likely, but additional information is needed) • No (perhaps, but additional information is needed) ***Instructor note:*** This adolescent appears to be very ill. It is important to perform a focused primary assessment and be prepared to interrupt the assessment to provide immediate intervention if signs of respiratory failure or shock are detected
	3	Tell students to focus on the primary assessment; then **resume video 2 clip**
	4	**When video pauses,** ask students to focus on the primary assessment (Airway [A], Breathing [B], Circulation [C], Disability [D], and Exposure [E]) Ask students: 1. **A:** Is the airway maintainable? • Yes 2. **B:** Is breathing adequate? • Yes • Tachypnea (respiratory rate: 27/min) • Breath sounds clear • SpO_2: 95% to 96% while receiving oxygen by nasal cannula 3. **C:** Is the child perfusing adequately? • No • Very pale • Weak central and peripheral pulses • Heart rate: 153 to 156/min (sinus tachycardia) • Hypotensive (blood pressure: 81/46 mm Hg) • Significantly delayed capillary refill: 6 to 7 seconds We've now identified a **life-threatening condition** that requires immediate intervention. What is the condition? [Hypotensive shock] What are the potential causes? [Dehydration, sepsis] We need to focus the remainder of the primary assessment on factors that will help us identify and treat the cause of the hypotensive shock.

(continued)

(continued)

	4. **D:** What's the child's level of consciousness?
	   • Lethargic response to verbal and auditory stimuli
	   • Glucose: 145 mg/dL
	5. **E:** What is the child's temperature?
	   • Febrile (temperature: 103.8°F/39.9°C)
	6. **E:** Are there any obvious signs of trauma?
	   • No obvious signs of trauma

5	Ask students:
	1. What is your assessment?
	   • Hypotensive distributive shock probably caused by sepsis
	   • ***Instructor note:*** Have students refer to the Pediatric Recognition of Shock Emergencies Flowchart in the *PALS Provider Manual*
	2. What interventions do you anticipate?
	   • Establish IV/IO access (the child may already have access established); administer bolus of 20 mL/kg isotonic crystalloid (the adult bolus of 500 mL can be used instead). Perform careful and frequent reassessments during and after fluid bolus administration; stop fluid bolus if signs of heart failure develop (worsening respiratory distress or development of rales or hepatomegaly)
	   • Administer empiric IV antibiotic therapy within the first hour of the development of shock symptoms
	   • Obtain blood cultures
	   • Administer additional fluid boluses as needed to treat shock. Perform frequent cardiorespiratory and neurologic reassessments with each isotonic crystalloid bolus
	   • Begin vasoactive drug infusion within the first hour of therapy if patient remains in shock despite fluid administration
	   • Consider glucocorticoid therapy (for adrenal insufficiency) if patient remains hypotensive despite fluid resuscitation and vasoactive infusions

Resume Video

Video will automatically pause on the patient.

Shock video case discussion 3: 18-month-old blonde girl with yellow pacifier—*cardiogenic shock*

	Instructor discussion
	Shock video case discussion 3: 18-month-old blonde girl with yellow pacifier— *cardiogenic shock*
1	***Instructor note:*** Read the following lead-in to students before beginning this section: Patient received bolus of 20 mL/kg of normal saline, and her work of breathing increased
2	Draw or tell students to reference and focus on the initial impression—PAT and the Primary Assessment section in the *PALS Provider Manual*; then play video 3 clip

(continued)

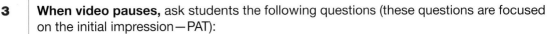

3 | **When video pauses,** ask students the following questions (these questions are focused on the initial impression—PAT):
Answers are provided to help guide discussion if students have difficulty answering any questions
1. What is the patient's appearance?
  • Lethargic
2. What is the patient's work of breathing?
  • Tachypneic
  • Retractions (suprasternal, intercostal, and subcostal)
3. What is this patient's color?
  • Flushed cheeks
  • Appears pink, but right thigh is mottled
4. Does this patient need immediate intervention?
  • Yes (likely, but additional information is needed)
  • No (possibly, but additional information is needed)
Instructor note: This child appears to be very ill. It is important to perform a focused primary assessment and be prepared to interrupt the assessment to provide immediate intervention if signs of respiratory failure or shock are detected

4 | Tell students to focus on the primary assessment; then **resume video 3 clip**

5 | **When video pauses,** ask students to focus on the primary assessment (Airway [A], Breathing [B], Circulation [C], Disability [D], and Exposure [E])
Ask students:
1. A: Is the airway maintainable?
  • Yes
2. B: Is breathing adequate?
  • Yes, with risk of deterioration
  • Tachypnea (respiratory rate: 76/min)
  • Retractions (suprasternal, intercostal, and subcostal)
  • Crackles bilaterally
  • Air movement is equal and adequate bilaterally
  • SpO$_2$: 96% to 98% while receiving oxygen by nasal cannula
3. C: Is the child perfusing adequately?
  • No
  • Pale
  • Mottled skin in lower extremities
  • Central pulses adequate; peripheral pulses weak
  • Heart rate: 153 to 156/min (sinus tachycardia)
  • Hypotensive (blood pressure: 67/37 mm Hg)
  • Capillary refill: 5 to 6 seconds
  • Hepatomegaly

We've now identified a **life-threatening condition** that requires immediate intervention. What is the condition? [Hypotensive shock and signs of heart failure, ie, hepatomegaly and pulmonary edema] What are the potential causes? [Myocardial failure]

We need to focus the remainder of the primary assessment on factors that will help us identify and treat the cause of the hypotensive cardiogenic shock

4. D: What's the child's level of consciousness?
  • Lethargic, but irritable when touched
5. E: What is the child's temperature?
  • Normothermic (temperature: 98.6°F/37°C)
6. E: Are there any obvious signs of trauma or infection?
  • No obvious signs of trauma; no rashes

(continued)

(continued)

6	Ask students:

1. What is your assessment?

- Hypotensive cardiogenic shock with increased respiratory distress after fluid bolus (Identify section of Systematic Approach Algorithm)
- ***Instructor note:*** Have students refer to "Cardiogenic Shock" in the *PALS Provider Manual,* a color-coded length-based tape, and appropriate drug doses. Encourage discussion on potential benefits and potential harm from bolus fluid administration and the need for inotrope or inodilator and possible vasoactive drugs in patients with cardiogenic shock with hepatomegaly and pulmonary edema

2. What interventions do you anticipate?

- Obtain consultation
- Hold additional IV fluid boluses. If additional boluses are needed later, smaller fluid boluses (ie, 5 to 10 mL/kg) should be administered over a longer period of time (eg, 10 to 20 minutes)
- Consider administration of diuretics

Instructor Note: **Optional Scenario for Advanced-Level Providers**

This scenario can be changed by decreasing the patient's oxygen saturation to 76% to illustrate unstable cardiogenic shock with worsening pulmonary edema. Encourage discussion on potential detrimental effects of positive pressure ventilation. Experienced providers may consider the use of continuous positive airway pressure/bilevel positive airway pressure if the child can be continuously and closely monitored and providers experienced in pediatric intubation are readily available

Instructor Notes

_____

_____

_____

_____

Next

Learning Station:
Vascular Access

Lesson 10C
Learning Station: Vascular Access

20 minutes

Learning Objective
- Perform early interventions for the treatment of shock

Instructor Tips
- Depending on each learner's experience and scope of practice, some students may be uncomfortable with IO insertion
  - Give these providers extra time to practice and encourage them to help them feel more comfortable and confident

Play IO Access Video
- Play the video

Students Practice
- Instructor should have 6 students in this station and perform the following tasks:
  - Have students practice IO insertion skills according to the skills station competency checklist
  - Ensure that each student can prepare equipment to administer an IV/IO bolus rapidly, including 3-way stopcock, syringes, and IV tubing
  - Ensure that each student can perform IO access correctly and confirm when needle has reached the marrow cavity
  - Provide corrective feedback during IO insertion, IV/IO fluid administration, and use of IV medications

Discussion
- Were there any specific elements that you found difficult?
- If you were asked to perform the same skills again, is there anything that you would do differently?
  - What?
  - Why?

Next

Management of
Arrhythmia Emergencies

Lesson 11A
Management of Arrhythmia Emergencies

15 minutes

Learning Objective

- Differentiate between unstable and stable patients with arrhythmias

Instructor Tips

- Ask students to use the *PALS Provider Manual* in this lesson to help further engage them and help with retention of information
- Make sure not to interrupt the video. If you have any comments to add, write them down and discuss them at the end of the video. Students do not learn well when they are trying to listen to 2 things at once
- **Before teaching this lesson, have your questions ready for sinus tachycardia, sinus bradycardia, supraventricular tachycardia, ventricular tachycardia, ventricular fibrillation, and asystole for discussion after the video**

Advise Students to Open the *PALS Provider Manual* to Part 11

Play Management of Arrhythmia Emergencies Video

- Play the video
- **Review the signs, symptoms, and treatments of arrhythmia emergencies**

Instructor Notes

_____

_____

_____

_____

Next

Arrhythmia Video Case Discussions

Lesson 11B
Arrhythmia Video Case Discussions

20 minutes

Learning Objective

- Describe clinical characteristics of instability in patients with arrhythmias

Instructor Tips

- During all video discussions, use the video titles to help you understand each case
  - Make sure to facilitate a full discussion that includes the PAT and primary assessment before disclosing the final diagnosis of the case
- After playing the video, be sure to provide a recap of what the video covered and what is next
- Encourage students to use their *PALS Provider Manual*, pocket reference cards, or ECC Handbook early on during the cases but to become less reliant on those resources as the cases progress
- When debriefing students
  - Ask open-ended questions to engage group discussion and allow for greater details
  - When answering a question, acknowledge the individual with eye contact, and then answer to the entire room, coming back to the questioner periodically

Play PALS Arrhythmia Case Discussions Video

Video will automatically pause on the patient.

Arrhythmia video case discussion 1: 13-year-old male adolescent with teddy bear—*OPA/bradycardia*

	Instructor discussion
	Arrhythmia video case discussion 1: 13-year-old male adolescent with teddy bear— *OPA/bradycardia*
1	Draw or tell students to reference and focus on the initial impression—PAT and the Primary Assessment section in the *PALS Provider Manual*; then play video 1 clip

2	**When video pauses,** ask students the following questions (these questions are focused on the initial impression—PAT): *Answers are provided to help guide discussion if students have difficulty answering any questions*
	 1. What is the patient's appearance?
	    • Unresponsive
	 2. What is the patient's work of breathing?
	    • Decreased
	    • Shallow
	 3. What is this patient's color?
	    • Pink, with heightened color in cheeks

(continued)

(continued)

4. Does this patient need immediate intervention?
- Yes (probably, but more information is needed)
- No (possibly, but more information is needed)

Instructor note: This child is unresponsive and appears to be very ill. It is important to perform a focused primary assessment and be prepared to interrupt the assessment to provide immediate intervention if signs of respiratory failure or shock are detected"

3	Tell students to focus on the primary assessment; then **resume video 1 clip**

4   **When video pauses,** ask students to focus on the primary assessment (Airway [A], Breathing [B], Circulation [C], Disability [D], and Exposure [E])
Ask students:

1. A: Is the airway maintainable?
- Yes, with an OPA in place

2. B: Is breathing adequate?
- No
- Hypoxemic (SpO$_2$: 80%)
- Respiratory rate: 6/min
- Respiratory failure
- Breath sounds clear

3. C: Is the child perfusing adequately?
- No
- Mottling on shoulders
- Central pulses weak; peripheral pulses absent
- Heart rate: 44 to 45/min (sinus bradycardia)
- Hypotensive (blood pressure: 63/33 mm Hg)
- Capillary refill: 6 seconds

We've now identified **life-threatening conditions** that require immediate intervention. What are the conditions? [Inadequate oxygenation and ventilation, bradycardia and hypotension, cardiopulmonary failure] What are the potential causes? [Hypoventilation and resultant hypoxia]

We need to focus the remainder of the primary assessment on factors that will help us identify and treat the cause of the cardiorespiratory failure

4. D: What's the child's level of consciousness?
- Unresponsive to painful stimuli
- Pupils 3 mm, sluggishly reactive
- Glucose: 190 mg/dL

5. E: What is the child's temperature?
- Temperature: 98.6°F/37.0°C

6. E: Are there any obvious signs of trauma?
- Possible signs of neck trauma

(continued)

(continued)

5	Ask students:
	1. What is your assessment?
	  • Cardiorespiratory failure, including inadequate oxygenation and ventilation (hypoventilation), and sinus bradycardia with poor perfusion
	  • *Instructor note:* Have students refer to the Pediatric Bradycardia With a Pulse and Poor Perfusion Algorithm in the *PALS Provider Manual* and appropriate drug doses
	2. What interventions do you anticipate?
	  • Provide immediate bag-mask ventilation with 100% oxygen; add chest compressions with ventilation if heart rate does not increase to 60/min or higher with adequate perfusion following effective bag-mask ventilation (Intervene section of Systematic Approach Algorithm)
	  • Follow Bradycardia Algorithm
	  • If bradycardia with poor perfusion persists despite these measures, epinephrine should be administered
	  • Administration of atropine should be considered if bradycardia is associated with increased vagal tone or primary atrioventricular block
	  • Consider external pacing if the patient's bradycardia persists
	  • H's and T's: Discuss the most likely etiology of this patient's bradycardia, which is hypoxia caused by hypoventilation
	
	***Instructor Note:* Optional Scenario for Advanced-Level Providers**
	
	This scenario can be changed by altering the patient's cardiac rhythm to third-degree AV block. Consider discussing external pacing and when to use atropine vs pacing

Resume Video

Video will automatically pause on the patient.

Arrhythmia video case discussion 2: 15-year-old male adolescent, post–heart surgery—
ventricular tachycardia

	Instructor discussion
	Arrhythmia video case discussion 2: 15-year-old male adolescent, post–heart surgery—*ventricular tachycardia*
1	Draw or tell students to reference and focus on the initial impression—PAT and the Primary Assessment section in the *PALS Provider Manual*. Then play video 2 clip

2	**When video pauses,** ask students the following questions (these questions are focused on the initial impression—PAT):
	Answers are provided to help guide discussion if students have difficulty answering any questions
	1. What is the patient's appearance?
	  • Unresponsive to touch
	2. What is the patient's work of breathing?
	  • Adequate respirations
	  • Good chest rise
	  • No increased work of breathing
	  • No retractions
	  • No nasal flaring

(continued)

(continued)

3. What is this patient's color?
   - Mild pallor to lips (otherwise color appears appropriate)
   - No mottling
   - No cyanosis
4. Does this patient need immediate intervention?
   - No

3	Tell students to focus on the primary assessment; then **resume video 2 clip**

4 — **When video pauses,** ask students to focus on the primary assessment (Airway [A], Breathing [B], Circulation [C], Disability [D], and Exposure [E])

Ask students:
1. **A:** Is the airway maintainable?
   - Yes
2. **B:** Is breathing adequate?
   - No
   - Breath sounds clear but decreased at bases bilaterally
   - Respiratory rate: 18/min
   - SpO_2: 92%
3. **C:** Is the child perfusing adequately?
   - Yes
   - Strong central pulses; peripheral pulses easily palpable
   - Heart rate: 156 to 163/min (ventricular tachycardia)
   - Blood pressure: 101/70 mm Hg
   - Capillary refill: 2 seconds
4. **D:** What's the child's level of consciousness?
   - Opens eyes to loud voice and touch, and then quickly falls back asleep
   - Pupils 3/3 and briskly reactive to light
   - Glucose: 110 mg/dL
5. **E:** What is the child's temperature?
   - Normothermic (98.2°F/36.8°C)
6. **E:** Are there any obvious signs of trauma?
   - Post–heart surgery with visible surgical incision

5 — Ask students:
1. What is your assessment?
   - Ventricular tachycardia (monomorphic) with a pulse and adequate perfusion (Identify section of Systematic Approach Algorithm)
   - ***Instructor note:*** Have students refer to the Pediatric Tachycardia With a Pulse and Adequate Perfusion Algorithm in the *PALS Provider Manual*, and appropriate drug doses
2. What interventions do you anticipate?
   - Administer oxygen
   - Obtain expert consultation. Because this child is stable, it's important to avoid making the child unstable with administration of antiarrhythmics that may cause complications. If this child becomes unstable (eg, significant hypotension, acutely altered mental status, or signs of shock such as diminished peripheral pulses and prolonged capillary refill), providers should prepare for synchronized cardioversion

Resume Video

Video will automatically pause on the patient.

Arrhythmia video case discussion 3: 3-year-old boy with yellow shirt who grins while having temperature taken—*supraventricular tachycardia*

	Instructor discussion
	Arrhythmia video case discussion 3: 3-year-old boy with yellow shirt who grins while having temperature taken. Mom noticed a rapid heart rate after he took his albuterol today—*supraventricular tachycardia*
1	Draw or tell students to reference and focus on the initial impression—PAT and the Primary Assessment section in the *PALS Provider Manual*. Then play video 3 clip
2	**When video pauses,** ask students the following questions (these questions are focused on the initial impression—PAT): *Answers are provided to help guide discussion if students have difficulty answering any questions* 1. What is the patient's appearance? • Alert and responsive 2. What is the patient's work of breathing? • Normal 3. What is this patient's color? • Lips, mucous membranes, and nail beds are pale pink 4. Is immediate intervention required? • No
3	Tell students to focus on the primary assessment; then **resume video 3 clip**
4	**When video pauses,** ask students to focus on the primary assessment (Airway [A], Breathing [B], Circulation [C], Disability [D], and Exposure [E]) Ask students: 1. **A:** Is the airway maintainable? • Yes 2. **B:** What is the patient's work of breathing? • No increased work of breathing • Breath sounds clear • SpO$_2$: 96% to 98% 3. **C:** Is the child perfusing adequately? • Yes • Normal central and peripheral pulses • Heart rate: 207 to 213/min (narrow-complex ventricular tachycardia) • Normotensive (blood pressure: 98/60 mm Hg) • Capillary refill: 2 seconds 4. **D:** What's the child's level of consciousness? • Alert • Pupils 3/3 equal and briskly reactive to light • Glucose: 110 mg/dL 5. **E:** What is the child's temperature? • Normothermic (temperature: 98.0°F/36.7°C) 6. **E:** Are there any obvious signs of trauma? 7. No obvious signs of trauma

(continued)

(continued)

5

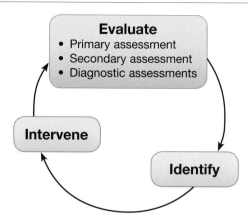

6 Ask students:

1. What is your assessment?
   - Supraventricular tachycardia with pulses and adequate perfusion
     - *Instructor note:* Have students refer to the Pediatric Tachycardia With a Pulse and Adequate Perfusion Algorithm in the *PALS Provider Manual*, a color-coded length-based tape, and appropriate drug dose and shock dose (joules) for synchronized cardioversion
   - Review H's and T's
2. What interventions do you anticipate?
   - Consider vagal maneuvers. Ask students to provide examples of vagal maneuvers (eg, child attempts to blow through a narrowed or obstructed straw)
   - Establish IV access. Administer adenosine using rapid bolus technique (ensure that students are able to describe this); you may give second dose (double the first dose) if the first dose is not effective. Ensure that a rapid bolus technique is used
   - If SVT persists despite adenosine administration, obtain expert consultation
   - Follow Pediatric Tachycardia With a Pulse and Adequate Perfusion Algorithm

Instructor Note: Optional Scenario for Advanced-Level Providers

This scenario can be changed by altering the patient's vital signs to indicate poor perfusion (and use of the Pediatric Tachycardia With a Pulse and Poor Perfusion Algorithm, with the need for synchronized cardioversion), or even change rhythm to pulseless ventricular tachycardia (Pediatric Cardiac Arrest Algorithm) and discuss defibrillation

Next
Learning Station: Rhythm Disturbances/Electrical Therapy

Lesson 11C
Learning Station:
Rhythm Disturbances/Electrical Therapy   25 minutes

Learning Objective

- Differentiate between unstable and stable patients with arrhythmias

Instructor Tips

- Familiarize students with all equipment before hands-on practice
- Depending on scope of practice, some students may appear to be uncomfortable performing the skills in this lesson
  - Give these providers extra time to practice and encourage them to help them feel more comfortable and confident

Discussion

- Use Rhythm Disturbances/Electrical Therapy Skills Station Competency Checklist
- Instructor should have 6 students in this station and should demonstrate how to
  - Apply ECG leads
  - Use the monitor and obtain a rhythm strip
  - Apply defibrillation/cardioversion electrode pads
  - Perform defibrillation and synchronized cardioversion
- Students will then practice the above skills
- Evaluate each student's ability to correctly perform these skills
- Verify that students can recognize selected rhythms and state the appropriate electrical therapy, if indicated, for each
- Record evaluation results on PALS Course Progress Checklist

Students Practice

This part of the lesson is designed to have the students demonstrate effective and safe use of the equipment (cardiac monitor and manual defibrillator) and to enable you to validate each student's skills

Gather students around the equipment and have each student demonstrate, one at a time.

Step	Ensure that each student is able to
1. Use of monitor	• Apply ECG leads properly • Turn on monitor and run a rhythm strip • Show how to properly operate the monitor

2. Rhythm recognition	• Recognize rhythms that require electrical therapy
	   – Ventricular tachycardia (defibrillation)
	   – Ventricular fibrillation (defibrillation)
	   – Supraventricular tachycardia, unstable (cardioversion)

(continued)

(continued)

3. Steps for defibrillation	• Select and position correct paddles/pads for infant or child • Set appropriate energy dose (2 to 4 J/kg) • Select appropriate mode: not synchronized • Charge • Clear • Press and hold shock buttons until energy is discharged
4. Steps for cardioversion	• Select and position correct paddles/pads for infant or child • Set appropriate energy dose (0.5 to 1 J/kg) • Select appropriate mode: synchronized • Charge • Clear • Press and hold shock buttons until energy is discharged

Indicate each student's evaluation on the PALS Course Progress Checklist

Discussion

- Were there any specific elements that you found difficult?
- Is there any piece of equipment that was either unfamiliar or different from what you are accustomed to?

Instructor Notes

_____

_____

_____

_____

Next

Management of Post–Cardiac Arrest Care

Lesson 12
Management of Post–Cardiac Arrest Care

15 minutes

Instructor Tips

- Ask students to use the *PALS Provider Manual* in this lesson to help further engage them and help with retention of information

- Make sure not to interrupt the video. If you have any comments to add, write them down and discuss them at the end of the video. Students do not learn well when they are trying to listen to 2 things at once

- **Before teaching this lesson, have your questions ready for airway, breathing, circulation, and temperature control**

Advise Students to Open the *PALS Provider Manual* to Part 12

Play Management of Post–Cardiac Arrest Care Video

- Play the video
- Briefly answer students' questions
- If there are no student questions, consider asking questions to highlight key concepts

Instructor Notes

_____

_____

_____

_____

_____

Next
Learning Station: Coping With Death (Optional)

Lesson 13
Learning Station:
Coping With Death (Optional)

20 minutes

Instructor Tips

- Remind students that if they have recently experienced the loss of a loved one, this video might be difficult to view

- **Participation in this lesson is not required to complete the PALS Course**

- Students may choose not to view this video at their discretion

Play Coping With Death Video (Optional)

- Address what students will learn from the video
- Play the video
- Answer students' questions

Discussion

- Discuss how the news of the patient's death could have been delivered more effectively
    - News was delivered in the hallway, with no privacy
    - Vague terms were used to describe the death
    - The words *dead* or *died* were never used
    - Physician left family for "another emergency"
    - Physician left family with no support and no one to answer their questions
- Ask if there are any questions

Instructor Notes

_____

_____

_____

_____

Next

Case Scenario Practice
With Simulations

Lesson 14
Case Scenario Practice
With Simulations

80 minutes (per group)

Instructor Tips

- Refer to the course agenda for additional information on which case scenarios to use for each day
- Scenarios have been grouped together from least to most complex
- Refer to the *PALS Instructor Manual* for all case scenarios
- This is the last opportunity to facilitate learning before the case scenario testing. Use this time to address critical areas where students may still be weak

Students Practice

- Students are required to do 2 practice scenarios as Team Leader, ensuring that all 4 scenarios in each group are covered
- Students should practice and demonstrate the following skills *as listed on the skills station competency checklist*

Learning Stations: Simulation/Debriefing

Note: **Use a stopwatch or timing device for each case simulation and debriefing.**

Simulation (10 minutes)	• **Set the stopwatch or timer for 10 minutes** • **Remove chairs from area—no one should be seated** • Ensure that each person has a designated role; rotate roles in subsequent patient simulations • Introduce case by reading the case scenario lead-in on the instructor case scenario designated for a particular simulation • Direct the Team Leader to begin managing the case in conjunction with the team • Provide information that is not obtainable from the manikin • Assess the performance of the Team Leader/team by using the actions listed on the instructor case scenario as a guide • Let the simulation continue without interruption for full 10 minutes • Stop the simulation after 10 minutes
Debriefing (10 minutes)	• Set the stopwatch or timer for 10 minutes • Ask the Timer/Recorder to review actions that occurred during the simulation • Debrief the team by using the debriefing tool on the back of the instructor case scenario • Have observers give feedback by using the skills station competency checklists

- Summarize key concepts of the case
- Use the PALS Course Progress Checklist as a guide to monitor students' performance

Structured and Supported Debriefing Process

Phase	Goal	Actions
Gather	Listen to students to understand what they think and how they feel about the simulation	• Request narrative from the Team Leader • Request clarifying or supplemental information from team
Analyze	Facilitate students' reflection on and analysis of their actions	• Review an accurate record of events • Report observations (both correct and incorrect steps) • Assist students in thoroughly reflecting on/examining performance during the simulation, as well as on their perceptions during the debriefing • Direct and/or redirect students during the debriefing to ensure continuous focus on session objectives
Summarize	Facilitate identification and review of lessons learned	• Summarize comments or statements from students • Have students identify positive aspects of team or individual behaviors • Have students identify areas of team or individual behaviors that require change or correction

Sample Course Rotation Schedule for 6 Students

20 minutes per case Team Role	First Case	Next Case
Team Leader	Student 1	Student 2
Airway	Student 2	Student 3
IV/IO/Medications	Student 3	Student 4
Monitor/Defibrillator	Student 4	Student 5
Compressor	Student 5	Student 6
Timer/Recorder	Student 6	Student 1

If <6 students, combine roles; if >6 students, include additional observer roles.

• Please see the course agenda for suggested scenarios; scenarios are grouped from least complex to most complex

• The order of the case scenarios is flexible; arrange case scenarios to best support your instructors

Instructor Notes

Next

Case Scenario Testing

Lesson 15
Case Scenario Testing

120 minutes

Instructor Tips

• In this station, the focus changes to assessment instead of facilitating learning. Students must perform the test from beginning to end. Do not interrupt students while they are completing the test. Address any deficiencies during remediation

• For evaluation purposes, students must complete the scenario without team member prompting

• **Conduct testing station cases in real time**

• Have students rotate through the testing stations

Test

With 6 students in the PALS case scenario test 1 and 6 students in the PALS case scenario test 2, perform the following tasks (instructor-to-student ratio is 1:6 for PALS case scenario tests 1 and 2):

• Instruct each student to select a case immediately before beginning his or her case scenario test

• Evaluate the competency of each student, one at a time, each functioning as Team Leader for his or her selected case

• Document the Team Leader's performance on the PALS case scenario testing checklist

• Do not coach or give hints during the test

• Make sure other students participate as team members

• Briefly provide feedback on the Team Leader's performance

• Indicate evaluation results on the PALS Course Progress Checklist

Case Scenario Test 1

Take no longer than 8 minutes to test and 2 minutes to give students feedback on their performance

• Test each student, one at a time, functioning as Team Leader; the student being tested may use a quick reference aid (eg, ECC Handbook, pocket reference card)

• Randomly assign test scenarios one at a time immediately before each test

Test 1: Case Scenario Selection

• There are 4 case scenarios for PALS case scenario test 1:

  – Supraventricular Tachycardia

  – Bradycardia

  – Asystole/Pulseless Electrical Activity

  – Ventricular Fibrillation/Pulseless Ventricular Tachycardia

- Write each of these case scenarios on a separate piece of paper or a card
- Immediately before each case scenario test, instruct the student being tested to randomly select a case scenario from the papers/cards
- Subsequent students select their test case scenarios from the remaining papers/cards
- Read the lead-in that matches the student's work environment (eg, nurse, EMT-P); provide information about the case in response to students' questions
- Do not help, coach, guide, lead, or give feedback to a student during the test; do not answer questions or give hints about what the student should do or not do during the test
- You may, however, ask a leading question to prompt a student to verbalize or state a required critical performance step when indicated on the case scenario testing checklist
- Give information during the test as requested (eg, vital signs, responses to therapy)
- The Timer/Recorder documents what happens during the case by writing on a flip chart or whiteboard
- Fill out the case scenario testing checklist for the appropriate case as you observe the student's performance
- For a student to pass the test, **all** critical action steps must be performed satisfactorily
- *Conduct a feedback debriefing session for a student who was tested in private at the end of the PALS case scenario test*
- Indicate evaluation results on the PALS Course Progress Checklist
- While the student is being debriefed, other students will reset the station
- Refer students who need remediation to the remediation lesson

Case Scenario Test 2

With 6 students in PALS case scenario test 2 and 6 students in PALS case scenario test 1, perform the following tasks:

- Instruct each student to select a case immediately before beginning his or her case scenario test
- Evaluate the competency of each student, one at a time, each functioning as Team Leader for his or her selected case
- Document the Team Leader's performance on the PALS case scenario testing checklist
- Do not coach or give hints during the test
- Make sure other students participate as team members
- Briefly provide feedback on the Team Leader's performance
- Indicate evaluation results on PALS Course Progress Checklist

Test 2: Case Scenario Selection

- There are 8 case scenarios for PALS case scenario test 2:
  - Upper Airway Obstruction
  - Lower Airway Obstruction
  - Lung Tissue Disease
  - Disordered Control of Breathing
  - Hypovolemic Shock
  - Obstructive Shock
  - Distributive Shock
  - Cardiogenic Shock
- Write each of these case scenarios on a separate piece of paper or a card
- Immediately before each case scenario test, instruct the student being tested to randomly select a case scenario from the papers/cards
- Subsequent students select their test case scenarios from the remaining papers/cards

Instructor Notes

_____

_____

_____

_____

Next
Exam

Lesson 16
Exam

60 minutes

Exam

All students must take the open-resource exam

- Distribute the open-resource exam
- Proctor the exam
- Collect and score each exam
  - Students must score 84% or better to pass the exam
- Review the answers by using the answer key with the students

Exam Details

- The exam is an open-resource exam

  Resources could include the *PALS Provider Manual*, either in printed form or as an eBook on a personal device; any notes the student took during the course; the ECC Handbook; the *2015 AHA Guidelines Update for CPR and ECC*; posters; etc. *Open resource* does not mean open discussion with other students or the instructor

- Students may not cooperate with or talk to each other during the exam
- When a student completes the exam, grade the exam
- Refer to the annotated answer key to discuss questions answered incorrectly
- Answer any questions
- Students who scored less than 84% need immediate remediation
  - Make sure the student understands the errors and corrects the answers
  - Give a second test or have the student orally go over each item that he or she got incorrect, showing understanding of incorrect items

Instructor Notes

_____

_____

_____

_____

Next

Remediation

Lesson REM
Remediation

For case scenario retesting, the instructor may play multiple team member roles, or other available students may be team members

Exam

- Review the course material for each student who needs remediation
- Retest students as necessary
- Give feedback
- Evaluate competency

Instructor Notes

PALS Update
Lesson Plans

Lesson PALS-Update
Course Introduction

Instructor Tips

- Knowing what you want to communicate, why it's important, and what you want to have happen as a result is critical to the success of your presentation
- Be willing to adjust your Lesson Plans to the students' learning needs
- Introductions: Use the class roster or other visual aids (flip chart, whiteboard) to help keep track of the students in the course (eg, name, scope of practice, workplace)

Discussion

In a large group, with all students, discuss the following:

- Introduce yourself and additional instructors, if needed
- Invite students to introduce themselves and ask them to provide the following information:
  - Name
  - Occupation
  - Specialty
  - Place of practice
- As students are introducing themselves, document occupation, specialty, etc; this will assist instructors when tailoring future case scenarios and lessons
- Explain that the course is interactive. Use of the
  - BLS skills testing checklists (2)
    - Child
    - Infant
  - Case scenario testing checklists (3)
    - Respiratory
    - Cardiac
    - Shock
- Explain that parts of the course are somewhat physically strenuous
  - For example, Lesson 4 involves CPR, which will require you to perform a number of compressions that could be physically strenuous
- Ask that anyone with a medical concern, such as knee or back problems, speak with one of the instructors
- Explain the layout of the building, including bathrooms and fire exits
- Advise students where AEDs can be found in the building
- Tell students to silence cell phones
  - If a call needs to be answered, tell students to answer in the hallway
- Tell the students, "We are scheduled to end at _____"
- **At no time was medical care delayed for the purpose of obtaining videos. All children received timely and appropriate medical care, and parents provided consent before recording**

3

- Be certain students understand major course concepts
  - Importance of high-quality CPR to patient survival
  - Integration of high-quality BLS with pediatric interventions and effective team dynamics
- Tell students that they will be taking their *PALS Provider Manual* with them to every station throughout the course
- Remind students about course completion requirements
  - **PALS course completion requirements**
    - Actively participate in, practice, and complete the skills stations and learning stations
    - Pass skills tests in child CPR and AED and infant CPR
    - Pass an exam with a minimum score of 84%
    - Perform satisfactorily as a Team Leader in both of the following:
      ○ A cardiac case scenario
      ○ Either a respiratory or a shock case scenario

Instructor Notes

Next

Life Is Why Activity
(Optional)

Lesson PALS-Update 1
Life Is Why™ Activity (Optional)

5 minutes

Instructor Tips

- Before facilitating this lesson, complete the Life Is Why activity in the Instructor Manual. Have your "_____ Is Why" prepared to share with students

- You can make additional copies of the Life Is Why activity from the Instructor Manual for students who do not bring their Provider Manual to class

Play Life Is Why Video

- Play the video (found in the video menu)

Discussion

- To engage the class, after viewing the Life Is Why video, take 2 to 3 minutes to share your Why with the class, based on your completed Life Is Why activity in the Instructor Manual

- Then, encourage students to participate in the following activity:

  - Have students find the "_____ Is Why" page in their Provider Manual and follow the directions. Tell students:

    - Complete this activity by filling in the blank with the word that describes your Why

    - Tell your family and friends about your "_____ Is Why," and ask them to discover their Why

AHA Life Is Why Icon

- Tell students that throughout their Provider Manual, they will find information that correlates what they are learning in this course to Life Is Why and the importance of cardiovascular care. This information is identified by the Life Is Why heart-and-torch icon

- Remind students that what they are learning today has an impact on the mission of the American Heart Association

Instructor Notes

Next
Science of Pediatric Resuscitation

Lesson PALS-Update 2
Science of Pediatric Resuscitation

Learning Objective

• Perform high-quality CPR per AHA BLS recommendations

Instructor Tips

• After playing the video, be sure to emphasize how this new information will fit in with the providers' clinical practice

• Assure students that this information will be reinforced throughout the course

• To optimize the content learned from the video, try to tie in science updates to what was learned in the video and how it can be used in the students' scope of practice

Play Science of Pediatric Resuscitation Video

• In a large group, play the video

Discussion

• Briefly answer students' questions (refer to the Summary of High-Quality CPR Components table on the next page)

• If there are no student questions, consider asking questions to highlight key concepts

(continued)

Summary of High-Quality CPR Components for BLS Providers— Comparison of Key Elements of Child and Infant BLS

Component	Adults and Adolescents	Children (Age 1 Year to Puberty)	Infants (Age Less Than 1 Year, Excluding Newborns)
Scene safety	Make sure the environment is safe for rescuers and the victim		
Recognition of cardiac arrest	Check for responsiveness No breathing or only gasping (ie, no normal breathing) No definite pulse felt within 10 seconds (Breathing and pulse check can be performed simultaneously in less than 10 seconds)		
Activation of emergency response system	If you are alone with no mobile phone, leave the victim to activate the emergency response system and get the AED before beginning CPR Otherwise, send someone and begin CPR immediately; use the AED as soon as it is available	***Witnessed collapse*** Follow steps for adults and adolescents on the left ***Unwitnessed collapse, single rescuer*** Give 2 minutes of CPR Leave the victim to activate the emergency response system and get the AED Return to the child or infant and resume CPR; use the AED as soon as it is available	
Compression-ventilation ratio *without advanced airway*	*1 or 2 rescuers* 30:2	*1 rescuer* 30:2 *2 or more rescuers* 15:2	
Compression-ventilation ratio *with advanced airway*	Continuous compressions at a rate of 100-120/min Give 1 breath every 6 seconds (10 breaths/min)		
Compression rate	100-120/min		
Compression depth	At least 2 inches (5 cm)*	At least one third AP diameter of chest About 2 inches (5 cm)	At least one third AP diameter of chest About 1½ inches (4 cm)
Hand placement	2 hands on the lower half of the breastbone (sternum)	2 hands or 1 hand (rescuer can use either method on small child) on the lower half of the breastbone (sternum)	*1 rescuer* 2 fingers in the center of the chest, just below the nipple line *2 or more rescuers* 2 thumb–encircling hands in the center of the chest, just below the nipple line
Chest recoil	Allow full recoil of chest after each compression; do not lean on the chest after each compression		
Minimizing interruptions	Limit interruptions in chest compressions to less than 10 seconds		

*Compression depth should be no more than 2.4 inches (6 cm).

Abbreviations: AED, automated external defibrillator; AP, anteroposterior; CPR, cardiopulmonary resuscitation.

(continued)

Instructor Notes

_____

_____

_____

_____

Next
Learning/Testing Station: Child High-Quality BLS Practice

Lesson PALS-Update 3A
Learning/Testing Station:
Child High-Quality BLS Practice

25 minutes

Learning Objective
- Recognize cardiopulmonary arrest early and begin CPR within 10 seconds

Instructor Tips
- Play the video without interruption; if you have additional comments, wait until the end of the video
- Consider using a stopwatch or timing device during testing to ensure accurate and objective assessments
- Familiarize yourself with the skills testing checklist (refer to "Part 3: Testing and Remediation" in the *PALS Instructor Manual* for information on how to use skills testing checklists)

Play Basic Life Support Video
- Play the video
- Video will instruct students to position themselves for practice and then pause automatically

Practice While Watching: Child 1-Rescuer CPR
- **Resume video**
- Ensure that students pay attention to the video as they practice CPR
- Use of directive feedback devices is recommended
- Give positive and corrective feedback
- Use a stopwatch or timer to familiarize students with being timed during compressions
- Tell students that they will practice with the Child High-Quality BLS testing video and will rotate roles
- Have students position themselves in front of manikins
  - 2 to 3 students per manikin
  - Each student must have a 1-way valve
- Emphasize the following concepts:
  - Students' shoulders should be positioned directly over the manikin's sternum with straight arms
  - Push hard, push fast (proper rate and depth)
    - Depress chest at least one third the diameter of the chest (5 cm in most children)
    - Rate of 100 to 120 compressions/min
  - Let the chest return to the normal position between compressions (recoil); no pressure should be applied to the chest during recoil (ie, do not lean on the patient)
  - Minimize the number and duration of compression interruptions
- Video will pause automatically; replay for practice or **resume video**

Practice While Watching: Bag-Mask Device for a Child

- **Resume video**
  - Students practice
  - Give correction and feedback
- Demonstrate appropriate ventilation rate and volume
  - Deliver 1 breath every 6 seconds
  - Deliver breath until chest rise is visible
- Video will pause automatically; replay for practice or **resume video**

Students Practice: AED

- Video will explain the use of an AED and then pause automatically for practice
- Instructor demonstrates correct AED use
- Answer any questions students have about AEDs
- Place students in groups to practice the use of an AED
- Confirm that each student can operate the AED effectively
- Video will pause automatically

Students Practice: Putting It All Together

- Students should practice compressions, bag-mask ventilation, and AED skills
- After practice, test students

Instructor Notes

Next

Learning/Testing Station:
Child High-Quality BLS
Testing—Testing Details

Lesson PALS-Update 3B
Learning/Testing Station: Child High-Quality BLS Testing—Testing Details

15 minutes

Instructor Tips

- Use a stopwatch or feedback device—which is highly recommended—during testing to ensure accurate and objective assessments

- Familiarize yourself with the Child CPR and AED Skills Testing Checklist (refer to "Part 3: Testing and Remediation" in the *PALS Instructor Manual* for information on how to use skills testing checklists)

- Complete the Child CPR and AED Skills Testing Checklist for each student during this portion of the lesson

---

Skills Testing

- **Test students one at a time**

- Ask students who are not testing to practice on another manikin

- Consider matching one of the scenarios on the skills testing checklist to each student's scope of practice

- Each student must demonstrate the entire sequence of 2-rescuer CPR and AED **without instructor prompting**

- Carefully observe the student being tested for appropriate

  - Compression rate (use a stopwatch)

  - Compression depth

    - For example, check the depth of compressions with a feedback device, which is highly recommended

- If a student is unsuccessful (based on checklist requirements), refer him or her for immediate remediation

  - Each student may retest 1 additional time during this station

  - If a student remains unsuccessful after a second attempt, ensure that the student receives formal remediation at the end of the course (refer to "Part 3: Testing and Remediation" in the *PALS Instructor Manual*)

- Complete the Child CPR and AED Skills Testing Checklist for each student

- Summarize the importance of high-quality CPR to patient survival

---

Instructor Notes

_____

_____

_____

_____

Next
Learning/Testing Station: Infant High-Quality BLS Practice

Learning Objective

- Recognize cardiopulmonary arrest early and begin CPR within 10 seconds

Instructor Tips

- Use a stopwatch or feedback device—which is highly recommended—during testing to ensure accurate and objective assessments
- Familiarize yourself with the Infant CPR Skills Testing Checklist (refer to "Part 3: Testing and Remediation" in the *PALS Instructor Manual* for information on how to use skills testing checklists)
- Complete the skills testing checklist for each student during this portion of the lesson

---

Play Basic Life Support Video

- **Play the video**
- Video will instruct students to position themselves for practice and then pause automatically

---

Practice While Watching: Infant Compressions

- Have students position themselves in front of manikins
  - 2 to 3 students per manikin
- Play the video
  - Ensure that students pay attention to the video as they practice CPR
  - Use of directive feedback devices is recommended
  - Give positive and corrective feedback
  - Use a stopwatch or timer to familiarize students with being timed during compressions
  - Tell students that they will practice with the High-Quality BLS testing video and will rotate roles
- Video will pause automatically; replay for practice or **resume video**

Practice While Watching: Infant 2-Rescuer CPR

- Play the video
  - Ensure that students pay attention to the video as they practice CPR
  - Use of directive feedback devices is recommended
  - Give positive and corrective feedback
  - Use a stopwatch or timer to familiarize students with being timed during compressions
  - Tell students that they will practice with the High-Quality BLS testing video and will rotate roles
- Have students position themselves in front of manikins
  - 2 to 3 students per manikin
- Video will pause automatically; replay for practice or **resume video**

Students Practice: Putting It All Together

- When video pauses, students will practice compressions along with bag-mask ventilation skills
- After practice, test students

Instructor Notes

Next
Learning/Testing Station: Infant High-Quality BLS Testing—Testing Details

Lesson PALS-Update 4B
Learning/Testing Station: Infant High-Quality BLS Testing—Testing Details

15 minutes

Instructor Tips

- Use a stopwatch or feedback device—which is highly recommended—during testing to ensure accurate and objective assessments
- Review the Infant CPR Skills Testing Checklist before testing students (refer to "Part 3: Testing and Remediation" in the *PALS Instructor Manual* for information on how to use skills testing checklists)
- Complete the skills testing checklist for each student while he or she is completing the test

---

Skills Testing

- **Test students one at a time**
- Ask students who are not testing to practice on another manikin
- Consider matching one of the scenarios on the skills testing checklist to your student's scope of practice
- Each student must demonstrate the entire sequence of 2-rescuer CPR **without instructor prompting**
- Carefully observe the student being tested for appropriate:
  - Compression rate (use a stopwatch)
  - Compression depth
    - For example, check the speed of chest compressions with a stopwatch or feedback device, which is highly recommended
- If a student is unsuccessful (based on checklist requirements), refer him or her for immediate remediation
  - Each student may retest 1 additional time during this station
  - If a student remains unsuccessful after a second attempt, ensure that the student receives formal remediation at the end of the course (refer to "Part 3: Testing and Remediation" in the *PALS Instructor Manual*)
- Complete the Infant CPR Skills Testing Checklist for each student
- Summarize the importance of high-quality CPR to patient survival

---

Instructor Notes

_____

_____

_____

Next
Learning/Testing Station: Child and Infant Choking (Optional)

Lesson PALS-Update 5
Learning/Testing Station: Child and Infant Choking (Optional)

20 minutes

Learning Objective

- Perform high-quality CPR per AHA BLS recommendations

Instructor Tips

- Play the video without interruption. If you have additional comments, wait until the end of the video

Play Relief of Choking Video

- **Play the video**
- Video will demonstrate choking interventions for children and infants

Practice While Watching: Relief of Choking in an Infant

- **Play the video**
- Ensure that students pay attention to the video as they practice choking intervention techniques
- Use of directive feedback devices is recommended
- Give positive and corrective feedback
- Tell students that they will practice infant choking interventions

Discussion: Debrief

- Were there any specific elements you found difficult?
- If you were asked to perform the same skills again, is there anything you would do differently?
  - What?
  - Why?

Instructor Notes

_____

_____

_____

_____

Next
Overview of Systematic Approach Model

Lesson PALS-Update 6
Overview of Systematic Approach Model

Learning Objective

- Differentiate between patients who do and do not require immediate intervention

Instructor Tips

- Ask students to use the *PALS Provider Manual* in this lesson to help further engage them and help with retention of information
- Draw or reference the PAT before presenting patient cases
- Make sure not to interrupt the video. If you have any comments to add, write them down and discuss them at the end of the video. Students do not learn well when they are trying to listen to 2 things at once
- **Consider watching the videos before teaching this lesson to become familiar with the content**

Instructor Note

When facilitating this lesson, keep in mind each element of the systematic approach is designed to lay the foundation for the next. Be intentional to not progress beyond the individual elements of the systematic approach; ie, don't progress into primary assessment information in the PAT case discussion videos

Ask Students to Open the *PALS Provider Manual* to Part 3

Play Systematic Approach Video

- Play the video
- The video automatically pauses on the patient for the instructor to identify the components of the PAT related to this patient
    - Video will discuss evaluate-identify-intervene, initial impression—PAT, and primary assessment
- Initial impression and primary assessment are the evaluation tools used to evaluate the patient, identify medical emergencies, and provide appropriate interventions
- The PAT and primary assessment are performed in a systematic order to address medical emergencies from most critical to least critical
- When you are performing the PAT and primary assessment, interventions must be provided as medical emergencies are identified **before** you proceed with the assessment (see instructor note about **life-threatening conditions**)
- Advise students to refer to the PAT in Part 3 of the *PALS Provider Manual* for the next 3 videos

Instructor Note: Life-Threatening Conditions

- If at any part of this sequence you find that a patient has a **life-threatening condition**, correction of those conditions takes precedence over establishing baseline vital sign measures, such as blood pressure or pulse oximetry. When the primary assessment is completed, and after life-threatening problems have been addressed, the healthcare provider proceeds to the secondary assessment

- Always remember that a **life-threatening condition** is present if the child is unresponsive or apneic; has inadequate or labored breathing; or is mottled, gray, pale, or cyanotic. If these are present, immediately call for help and begin lifesaving treatment. If there is no **life-threatening condition**, you proceed with the primary assessment

Evaluate-Identify-Intervene Algorithm

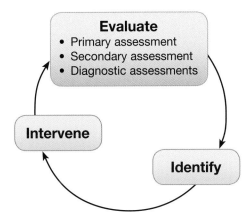

Initial Impression—Pediatric Assessment Triangle

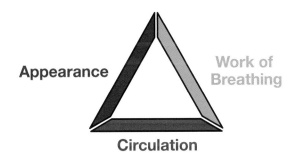

Initial Impression—Pediatric Assessment Triangle*
Appearance   From the doorway, your initial observation of the patient
Caregiver observes   • Abnormal tone   • Decreased interaction   • Inconsolable   • Abnormal look/gaze   • Abnormal speech/cry

(continued)

(continued)

Work of Breathing

- Abnormal audible sounds
- Abnormal positioning
- Retractions or use of accessory muscles
- Nasal flaring
- Apnea/gasping
- Absent, inadequate, or increased respiratory effort

Circulation to the Skin

- Pallor
- Mottling
- Dusky
- Cyanosis
- Bruising or petechiae

*If the patient is unresponsive, not breathing, or only gasping, initiate the BLS algorithm. Students can refer to Part 2 of the *PALS Provider Manual*.

Video will automatically pause on the patient.

Systematic Approach video 1: Blonde, 18-month-old child with pacifier

	Instructor discussion
	Systematic Approach video 1: Blonde, 18-month-old child with pacifier
1	Draw or tell students to reference and focus on the initial impression—PAT; then play video 1 clip

2	**When video pauses,** ask students the following questions (these questions are focused on the initial impression): *Answers are provided to help guide discussion if students have difficulty answering any questions*
	 1. What is the patient's appearance?
	   • Awake but decreased interaction
	 2. What is the patient's work of breathing?
	   • Increased work of breathing
	   • Tachypnea
	   • Retractions (suprasternal, intercostal, and subcostal)
	   • Nasal flaring
	   • Abdominal breathing
	 3. What is this patient's color?
	   • Pale
	 4. Does this patient need immediate intervention?
	   • Yes; this infant looks ill and, despite oxygen administration, has tachypnea and increased work of breathing
	 Instructor note: This child appears to be very ill. It is important to perform a focused primary assessment and be prepared to interrupt the assessment to provide immediate intervention if signs of respiratory failure or shock are detected

Resume Video

Video will automatically pause on the patient.

Systematic Approach video 2: 3-year-old child in yellow shirt

	Instructor discussion
	Systematic Approach video 2: 3-year-old child in yellow shirt
1	Draw or tell students to reference and focus on the initial impression—PAT; then play video 2 clip

2	**When video pauses,** ask students the following questions (these questions are focused on the initial impression):
	Answers are provided to help guide discussion if students have difficulty answering any questions
	1. What is the patient's appearance?
	  • Increased interaction
	2. What is the patient's work of breathing?
	  • No abnormal/audible breath sounds
	  • Normal position
	  • No nasal flaring
	3. What is this patient's color?
	  • Pink mucous membranes
	4. Does this patient need immediate intervention?
	  • No

Resume Video

Video will automatically pause on the patient.

Systematic Approach video 3: Infant in car seat

	Instructor discussion
	Systematic Approach video 3: Infant in car seat
1	Draw or tell students to reference and focus on the initial impression—PAT; then play video 3 clip

2	**When video pauses,** ask students the following questions (these questions are focused on the initial impression):
	Answers are provided to help guide discussion if students have difficulty answering any questions
	1. What is the patient's appearance?
	  • Decreased interaction
	  • Altered level of consciousness
	2. What is the patient's work of breathing?
	  • Increased work of breathing
	  • Abdominal breathing
	  • Abnormal audible inspiratory sounds (stridor)
	3. What is this patient's color?
	  • Pale to gray
	4. Does this patient need immediate intervention?
	  • Yes; the stridor indicates upper airway obstruction, and the pale, gray color likely indicates hypoxemia. The infant should be positioned to open the airway, and oxygen should be administered while additional assessment is performed

Instructor Notes

_____

_____

_____

_____

Next

Team Dynamics

Lesson PALS-Update 7
Team Dynamics

Learning Objective
- Apply team dynamics

Instructor Tips
- Clearly communicate the objective of this Lesson Plan to help students gain a better understanding of the lesson
- This Team Dynamics lesson is a great way to further engage your students
  - Change the inflection in your voice and also change your pace to help change the energy level in the room

---

Ask Students to Open the *PALS Provider Manual* to Part 5

Play Team Dynamics Video
- Play the video
- Video will automatically pause after Poor Team Dynamics

Discussion
- When video pauses, ask students the following:
  - What poor team dynamics were observed?
  - What behaviors were observed?

Resume Video
- Refer to table below to help identify effective team behaviors
- Elements of effective team dynamics
  - Roles
    - Clear roles and responsibilities
    - Knowing your limitations
    - Constructive intervention
  - What to communicate
    - Knowledge sharing
    - Summarizing and reevaluation
  - How to communicate
    - Closed-loop communication
    - Clear messages
    - Mutual respect

- Remind students that they will be functioning as Team Leaders and other roles in the learning and testing stations, and they will need to apply these concepts

Element	Effective Team Dynamics: Team Leader	Effective Team Dynamics: Team Members
1. Clear roles and responsibilities	• Clearly define all roles of team members in the clinical setting • Assign roles and responsibilities according to competence and the scope of practice of each team member • Distribute assignments evenly so that resources (skills) of team members are used as efficiently and effectively as possible	• Seek out and perform tasks that are clearly defined and appropriate to level of competence • Inform the Team Leader if the role or requested task is too difficult based on experience or competence • Be prepared to assist with tasks as needed
2. Knowing your limitations	• Call for assistance early rather than waiting until the patient deteriorates and it is too late to get the help needed • Ask other team members to help if one team member is having difficulty completing tasks • Seek advice from more experienced personnel when the patient's condition worsens despite initial treatment	
3. Constructive intervention	• Intervene if a team member is preparing to perform an incorrect action • Take corrective action to ensure that team members are performing the correct tasks in the appropriate sequence • Reassign a team member if that team member is not able to perform assigned tasks	• Ask the Team Leader or a team member to verify an action if you think a team member is about to make a mistake • Suggest an alternative drug, drug dose, or therapy if you observe an error in the drug, drug dose, or therapy ordered or prepared for administration
4. Knowledge sharing	• Encourage an environment of information sharing, and ask for suggestions if uncertain of the next best interventions • Ask for opinions and suggestions from team members about reversible causes of arrest and factors that may be limiting the effectiveness of the resuscitation attempt • Ask if anything has been overlooked (eg, IV access should have been obtained or drugs should have been administered) • Consider all clinical signs that are relevant to treatment	• Share information with other team members • Try to identify factors that may be limiting the effectiveness of the resuscitation attempt

(continued)

5. Summarizing and reevaluation	• Ask for suggestions from team members about differential diagnoses and factors that may be contributing to unsuccessful resuscitative efforts • Frequently review the drugs and treatments administered and the patient's response with the team • Change the treatment strategy when new information or patient response (or failure to respond) suggests the need for such a change • Inform arriving personnel of the patient's current status and plans for further action	• Clearly draw attention to significant changes in the patient's clinical condition and increase monitoring frequency (eg, blood pressure measurements) when the patient's condition deteriorates
6. Closed-loop communication	• Listen for verbal confirmation that requests are heard and understood • Await confirmation that the previous task has been completed (eg, "Vascular access in place") before assigning another task • Confirm receipt of a completed assignment (eg, "Good, now that the IV is in, give 1 mg of epinephrine")	• Confirm that the request is heard and understood (eg, "I'll start the IV") • Inform the Team Leader when a task begins or ends (eg, "The IV is in") • Verify orders for drugs or other treatments before administration (eg, "Did you want the 5 mg/kg of IV amiodarone given now?")
7. Clear messages	• Provide clear messages and orders to specific team members • Encourage team members to speak clearly and distinctly • Request clarification of any ambiguous messages • Speak in a calm and normal tone of voice • Outline next steps so the team can understand/anticipate what you will need next	• Repeat the medication order • Clarify an order if it is ambiguous or not understood
8. Mutual respect	• Speak in a respectful, controlled tone of voice • Provide feedback to team members • Intervene if team members begin to raise their voices or speak disrespectfully • Remember, all team members are trying to perform well despite the stress present during the attempted resuscitation	• Speak in friendly, controlled tone of voice • Remember, the Team Leader and all team members are trying to perform well despite the stress present during the attempted resuscitation

Roles and Responsibilities of Team Dynamics

Positions for 6-Person High-Performance Teams*

Resuscitation Triangle Roles

Compressor
- Assesses the patient
- Does 5 cycles of chest compressions
- Alternates with AED/Monitor/Defibrillator every 5 cycles or 2 minutes (or earlier if signs of fatigue set in)

AED/Monitor/Defibrillator
- Brings and operates the AED/monitor/defibrillator
- Alternates with Compressor every 5 cycles or 2 minutes (or earlier if signs of fatigue set in), ideally during rhythm analysis
- If a monitor is present, places it in a position where it can be seen by the Team Leader (and most of the team)

Airway
- Opens the airway
- Provides bag-mask ventilation
- Inserts airway adjuncts as appropriate

The team owns the code. No team member leaves the triangle except to protect his or her safety.

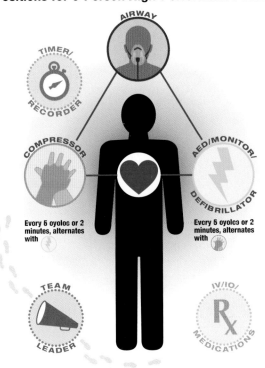

Every 5 cycles or 2 minutes, alternates with

Every 5 cycles or 2 minutes, alternates with

*This is a suggested team formation. Roles may be adapted to local protocol.

Leadership Roles

Team Leader
- **Every resuscitation team must have a defined leader**
- Assigns roles to team members
- Makes treatment decisions
- Provides feedback to the rest of the team as needed
- Assumes responsibility for roles not assigned

IV/IO/Medications
- An ACLS provider role
- Initiates IV/IO access
- Administers medications

Timer/Recorder
- Records the time of interventions and medications (and announces when these are next due)
- Records the frequency and duration of interruptions in compressions
- Communicates these to the Team Leader (and the rest of the team)

Discussion

- When video ends, ask students the following questions:
  - What good team dynamics were observed?
  - What behaviors were observed?

Instructor Notes

Next

Management of Post–Cardiac Arrest Care

Lesson PALS-Update 8
Management of Post–Cardiac Arrest Care

15 minutes

Learning Objective

- Implement post–cardiac arrest management

Instructor Tips

- Ask students to use the *PALS Provider Manual* in this lesson to help further engage them and help with retention of information

- Make sure not to interrupt the video. If you have any comments to add, write them down and discuss them at the end of the video. Students do not learn well when they are trying to listen to 2 things at once

- **Before teaching this lesson, have your questions ready for airway, breathing, circulation, and temperature control**

Advise Students to Open the *PALS Provider Manual* to Part 12

Play Management of Post–Cardiac Arrest Care Video

- Play the video
- Answer students' questions

Instructor Notes

_____

_____

_____

_____

Next
Learning Station: Coping With Death (Optional)

Lesson PALS-Update 9
Learning Station:
Coping With Death (Optional)

20 minutes

Instructor Tips

- Remind students that if they have recently experienced the loss of a loved one, this video might be difficult to view

- **Participation in this lesson is not required to complete the PALS Course**

- Students may choose not to view this video at their discretion

Play Coping With Death Video (Optional)

- Address what students will learn from the video
- Play the video
- Answer students' questions

Discussion

- Discuss how the news of the patient's death could have been delivered more effectively
    - News was delivered in the hallway, with no privacy
    - Vague terms were used to describe the death
    - The words *dead* or *died* were never used
    - Physician left family for "another emergency"
    - Physician left family with no support and no one to answer their questions
- Ask if there are any questions

Instructor Notes

_____

_____

_____

_____

Next
Case Scenario Practice With Simulations

Lesson PALS-Update 10
Case Scenario Practice With Simulations   120 minutes

Instructor Tips

- Refer to the course agenda for additional information on which case scenarios to use for each day
- Scenarios have been grouped together from least to most complex
- Refer to the *PALS Instructor Manual* for all case scenarios

Students Practice

- Students are required to do 1 practice scenario
- Instructor may require student to do additional scenario based on student's performance on first scenario
- Students should practice and demonstrate the following skills *as listed on the skills station competency checklist*

Learning Stations: Simulation/Debriefing

Note: **Use a stopwatch or timing device for each case simulation and debriefing.**

Simulation (10 minutes)	• **Set the stopwatch or timer for 10 minutes** • **Remove chairs from area—no one should be seated** • Ensure that each person has a designated role; rotate roles in subsequent patient simulations • Introduce the case by reading the case scenario lead-in on the instructor case scenario designated for a particular simulation • Direct the Team Leader to begin managing the case in conjunction with the team • Provide information that is not obtainable from the manikin • Assess the performance of the Team Leader/team by using the actions listed on the instructor case scenario as a guide • Let the simulation continue without interruption for full 10 minutes • Stop the simulation after 10 minutes
Debriefing (10 minutes)	• Set the stopwatch or timer for 10 minutes • Ask the Timer/Recorder to review actions that occurred during the simulation • Debrief the team by using the debriefing tool on the back of the instructor case scenario • Have observers give feedback by using the skills station competency checklists

- Summarize key concepts of the case
- Use the PALS Course Progress Checklist as a guide to monitor students' performance

Sample Course Rotation Schedule for 6 Students

20 minutes per case	First Case	Next Case
Team Role		
Team Leader	Student 1	Student 2
Airway	Student 2	Student 3
IV/IO/Medications	Student 3	Student 4
Monitor/Defibrillator	Student 4	Student 5
Compressor	Student 5	Student 6
Timer/Recorder	Student 6	Student 1

If <6 students, combine roles; if >6 students, include additional observer roles.

- A repository of instructor case scenarios has been created for each of the case scenarios to allow instructors to challenge students related to their scope of practice and level of experience. The case scenarios contain the information that you will need to facilitate the case discussions and case simulations. Each scenario includes a debriefing tool on the back that is specific to that particular scenario

- Please see course agenda for suggested scenarios; scenarios are grouped from least complex to most complex

- The order of the case scenarios is flexible; arrange case scenarios to best support your instructors

Instructor Notes

Next
Case Scenario Testing

Lesson PALS-Update 11
Case Scenario Testing

- Demonstrate competency in management of arrhythmia and shock or respiratory emergencies

Instructor Tips

- In this station, the focus changes to assessment instead of facilitating learning. Students must perform the test from beginning to end. Do not interrupt students while they are completing the test. Address any deficiencies during remediation
- For evaluation purposes, students must complete the scenario without team member prompting
- **Conduct testing station cases in real time**
- Have students rotate through the testing stations

Test

With 6 students in PALS case scenario test 1 and 6 students in PALS case scenario test 2, perform the following tasks (instructor-to-student ratio is 1:6 for PALS case scenario tests 1 and 2):

- Instruct each student to select a case immediately before beginning his or her case scenario test
- Evaluate the competency of each student, one at a time, each functioning as Team Leader for his or her selected case
- Document the Team Leader's performance on the PALS case scenario testing checklist
- Do not coach or give hints during the test
- Make sure other students participate as team members
- Briefly provide feedback on the Team Leader's performance
- Indicate evaluation results on the PALS Course Progress Checklist

Case Scenario Test 1

Take no longer than 8 minutes to test and 2 minutes to give students feedback on their performance

- Test each student, one at a time, functioning as Team Leader; the student being tested may use a quick reference aid (eg, ECC Handbook, pocket reference card)
- Randomly assign test scenarios one at a time immediately before each test

Test 1: Case Scenario Selection

- There are 4 case scenarios for PALS case scenario test 1:
  - Supraventricular Tachycardia
  - Bradycardia
  - Asystole/Pulseless Electrical Activity
  - Ventricular Fibrillation/Pulseless Ventricular Tachycardia

PALS Update   **29**   © 2016 American Heart Association

- Write each of these case scenarios on a separate piece of paper or a card
- Immediately before each case scenario test, instruct the student being tested to randomly select a case scenario from the papers/cards
- Subsequent students select their test case scenarios from the remaining papers/cards
- Read the lead-in that matches the student's work environment (eg, nurse, EMT-P); provide information about the case in response to students' questions
- Do not help, coach, guide, lead, or give feedback to a student during the test; do not answer questions or give hints about what the student should do or not do during the test
- You may, however, ask a leading question to prompt a student to verbalize or state a required critical performance step when indicated on the case scenario testing checklist
- Give information during the test as requested (eg, vital signs, responses to therapy)
- The Timer/Recorder documents what happens during the case by writing on a flip chart or whiteboard
- Fill out the case scenario testing checklist for the appropriate case as you observe the student's performance
- For a student to pass the test, **all** critical action steps must be performed satisfactorily
- *Conduct a feedback debriefing session for a student who was tested in private at the end of the PALS case scenario test*
- Indicate evaluation results on the PALS Course Progress Checklist
- While the student is being debriefed, other students will reset the station
- Refer students who need remediation to the remediation lesson

Case Scenario Test 2

With 6 students in PALS case scenario test 2 and 6 students in PALS case scenario test 1, perform the following tasks:

- Instruct each student to select a case immediately before beginning his or her case scenario test
- Evaluate the competency of each student, one at a time, each functioning as Team Leader for his or her selected case
- Document the Team Leader's performance on the PALS case scenario testing checklist
- Do not coach or give hints during the test
- Make sure other students participate as team members
- Briefly provide feedback on the Team Leader's performance
- Indicate evaluation results on PALS Course Progress Checklist

Test 2: Case Scenario Selection

- There are 8 case scenarios for PALS case scenario test 2
  - Upper Airway Obstruction
  - Lower Airway Obstruction
  - Lung Tissue Disease
  - Disordered Control of Breathing
  - Hypovolemic Shock

- Obstructive Shock
- Distributive Shock
- Cardiogenic Shock

- Write each of these case scenarios on a separate piece of paper or a card
- Immediately before each case scenario test, instruct the student being tested to randomly select a case scenario from the papers/cards
- Subsequent students select their test case scenarios from the remaining papers/cards

Instructor Notes

Next

Exam

Exam

All students must take the open-resource exam

- Distribute the open-resource exam
- Proctor the exam
- Collect and score each exam
  - Students must score 84% or better to pass the exam
- Review the answers by using the answer key with the students

Exam Details

- The exam is an open-resource exam
  - Resources could include the Provider Manual, either in printed form or as an eBook on a personal device; any notes the student took during the course; the ECC Handbook; the *2015 AHA Guidelines Update for CPR and ECC;* posters; etc. *Open resource* does not mean open discussion with other students or the instructor
- Students may not cooperate with or talk to each other during the exam
- When a student completes the exam, grade the exam
- Refer to the annotated answer key to discuss questions answered incorrectly
- Answer any questions
- Students who scored less than 84% need immediate remediation
  - Make sure the student understands the errors and corrects the answers
  - Give a second test or have the student orally go over each item that he or she got incorrect, showing understanding of incorrect items

Instructor Notes

Next
Remediation

Lesson PALS-Update REM
Remediation

For case scenario retesting, the instructor may play multiple team member roles, or other available students may be team members

Exam

- Review the course material for each student who needs remediation
- Retest students as necessary
- Give feedback
- Evaluate competency

Instructor Notes

Instructor Notes

HeartCode®
PALS Lesson Plans

Lesson PALS-HeartCode
Course Introduction

Instructor Tips

- Knowing what you want to communicate, why it's important, and what you want to have happen as a result is critical to the success of your presentation
- Be willing to adjust your Lesson Plans to the students' learning needs
- Introductions: Use the class roster or other visual aids (flip chart, whiteboard) to help keep track of the students in the course (eg, name, scope of practice, workplace)

Discussion

In a large group, with all students, discuss the following:

- Introduce yourself and additional instructors, if needed
- Invite students to introduce themselves and ask them to provide the following information:
  - Name
  - Occupation
  - Specialty
  - Place of practice
- As students are introducing themselves, document occupation, specialty, etc; this will assist instructors when tailoring future case scenarios and lessons

- Explain that the course is interactive, and discuss use of the following checklists:
  - BLS skills testing checklists (2)
    - Child
    - Infant
  - Learning station competency checklists (3)
    - Respiratory
    - Cardiac
    - Shock
  - Case scenario testing checklists (3)
    - Respiratory
    - Cardiac
    - Shock
- Explain that parts of the course are somewhat physically strenuous
  - For example, Lesson PALS-HC 2 involves CPR, which will require you to perform a number of compressions that could be physically strenuous
- Ask that anyone with a medical concern, such as knee or back problems, speak with one of the instructors

- Explain the layout of the building, including bathrooms and fire exits
- Advise students where AEDs can be found in the building
- Tell students to silence cell phones
  - If a call needs to be answered, tell students to answer in the hallway
- Tell the students, "We are scheduled to end at _____"

Instructor Notes

Next

Life Is Why Activity
(Optional)

Lesson PALS-HeartCode 1
Life Is Why™ Activity (Optional)
5 minutes

Instructor Tips

- Before facilitating this lesson, complete the Life Is Why activity in the Instructor Manual. Have your "_____ Is Why" prepared to share with students

- You can make additional copies of the Life Is Why activity from the Instructor Manual for students who do not bring their Provider Manual to class

Play Life Is Why Video

- Play the video (found in the video menu)

Discussion

- To engage the class, after viewing the Life Is Why video, take 2 to 3 minutes to share your Why with the class, based on your completed Life Is Why activity in the Instructor Manual

- Then, encourage students to participate in the following activity:

  - Have students find the "_____ Is Why" page in their Provider Manual and follow the directions. Tell students:

    - Complete this activity by filling in the blank with the word that describes your Why

    - Tell your family and friends about your "_____ Is Why," and ask them to discover their Why

AHA Life Is Why Icon

- Tell students that throughout their Provider Manual, they will find information that correlates what they are learning in this course to Life Is Why and the importance of cardiovascular care. This information is identified by the Life Is Why heart-and-torch icon

- Remind students that what they are learning today has an impact on the mission of the American Heart Association

Instructor Notes

_____

_____

_____

_____

Next
Learning/Testing Station: Child High-Quality BLS Practice

Learning Objective

- Recognize cardiopulmonary arrest early and begin CPR within 10 seconds

Instructor Tips

- Play the video without interruption; if you have additional comments, wait until the end of the video
- Consider using a stopwatch or timing device during testing to ensure accurate and objective assessments
- Familiarize yourself with the skills testing checklist (refer to "Part 3: Testing and Remediation" in the *PALS Instructor Manual* for information on how to use skills testing checklists)

Play Basic Life Support Video

- Based on students' experience, the instructor can choose to play the video or have students move directly into practice while watching
- Play the video
- Video will instruct students to position themselves for practice

Practice While Watching: Child 1-Rescuer CPR

- Ensure that students pay attention to the video as they practice CPR
- Use of directive feedback devices is recommended
- Give positive and corrective feedback
- Use a stopwatch or timer to familiarize students with being timed during compressions
- Tell students that they will practice with the Child High-Quality BLS testing video and will rotate roles
- Have students position themselves in front of manikins
  - 2 to 3 students per manikin
  - Each student must have a 1-way valve
- Emphasize the following concepts:
  - Students' shoulders should be positioned directly over the manikin's sternum with straight arms
  - Push hard, push fast (proper rate and depth)
    - Depress chest at least one third the diameter of the chest (5 cm in most children)
    - Rate of 100 to 120 compressions/min
  - Let the chest return to the normal position between compressions (recoil); no pressure should be applied to the chest during recoil (ie, do not lean on the patient)
  - Minimize the number and duration of compression interruptions
- Video will pause automatically; replay for practice or **resume video**

Practice While Watching: Bag-Mask Device for a Child

- Resume video
  - Students practice
  - Give correction and feedback
- Demonstrate appropriate ventilation rate and volume
  - Deliver 1 breath every 6 seconds
  - Deliver breath until chest rise is visible
- Video will pause automatically; replay for practice or **resume video**

Students Practice: AED

- Video will explain the use of an AED and then pause automatically for practice
- Instructor demonstrates correct AED use
- Answer any questions students have about AEDs
- Place students in groups to practice the use of an AED
- Confirm that each student can operate the AED effectively

Students Practice: Putting It All Together

- Students should practice compressions, bag-mask ventilation, and AED skills
- After practice, test students

Instructor Notes

Next

Learning/Testing Station:
Child High-Quality BLS
Testing—Testing Details

Lesson PALS-HeartCode 2B
Learning/Testing Station: Child High-Quality BLS Testing—Testing Details

15 minutes

Instructor Tips

- Use a stopwatch or feedback device—which is highly recommended—during testing to ensure accurate and objective assessments

- Familiarize yourself with the Child CPR and AED Skills Testing Checklist (refer to "Part 3: Testing and Remediation" in the *PALS Instructor Manual* for information on how to use skills testing checklists)

- Complete the Child CPR and AED Skills Testing Checklist for each student during this portion of the lesson

---

Skills Testing

- **Test students one at a time**

- Ask students who are not testing to practice on another manikin

- Consider matching one of the scenarios on the skills testing checklist to each student's scope of practice

- Each student must demonstrate the entire sequence of 2-rescuer CPR and AED **without instructor prompting**

- Carefully observe the student being tested for appropriate
  - Compression rate (use a stopwatch)
  - Compression depth
    - For example, check the depth of compressions with a feedback device, which is highly recommended

- If a student is unsuccessful (based on checklist requirements), refer him or her for immediate remediation
  - Each student may retest 1 additional time during this station
  - If a student remains unsuccessful after a second attempt, ensure that the student receives formal remediation at the end of the course (refer to "Part 3: Testing and Remediation" in the *PALS Instructor Manual*)

- Complete the Child CPR and AED Skills Testing Checklist for each student

- Summarize the importance of high-quality CPR to patient survival

---

Instructor Notes

Next
Learning/Testing Station: Infant High-Quality BLS Practice

Lesson PALS-HeartCode 3A
Learning/Testing Station:
Infant High-Quality BLS Practice

20 minutes

Instructor Tips

- Use a stopwatch or feedback device—which is highly recommended—during testing to ensure accurate and objective assessments
- Familiarize yourself with the Infant CPR Skills Testing Checklist (refer to "Part 3: Testing and Remediation" in the *PALS Instructor Manual* for information on how to use skills testing checklists)
- Complete the skills testing checklist for each student during this portion of the lesson

Play Basic Life Support Video

- Based on students' experience, the instructor can choose to play the video or have students move directly into practice while watching.
- **Play the video**
- Video will instruct students to position themselves for practice and then pause automatically

Practice While Watching: Infant Compressions

- Play the video
  - Ensure that students pay attention to the video as they practice CPR
  - Use of directive feedback devices is recommended
  - Give positive and corrective feedback
  - Use a stopwatch or timer to familiarize students with being timed during compressions
  - Tell students that they will practice with the High-Quality BLS testing video and will rotate roles
- Have students position themselves in front of manikins
  - 2 to 3 students per manikin

Practice While Watching: Infant 2-Rescuer CPR

- Play the video
  - Ensure that students pay attention to the video as they practice CPR
  - Use of directive feedback devices is recommended
  - Give positive and corrective feedback
  - Use a stopwatch or timer to familiarize students with being timed during compressions
  - Tell students that they will practice with the High-Quality BLS testing video and will rotate roles

- Have students position themselves in front of manikins
  - 2 to 3 students per manikin

Students Practice: Putting It All Together
- Students will practice compressions along with bag-mask ventilation skills
- After practice, test students

Instructor Notes

Next
Learning/Testing Station:
Infant High-Quality BLS
Testing—Testing Details

Lesson PALS-HeartCode 3B
Learning/Testing Station: Infant
High-Quality BLS Testing—Testing Details   15 minutes

Instructor Tips

- Use a stopwatch or feedback device—which is highly recommended—during testing to ensure accurate and objective assessments

- Review the Infant CPR Skills Testing Checklist before testing students (refer to "Part 3: Testing and Remediation" in the *PALS Instructor Manual* for information on how to use skills testing checklists)

- Complete the skills testing checklist for each student while he or she is completing the test

---

Skills Testing

- **Test students one at a time**

- Ask students who are not testing to practice on another manikin

- Consider matching one of the scenarios on the skills testing checklist to your student's scope of practice

- Each student must demonstrate the entire sequence of 2-rescuer CPR **without instructor prompting**

- Carefully observe the student being tested for appropriate

    - Compression rate (use a stopwatch)

    - Compression depth

        - For example, check the speed of chest compressions with a stopwatch or feedback device, which is highly recommended

- If a student is unsuccessful (based on checklist requirements), refer him or her for immediate remediation

    - Each student may retest 1 additional time during this station

    - If a student remains unsuccessful after a second attempt, ensure that the student receives formal remediation at the end of the course (refer to "Part 3: Testing and Remediation" in the *PALS Instructor Manual*)

- Complete the Infant CPR Skills Testing Checklist for each student

- Summarize the importance of high-quality CPR to patient survival

---

Instructor Notes

_____

_____

_____

Next
Learning/Testing Station: Child and Infant Choking (Optional)

Lesson PALS-HeartCode 4
Learning/Testing Station:
Child and Infant Choking (Optional)

20 minutes

Learning Objective
• Perform high-quality CPR per AHA BLS recommendations

Instructor Tips
• Play the video without interruption; if you have additional comments, wait until the end of the video

Play Relief of Choking Video
• **Play the video**
  • Video will demonstrate choking interventions for children and infants

Practice While Watching: Relief of Choking in an Infant
• **Play the video**
  • Ensure that students pay attention to the video as they practice choking intervention techniques
  • Use of directive feedback devices is recommended
  • Give positive and corrective feedback
  • Tell students that they will practice infant choking interventions

Discussion: Debrief
  • Were there any specific elements you found difficult?
  • If you were asked to perform the same skills again, is there anything you would do differently?
    – What?
    – Why?

Instructor Notes

Next

Learning Station: Airway Management

Learning Objective

- Perform early interventions for respiratory distress and failure

Instructor Tips

- Encourage students to use their Pocket Reference Cards or ECC Handbook early on during the cases but to become less reliant on those resources as the cases progress.
- When debriefing students
  - Ask your audience open-ended questions that focus on their perspective to engage their minds and increase energy focus

Students Practice

- Have students position themselves in front of manikins
- Students will complete respiratory skills check and demonstrate the following skills as listed on the skills station competency checklist (use Airway Management Skills Station Competency Checklist):
  - Verbalizes difference between high-flow and low-flow O_2 delivery systems
  - Verbalizes maximum nasal cannula flow rate (4 L/min)
  - Opens airway by using head tilt–chin lift and jaw-thrust maneuvers
  - After ROSC from cardiac arrest, titrates FIO_2 to maintain oxygen saturation at 94% to 99%
  - Verbalizes different indications for an OPA
  - Selects correct size OPA
  - Inserts OPA correctly
  - Evaluates breathing after insertion of an OPA
  - Suctions with an OPA in place; states suctioning not to exceed 10 seconds
  - Selects correct mask size for ventilations
  - Attaches bag-mask device, creates seal by using the E-C clamp technique, opens airway, and ventilates effectively
  - Gives 2 breaths (approximately 1 second for each) causing chest rise with bag-mask device
- Provide feedback as needed
- Record evaluation results on the PALS Course Progress Checklist

Next
Learning Station: Vascular Access

Learning Objective

• Perform early interventions for the treatment of shock

Instructor Tips

• Depending on each learner's experience and scope of practice, some students may be uncomfortable with IO insertion

– Give these providers extra time to practice and encourage them to help them feel more comfortable and confident

Play IO Access Video

• Based on students' experience, this video may be optional. This is the same IO video displayed in the online course

• Play the video

Students Practice

• Instructor should have 6 students in this station and perform the following tasks:

– Have students practice IO insertion skills according to the Vascular Access Skills Station Competency Checklist

– Ensure that each student can prepare equipment to administer an IV/IO bolus rapidly, including 3-way stopcock, syringes, and IV tubing

– Ensure that each student can perform IO access correctly and confirm when the needle has reached the marrow cavity

– Provide corrective feedback during IO insertion, IV/IO fluid administration, and use of IV medications

– Record evaluation results on the PALS Course Progress Checklist

Discussion

• Were there any specific elements that you found difficult?

• If you were asked to perform the same skills again, is there anything that you would do differently?

– What?

– Why?

Next

Learning Station: Rhythm Disturbances/Electrical Therapy

Lesson PALS-HeartCode 7
Learning Station:
Rhythm Disturbances/Electrical Therapy   25 minutes

Learning Objective

- Differentiate between unstable and stable patients with arrhythmias

Instructor Tips

- Familiarize students with all equipment before hands-on practice
- Depending on their scope of practice, some students may appear to be uncomfortable performing the skills in this lesson
  - Give these providers extra time to practice and encourage them to help them feel more comfortable and confident

Discussion

- Use the Rhythm Disturbances/Electrical Therapy Skills Station Competency Checklist
- Instructor should have 6 students in this station and should demonstrate how to
  - Apply ECG leads
  - Use the monitor and obtain a rhythm strip
  - Apply defibrillation/cardioversion electrode pads
  - Perform defibrillation and synchronized cardioversion
- Students will then practice the above skills
- Evaluate each student's ability to correctly perform these skills
- Verify that students can recognize the selected rhythms and state the appropriate electrical therapy, if indicated, for each
- Record evaluation results on the PALS Course Progress Checklist

Students Practice

This part of the lesson is designed to have the students demonstrate effective and safe use of the equipment (cardiac monitor and manual defibrillator) and to enable you to validate each student's skills

Gather students around the equipment and have each student demonstrate, one at a time.

Step	Ensure that each student is able to
1. Use of monitor	• Apply ECG leads properly • Turn on the monitor and run a rhythm strip • Show how to properly operate the monitor
2. Rhythm recognition	• Recognize rhythms that require electrical therapy 　– Ventricular tachycardia (defibrillation) 　– Ventricular fibrillation (defibrillation) 　– Supraventricular tachycardia, unstable (cardioversion)

(continued)

(continued)

3. Steps for defibrillation	• Select and position the correct paddles/pads for an infant or a child • Set the appropriate energy dose (2 to 4 J/kg). • Select the appropriate mode: not synchronized • Charge • Clear • Press and hold the shock buttons until energy is discharged
4. Steps for cardioversion	• Select and position the correct paddles/pads for an infant or a child • Set the appropriate energy dose (0.5 to 1 J/kg) • Select the appropriate mode: synchronized • Charge • Clear • Press and hold the shock buttons until energy is discharged

Indicate each student's evaluation on the PALS Course Progress Checklist

Discussion

- Were there any specific elements that you found difficult?
- Is there any piece of equipment that was either unfamiliar or different from what you are accustomed to?

Instructor Notes

_____

_____

_____

_____

Next
Case Scenario Testing (Optional)

Lesson PALS-HeartCode 8
Case Scenario Testing (Optional)

120 minutes

- Demonstrate competency in the management of arrhythmia and shock or respiratory emergencies

Instructor Tips

- In this station, the focus changes to assessment instead of facilitating learning. Students must perform the test from beginning to end. Do not interrupt students while they are completing the test. Address any deficiencies during remediation
- For evaluation purposes, students must complete the scenario without team member prompting
- **Conduct testing station cases in real time**
- Have students rotate through the testing stations

Test

With 6 students in the PALS case scenario test 1 and 6 students in the PALS case scenario test 2, perform the following tasks (instructor-to-student ratio is 1:6 for PALS case scenario tests 1 and 2):

- Instruct each student to select a case immediately before beginning his or her case scenario test
- Evaluate the competency of each student, one at a time, each functioning as Team Leader for his or her selected case
- Document the Team Leader's performance on the appropriate case scenario testing checklist
- Do not coach or give hints during the test
- Make sure other students participate as team members
- Briefly provide feedback on the Team Leader's performance
- Indicate evaluation results on the PALS Course Progress Checklist

Case Scenario Test 1

Take no longer than 8 minutes to test and 2 minutes to give students feedback on their performance

- Test each student, one at a time, functioning as Team Leader; the student being tested may use a quick reference aid (eg, ECC Handbook, pocket reference card)
- Randomly assign test scenarios one at a time immediately before each test

Test 1: Case Scenario Selection

- There are 4 case scenarios for PALS case scenario test 1:
  - Supraventricular Tachycardia
  - Bradycardia
  - Asystole/Pulseless Electrical Activity
  - Ventricular Fibrillation/Pulseless Ventricular Tachycardia
- Write each of these case scenarios on a separate piece of paper or a card
- Immediately before each case scenario test, instruct the student being tested to randomly select a case scenario from the papers/cards
- Subsequent students select their test case scenarios from the remaining papers/cards
- Read the lead-in that matches the student's work environment (eg, nurse, EMT-P); provide information about the case in response to students' questions
- Do not help, coach, guide, lead, or give feedback to a student during the test; do not answer questions or give hints about what the student should do or not do during the test
- You may, however, ask a leading question to prompt a student to verbalize or state a required critical performance step when indicated on the case scenario testing checklist
- Give information during the test as requested (eg, vital signs, responses to therapy)
- The Timer/Recorder documents what happens during the case by writing on a flip chart or whiteboard
- Fill out the case scenario testing checklist for the appropriate case as you observe the student's performance
- For a student to pass the test, **all** critical action steps must be performed satisfactorily
- *Conduct a feedback debriefing session for a student who was tested in private at the end of the PALS case scenario test*
- Indicate evaluation results on the PALS Course Progress Checklist
- While the student is being debriefed, other students will reset the station
- Refer students who need remediation to the remediation lesson

Case Scenario Test 2

With 6 students in PALS case scenario test 2 and 6 students in PALS case scenario test 1, perform the following tasks:

- Instruct each student to select a case immediately before beginning his or her case scenario test
- Evaluate the competency of each student, one at a time, each functioning as Team Leader for his or her selected case
- Document the Team Leader's performance on the appropriate case scenario testing checklist
- Do not coach or give hints during the test
- Make sure other students participate as team members
- Briefly provide feedback on the Team Leader's performance
- Indicate evaluation results on PALS Course Progress Checklist

Test 2: Case Scenario Selection

- There are 8 case scenarios for PALS case scenario test 2:
  - Upper Airway Obstruction
  - Lower Airway Obstruction
  - Lung Tissue Disease
  - Disordered Control of Breathing
  - Hypovolemic Shock
  - Obstructive Shock
  - Distributive Shock
  - Cardiogenic Shock
- Write each of these case scenarios on a separate piece of paper or a card
- Immediately before each case scenario test, instruct the student being tested to randomly select a case scenario from the papers/cards
- Subsequent students select their test case scenarios from the remaining papers/cards

Instructor Notes

Instructor Notes

Instructor Notes

Instructor Notes